CURRENT TOPICS IN GASTRITIS - 2012

Edited by **Gyula Mózsik**

Current Topics in Gastritis - 2012
http://dx.doi.org/10.5772/46056
Edited by Gyula Mózsik

Contributors

Alejandro H. Corvalan, Gonzalo Carrasco, Kathleen Saavedra, Bruna Maria Roesler, José Murilo Zeitune, Shotaro Enomoto, Kiron Moy Das, Jiro Watari, Kentaro Moriichi, Hiroki Tanabe, Mikihiro Fujiya, Hiroto Miwa, Yutaka Kohgo, Gonzalo Castillo-Rojas, German Aguilar- Gutierrez, Eduardo Mucito-Varela, Stephanie E. Morales-Guerrero, Yolanda López-Vidal, Mohamed Elseweidy, Hanan Alshenawy, Zheming Lu, Dajun Deng, Gyula Mozsik, Jozsef Czimmer, Imre Laszlo Szabo, Janos Szolcsanyi, Kata Cseko, Paolo Arcari, S. Swarnakar, Achariya - Sailasuta

Published by InTech

Janeza Trdine 9, 51000 Rijeka, Croatia

Copyright © 2013 InTech

Notice

Publishing Process Manager Marija Radja
Technical Editor InTech DTP team
Cover InTech Design team

Additional hard copies can be obtained from orders@intechopen.com

Current Topics in Gastritis - 2012, Edited by Gyula Mózsik
p. cm.
ISBN 978-953-51-0907-5

For EU product safety concerns:
IN TECH d.o.o., Prolaz Marije Krucifikse Kozulić 3, 51000 Rijeka, Croatia,
info@intechopen.com or visit our website at intechopen.com.

Meet the editor

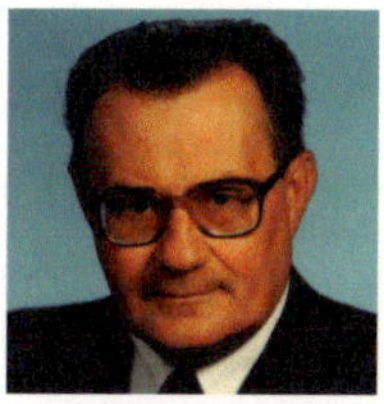

Dr Gyula Mózsik is a physician (internist, gastroenterologist, clinical pharmacologist). He gratuated at Debrecen University (1962) and worked at the First Department of Medicine of Pécs University, Hungary. He was a head of this Department (1993-2013). He also studied at Oslo University (Department of Pharmacology and Department of Medicine in 1969-1970 and at Harvard Medical School (Boston, USA) in 1985.He received Ph.D. (1970) and D.Sc. (1977) in medical sciences.He organized 42 national or international congresses and/or symposia and gave more than 700 lectures, published more than 350 peer reviewed papers, 190 book chapters and published 18 monographs and 28 edited books.Twelve of his pupils have been apointed as full professors.He is a members of 18 national and international scientific societies, scientific boards.His research fields are experimental and clinical gastroenterology, pharmacology, nutrition and clinical biochemistry.

Contents

Preface

Homeostasis of living organisms is extremelly well regulated by various physiological, hormonal, nutritional, immunological, genetic etc. pathways. We have learnt a lot about these mechanisms during last decades, however, some details remaine to be unknown.

The gastric mucosa's function is regulated by many intrinsic (neural, hormonal, immunological, genetic etc. regulations) and extrinsic (different foods or food components, xenobiotics, chemical agents, physical actions) factors, that directly reach the gastric mucosa in both healthy subjects and in patients with gastrointestinal or other diseases.

The gastric mucosa is able to reply to these endogenonous and exogenous actions by active and passive (dominantly metabolic) pathways. Many experimental works and clinical observations clearly indicate that the macroscopic (and in somewhat microscopic) features of the gastric mucosa to different endogenous and exogenous aggresive agents are very similar. The inflammation, as the general reaction, of gastric mucosa seems to be the same.

The role of inflammation in the development of different diseases was suggested by Hyppocrates (B.C. 460-377), who stated that the changes in the blood flow and other body fluids are caused by local irritations of organs („ubi stimulus, idi fluxus"). The appearence of classical inflammation were given by Aulus Cornelius Celsus (B.C. 25- A.C. 50) as „tumor,calor,dolor, rubor" and Claudius Galenos (A.C. 129-200/201) gave the last basic parameter of the inflammation as „functio laesa" to the previously mentinoned characteristic medical phenomena.These terminological questions were accepted by Wirchow in the 19th centrury, and many other famous researchers in our days.

Gastritis, as the inflammatory process (or processes), in the gastric mucosa is (are) a pathomorphological appearance(s) of inflammation in the gastric mucosa. Acute and chronic gastritis can be differentiated on the basis of the development and process of the diseases. Chronic gastritis may be caused by different factors such as many chemical, bacterial, viral, physical agents, and one of these is Helicobacter pylori infection, bacterial owergrowth in a hypochlrohydric stomach, autoimmune mechanisms, or chemical agents such as long-term nonsteroidal antinflammatory drug (NSAID) treatment and bile reflux.

Nowadays, the importance of Helicobacter pylori infection is increasing . Many of references in the literature used to emphasize the presence of Helicobacter pylori in patients with chronic atrophic gastritis with and without the development of gastric cancer.

This bacterium is highly prevalent in many countries and increases the risk for development of gastric and duodenal ulcer diseases, gastric cancer and gastric mucosa-associated lymphoid tissue lymphoma.

So the gastritis (as a pathomorphological event) does not represent a clinically uniform entity (as it can be clearly suggested from the difinition of inflammation). Of course, many mechanisms are involved in the development of chronic gastritis, produced by different intrinsic and extrinsic factors (including also the genetic backgrounds).

One of the main questions of chronic atrophic gastric is in which pathway(s) leads(lead) to the development of gastric cancer. Because everyone (after Marshall and Warren received the Nobel price in 2005) suggested that the Helicobacter pylori is a main etiological factor in development of gastric and dudenal ulcer, MALToma, gastric cancer and many other non gastrointestinally located disorders. Researchers' attention was focussed dominantly to the questions of Helicobacter pyloric infection (including the infection, its population spreading out, antibacterial treatment), meanwhile we have forgotten results of the previously carried research observations.

The „functio laesa" clinically detactable by the measuremens of gastric basal (basal acid output, BAO) and maximal (maximal acid output, MAO) can be obtained without application of any gastric stimulatory agens or with supermaximal doses of pentagastrin or histamine. Unfortunately, these types of measurements disappeared from the everyday medical practice. We studied the changes of gastric basal and maximal acid secretiory responses in duodenal ulcer pateints on dependence of patients' age and on time period after the onset of patients' complaints (number of patients was 120). We suprisingly registrated that the value of basal acid output significantly increased (not decreased) by increase of the patients' age and by increased time period after the onset of complaints, meanwhile the maximal acid secretory reponses remained unchaged by the patients' age increase or by time period after onset of complaints in patients with duodenal ulcer. This study was carried out in 1980' s. It is also true that we had no knowledge about the infection rate of gastric mucosa with Helicobacter pylori in patients with duodenal ulcer, however, we now know well the infection rate is near 100 per cent in these patients. The editor of this book has been working from 1962 in this field (including clinical research, experimental and clinical biochemical and molecular pharmacology, experimental and clinical clinical pharmacology, experimental and clinical clinical nutrition, clinical biochemistry, as internist, gastroenterologist, clinical pharmalogist) and participated in many different internationally accepted research processes. The editor's main dilemma is in why he newer could registrate the apperance of gastric cancer in patients who originally suffered from classical duodenal ulcer, really increased in before and after Helicobacter pylori era? The editor of this book never saw patients with gastric cancer, who originally suffered from classical duodenal ulcer (not in erosions) from 1962 to 2012. So, consequently the question is what is really the role of Helicobacter pylori infection in the development of different gastrointestinal (and many other extragastrointestinal located) diseases. In other words, is the presence of Helicobater pylori really a common main etiological agent for the development of gastric cancer, or only one of the factor shown in the development of these above mentioned diseases? However it can also be true that the groups of patients with gastric, duodenal ulcer and gastric cancer are not uniform. Marketing of the proton pump inhibitors plus antibiotics does not respresent a neutral economical position in the world (this is not a medical question).

This book is diveded into following sections : history of gastritis: from morphology to etiology and prognosis; animal models with a special strain of Helicobacter pylori in animal experimental circumstances;epidemiology of gastritis; afferent vagal neural pathway in the development and healing of chronic gastritis in patients;diagnostric backgrounds; molecular pathology; biochemistry and genetics involved in the pathways from Helicobacter pylori infection to gastric cancer.

Szabó et al. (Pécs, Hungary) offer an literure review on the permanently used terminology „gastritis" in the last 150 years. It is clear that the clinical pictures of gastritis changed together with scientific backgrounds of gastritis. The morphology (macroscopic and microscopic) had been emphasized earlier and now the etiological backgrounds, together with the their prognostic aspects are emphasised.

Sailasuta et al. (Chiangmai, Thailand) demonstrate the role of Helicobacter family (genus Helicobacter spp.) as couses of the diseases in domestic animals. Earlier, just the Mongolian gerbil was used in the experimental results to study the H. pylori induced gastric mucosal damage, including the pathway(s) from H. pylori infection to development of gastric cancer. This paper indicates the pathogenesis, diagnostic testing and treatment in veterinary medicine, which can help to understand the human problems.

Elseweidy (Zagazig, Egypt) details some epidemiological problems of gastritis (induced by H. pylori infection) and emphysise the roles of measurements of pepsinogen 1 and 11 (pg 1,11), gastric G17 and H. pylori antibodies (apperaring in fraction of IgM) as possibility to take difference between the Hp-related vs. non Hp-related gastritis.

Czimmer et al. (Pécs, Hungary) present results of clinical research on the possible role of capsaicin-sensitive afferent fibres of vagal nerve in the development of chronic gastritis. They proved that the increased expression of capsacin receptor (TRPV1) and calcitonin gene-raleted peptide (CGRP) in the gastric mucosa of patients with chronic gastritis, but no change was obtained in the substance P (SP). These changes were the same in the gastric mucosa of patients with H. pylori positive chronic gastritis. Surprizingly , increased expression of capsaicin receptor and CGRP remained unchanged after successful eradication treatment. These observations clearly indicated gastric mucosal protective role of capsaicin-sensitive neural pathway of afferent fibres of vagal nerve, which differs from the eradication treatment, in the gastric mucosa of patients with chronic gastritis.Probably the role of capsaicin receptor and CGRP differs from that of SP in these processes of humans.

Corvalan et al. (Santiago, Chile) attempt to summarize and integrate our current knowledge of the genetic as well as epigenetic bases of the dynamic process of chronic gastritis, and detail the so-called multistep cascade of gastric cancer.

Watari et al. (Nishinomiya, Japan and New Brunswick, USA) present the potential roles of biomarkers (microsatellite instability and chromosome instability) in the process of development of gastric cancer, detailed the steps of DNA hypermethylation and hypomethylation. According to the authors these biomarkers are predictive markers in the development of synchronous or metachronous gastric cancer after the H. pylori infection.

Zheming et Dajum (Beijing, China) studied the steps of DNA methylation changes in the progression of gastritis to gastric cancer. They indicated that the H. pylori induces methylation through the production of IL-1β, so the DNA methylation is one of ideal candidate biomarkers for detection of initiated cells in the precancerous lesions, assessment of cancer risk, and prediction of chemotherapy responses or clinical outcomes. On the other hand, the intrinsic reversibility of epigenic alterations enables them as promising targets for the development of novel strategies for cancer prevention and treatment.

Alshenawy and Alshafey (Tanta, Egypt) demonstrated in patients that the activity of chronic gastritis correlated with H. pylori infection, and on the other hand, p53 and c-Myc expression were correlated positively with the grade of chronic gastritis. It was also important that after eradication treatment of H. pylori infection, the activity of gastritis decreased together with the decrease of p53 and c-Myc in patients.

Enomoto et al. (Wakayama, Japan) decribe the diagnosis of gastric cancer risk with DNA methylation as an indicator in gastric mucosa tissue samples obtained by biopsy, and thes studies were carried out as molecular biological gastric cancer risk marker. They also studied serum pepsinogen as a risk marker. These studies were during the H. pylori infection and after eradication treatment (eg. H. pylori negative status) The article indicated that DNA methylation level of certain genes was associated with H. pylori infection and involved in the formation of epigenetic field for characterization. The serum level of pepsinogen and/or H.pylori antibody levels provide as index of cancer development. The author have the opinion that these markers of gastric cancer can be objectively determined in each individual with H. pylori related chronic gastritis.

Morales-Guerrero et al. summarizes the problems of highly virulent H. pylori strains harbor a (cytotoxin-associated genes) pathogenicity island an (Cag-PAI) that endodesproteins that are components of atype IV secretion system (T4SS) apparatus and its best characterized marker, the CagA effector protetin into the host target cells. The paper summarizes (in a form of review paper) the recent advances of host cell signaling cascade activities of the bacterial phosphorylation-dependent and phosphorylation-independent oncoprotein CagA and the T4SS together with including the actin cytoskeleton rearrrangements, induction of membrane dynamics and the dysruption of cell-to-cell junctions; and on the other hand, pro-inflammatory, proliferative and anti-apoptotic nuclear responses as well as their contribution to the activation of these signaling cascades to development int the gastric mucosa.

Banerjee et al. (Kolkata, India) gave a review paper to decode the mechanisms behind homing of the bacteria by modulating the host immune system that resulted in the induction and activation of matrix metalloproteinases. According to the authors, a cross talk exists between T helper cells and matrix metalloproteinases during the H. pylori infection, which may open up new therapeutic strategy in a better direction.

Roesler and Zeitune (São Paulo, Brasil) analyze the imprtance of cagPAI of H. pylori infected patients in the development of early and advanced gastric adenocarcinoma in patients with H. pylori-induced chronic gastritis. For both groups, advanced and early gastric adenocarcinoma, the most frequent genotype was cagA+cagT (62 percent versus 35 percent, respectively). However, when the authors compared the results in the two groups, they found a statistically significance in relation to cagA+cagT+ and cagA+cagT strains. Morever, the phenotype cagA+cagT occured with higher frequency in the advanced cancer group. The authors suggest that cagA gene positivity in independent from its polymorphisms, and it probably depends on the virulance factor for the development of most severe gastric diseases (like as gastric cancer).

Altieri et al. (Naples, Italy) offer an excellent review on the molecular pathology, biochemistry and genetics on genes, proteins and factors invoved in the gastric carcinogenesis based on currently available literature. Carcogenesis is a consequence of the multistep process involving different genetic and epigenetic changes in numerous genes. The majority of genetic alterations contributing to the malignant transformation were observed in growth regulatory genes, and in genes involved in cell cycle. According to the authors, the molecular mechanisms involved in carcinogensis of intestinal type differs from those prevaling in the development of diffuse one.

After giving a short review of the book chapters, it is clearly visible that this book provides an updated set of information on gastris.

The editor is sure that all our readers - experts, researchers (clinicians, gastroenterologists, pathologists, microbiologists, biochemists, genetists, oncologists, researchers working in the field of molecular levels) will be enriched by new information.

The editor wishes to express his thankfulness for the excellent work of the contributing authors. Without their help this book would not be possible. The editor is especially thankful on the excellent support given by Ms. Ivona Lovric and Ms. Marija Radja from the InTech Open Access Publisher

Dr Gyula Mózsik
Professor of Medicine
First Depatment of Medicine,
Medical and Health Centre,
University of Pécs,
Pécs, Hungary

Section 1

History of Gastritis: From Morphology to Etiology and Prognosis

Chapter 1

Diagnosis of Gastritis – Review from Early Pathological Evaluation to Present Day Management

Imre Laszlo Szabo, Kata Cseko, Jozsef Czimmer and Gyula Mozsik

Additional information is available at the end of the chapter

http://dx.doi.org/10.5772/52884

1. Introduction

The gastritis is an inflammatory condition of the gastric mucosa characterized by existence of elementary histological alternations. However these structural changes observed by the pioneer of gastric histology were noted more than a century ago, their etiology and proper interpretation for clinical practice required much longer time.

The ancient Egyptians wrote that the diseases of internal organs are difficult to detect even in well-preserved bodies, hence they were not able to comprehend outstanding discoveries on the stomach as they did on other organ diseases. The first major discovery in the field of gastric diseases was the description of gastric cancer by the Persian Avicenna around 1000 (quoted by Rugge et al, 2003). At the same time the discoveries of non-neoplastic gastric diseases, especially gastritis, was really elusive for quite a long time due to less macroscopic features and to post-mortem alternations. The inflammation of the inner lining of the stomach was first noted as "gastritis" by a German physician, Georg Ernst Stahl in 1728 (quoted by Bock, 1974). Italian anatomical pathologist Giovanni Battista Morgagni further described the signs of gastric inflammation. He gave the first classical description of an erosive or ulcerating gastritis. He stated that some of the erosions can become gangrenous, and described corrosive gastritis as it was the most well-known gastritis form of that time due high number of lye intoxication. French physician, François-Joseph-Victor Broussais gathering information by autopsy of dead French soldiers between 1808 and 1831, described common chronic gastritis as he called "Gastritides", and sometimes got delusive conclusions as gastritis was the cause of ascites and other diseases, like typhoid fever and meningitis (Bock, 1974). Jones Handfield and Wilson Fox (1854) described microscopic changes of mucous membrane in gastric inflammation, which exists in diffuse and segmental forms. Not much later another British physician, William Brinton (1859) emphasized the symptomatic and microscopic differences of acut, subacute and chronic gastritis in his medical book entitled "Diseases of Stomach", and described haemorrhagic erosion and follicular ulceration. Meanwhile Baron Carl von Rokitansky besides his major discoveries was the first to note hypertrophic gastritis in 1855. The next major footstep was done by Samuel Fenwick in 1870, who noted the presence of glandular atrophy due to gastric inflammation when classifying gastric lesions and anatomical alternations of the gastric mucosa (Fenwick, 1870). He also discovered that pernicious anaemia is associated with gastric mucosal atrophy. German surgeon, Georg Ernst Konjetzny using surgical specimens showed first that both gastric ulcer and gastric cancer are either secondary diseases or are associated in their pathogenesis to chronic gastric inflammation. Shields Warren and Willam A. Meissner described intestinal metaplasia of the stomach. They noted intestinal metaplasia as a feature of chronic gastritis, and found seldom extensive in duodenal ulcer patients, while it was extensive in stomachs removed due to carcinoma (Warren & Meissner, 1944; Rugge et al, 2003).

2. *In vivo* diagnosis of gastritis – Introduction of gastroscopy

In vivo diagnosis of gastritis got a huge drive with the development of routine gastroscopy. By the 1950's, Rudolf Schindler's part-flexible endoscopes became very common making rigid endoscopes to disappear. From 1960's, the commercial introduction of flexible endoscopes gave easy access for gastric biopsy and diagnosis of gastritis (Palmer, 1956). By the use of biopsy based histology Schindler gave overview of gastritis in his monograph entitled 'Gastritis' in 1947, he divided inflammation into 'superficial', 'atrophic' and 'hypertrophic' gastritis chronica (Schindler, 1947). Cheli and Dobero in 1958 differentiated 'superficial', 'interstitial' and 'atrophic gastritis' in the terminology of gastric inflammatory lesions (Cheli & Dobero, 1956). Up to his time classifications lack topography, but in 1972, Whitehead distinguished antral, fonical, corporal and pyloric region inflammation based on classical pathomorphology. Whitehead divided chronic gastritis into 'superficial' and 'atrophic', both 'active' or 'in-active' based on the presence of granulocyte infiltration in epithelium and interstitium beside the inflammatory infiltration of lamina propria from lymphocytes and plasmatic cells (Whitehead et al, 1972). He suggested the use of a mild-moderate-severe scale to evaluate the atrophy. He also introduced the evaluation of intestinal and pseudopyloric metaplasia into everyday pathological assessment.

Based on recent research data, Robert G. Strickland and Ian R. MacKay proposed the classification of gastritis based on additional factors just beside just histology and topography (Strickland & Mackay, 1973). They suggested that immunological and etiological data should be included along with pathomorphological and topographic parameters; gastric parietal cell antibody and serum level of gastrin have to be seen to get better classification of chronic gastritis. They used the term 'Type A gastritis' for gastric corporal inflammation mostly corresponding to pernicious anaemia, and 'Type B' for antral gastritis suspected to be induced by duodeno-gastric reflux according to some thoughts. In 1975 George B Jerzy Glass and Capecomorin S. Pitchumoni added the 'Type AB' to the classification. This term was aimed to be used for extended gastritis observed in corpus to pre-pyloric region (Glass & Pitchumoni, 1975). Those cases were named 'AB-plus' where antibody positivity was also founds against parietal cells. In 1980, the classification was further modified by Correa dividing chronic gastritis into autoimmune chronic gastritis with pernicious anaemia, 'hypersecretory' and 'environmental' forms. He described the gastritis accompanying ulcer to hypersecretory. All the rest of gastritis was called environmental, which are mostly due to diet and geographic localization (Correa, 1980). Later as more data were known from histological assessments, he changed his classification for 'diffuse antral', 'diffuse corporal' and 'multifocal' gastritis. By seeing his nomenclature, sometimes showing etiology, sometimes reflecting topography, we are able to see the controversy existed between pathologist and clinicians in the field of gastritis at that time. The extensiveness in topography along with histological and etiologic features were not to be combined in an uniformed nomenclature, even Correa in 1988 returned to his previous version of classification (Correa, 1988). Later, he went to different direction by dividing gastritis into two major categories of 'atrophic' and 'non-atrophic' gastritis.

The next major step was added by Judith I. Wyatt and Michael F. Dixon by the introduction of 'type C' gastritis for chemical (drug)-induced inflammation of gastric mucosa (Wyatt & Dixon, 1988). Two years later, examining 316 patients Sobala confirmed that most of reflux gastritis in intact (non-operated) stomach is not due to bile reflux but rather NSAID use. According to their proposition the term 'type C' or 'chemical' gastritis might be used for condition caused by both etiology (Sobala et al, 1990).

3. Modern time – Development of the Sydney system

Modern aspects of gastritis classification and knowledge of its biological course and consequences were relatively well-known at the time when *Helicobacter pylori* (*H. pylori*) was discovered by Robin Warren and Barry Marshall in 1982 (Warren & Marshall, 1983). Their discovery showed that the commonest form of gastritis is simply an infectious disease caused by an otherwise known pathogen. At that time gastroenterologist and pathologist had limited knowledge on even simple aspects of this chronic bacterial inflammation of gastric mucosa and the classification system used was confusing and differing from county to another. Very soon considerable amount of data became known about *H. pylori*, its disease associations and their natural courses by many physicians, microbiologist and basic researchers entering the field. As a consequence in the late 1980's several pre-meeting of Working Party (Anthony Axon, Wladimir Bogomoletz, Michael F. Dixon, Steart Goodwin, Jules Haot, Konrad L. Heilmann, Adrian Lee, Barry Marshall, George Misiewicz, Ashley Price, Penti Sipponen, Enrico Solcia, Manfred Stolte, Robert Strickland, Guido Tytgat) was set up to review the biology and natural course of chronic gastritis and to propose a new classification for gastritis by the leadership of George Misiewicz and Guido Tytgat. The working party actually consisted of two groups mainly working parallel to another: as a pathological group and a clinical group (Sipponen & Price, 2011). Based on new etiological facts and data collected, a new system of classification was presented at the World Congress of Gastroenterology held in Sydney, Australia in 1990, and subsequently published as six papers in the *Journal Gastroenterology and Hepatology*. The existence of the two Working Parties reflects on the histological and endoscopic division of Sydney System. The histological division of Sydney System intended to be a practical guideline showing which of the morphological features of gastritis in endoscopic biopsy specimens should be documented (Price, 1991). Type, severity and extent of gastric inflammation linked to possible etiology should be detailed according to a chart designed (see Fig. 1). The Sydney System declared the routine biopsy sampling protocol, the number of biopsies should be taken, the biopsies' proper localisation (two from antrum and two from corpus, both from anterior and posterior walls) and sample fixation in adequately labelled separate containers (Misiewicz et al, 1990; Price & Misiewicz, 1991). Many pathologist think to these last as the most important conclusions of the system. The system also established a four-level scale for defining severity (extent) of pathomorphological elements.

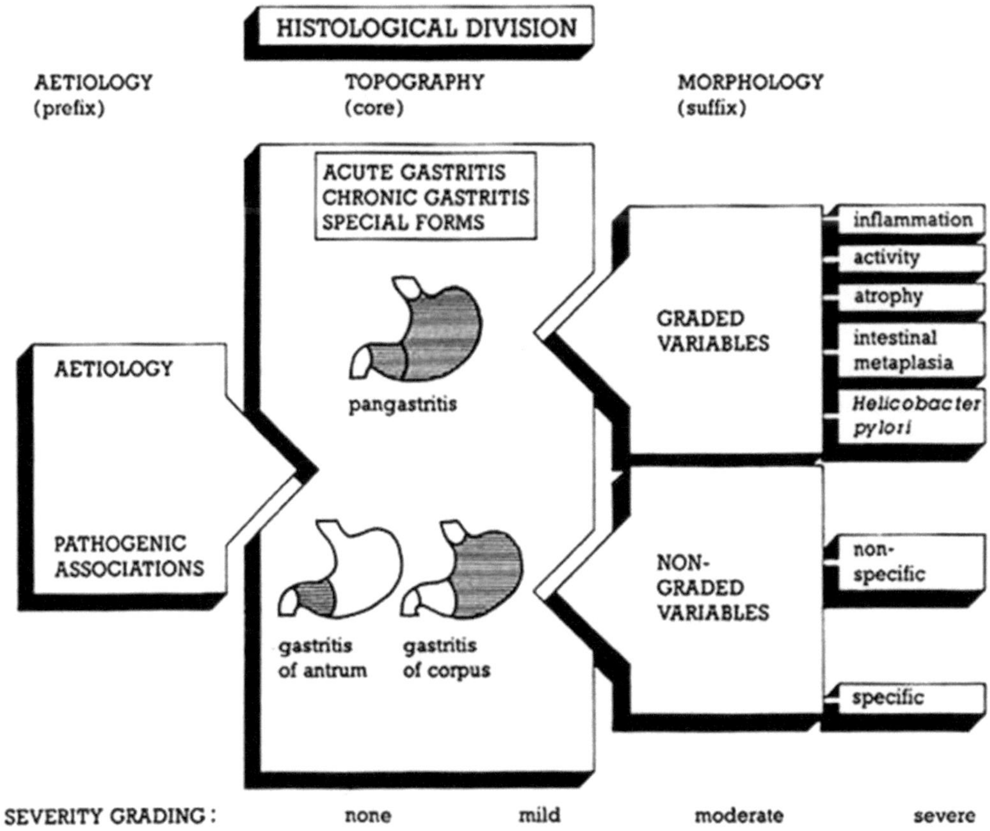

Figure 1. Chart designed for the histological division of the original Sydney System as presented to the World Congress of Gastroenterology. Published in Journal of Gastroenterology and Hepatology in 1991. Describes the nomenclature should be used in histological reporting of gastritis. Adopted etiological suffix phrases to topography and morphological features with grading suffixes to be documented in endoscopic biopsy reporting.

Year	Author/Classification	Comment
1728	Stahl	'Gastritis' defined (quoted by Bock, 1974)
1771	Morgagni	'Erosive' and 'ulcerating gastritis'' described (Crawford et al, 1932)
1859	William Brinton	Acute, subacute and chronic gastritis differentiated □
1855	Rokitansky	Hypertrophic gastritis described (quoted by Vaugham, 1945).
1870	Fenwik	Gastric atrophy described □
1944	Warren & Meissner	Intestinal metaplasia described □
1947	Wood	First gastric biopsy, 'Gastritis' defined (Wood et al, 1949)
1956	Cheli & Dobero ¤	Superficial, Interstitial and Atrophic gastritis □
1956	Eder-Palmer ∇	Introduction of flexible fibre optic endoscope (Palmer, 1956)
1972	Whitehead ¤	Superficial, Atrophic, both 'Active' or 'In-active'. Type and Stage of activity. Presence and type of metaplasia □
1973	Strickland & MacKay ¤	A (autoimmune) PCA+ in 95% and IFA+ in 75%, B (nonautoimmune = environmental) □
1975	Pitchumoni ¤	A (autoimmune-corpus), B (antrum), AB (both antrum and corpus) PCA+ or - (Glass & Pitchumoni, 1975)
1980	Correa ¤	Autoimmune, Hypersecretory, Environmental □
1988	Correa ¤	Diffuse corporal (autoimmune), Chr. diffuse antral, Multifocal environmental, Chr. Superficial, Lymphocytic, Postgastrectomy □
1989	Owen ¤	Chr. non-specific type A, Chr. non-specific type B □
1990	Yardley ¤	H. pylori gastritis, Metaplastic atrophic (type A, autoimmune), Metaplastic atrophic (type B), Lymphocytic, Chemical □
1990	Dixon ¤	'Type C' proposed to reactive gastric lesions □
1990	Sobala	Reflux gastritis defined as type C gastritis □
1990	Sydney ¤	Nonatrophic, Atrophic (Autoimmune, Multifocal), Special forms. Four-level scale, proper biopsy sampling & handling, standard reporting aiming etiology (Misiewicz et al, 1990)
1994	Appelman ¤	Acute or Chronic; Helicobacter type, Atrophic (type A, type B), Lymphocytic, Focal & miscellaneous, Chemical gastropathies □
1996	Up-dated Sydney ¤	Biopsy location changed from anterior and posterior wall to greater and lesser curvature (Dixon et al, 1996)
2000	Padova ¤	Classification of dysplasia and related lesions (Rugge et al, 2000)
2005	OLGA ¤	Classification of grading mucosal atrophy (Rugge et al, 2005b)

◦ Classification (system) ∇ Manufacturer □ See ref. under same name and year

Table 1. History of Classification of Gastritis.

The Sydney System which actually allowed statements to be made on etiology, topography and morphology of gastritis for the first time, was not accepted everywhere immediately, especially in the United States. The main criticism was that the some of the commonly used descriptive names were not enabled into the system, like the 'multifocal atrophic gastritis' or 'diffuse antral gastritis'. Although, by that time it was already accepted that the Sydney System was not designed to be the textbook of gastric pathology, but to be a guide for standard methology of reporting. Correa and Yardley criticized the system for missing out certain types of the gastritis and well as it is not a 'classification' (Correa & Yardley, 1992). Consequently, a new system needed to gain wider acceptance.

In 1994, a two-day consensus meeting was held in Houston. After this another consensus report, "Up-dated Sydney System" was published in 1997 (Dixon et al, 1996). Original classification of gastritis dividing into acute, chronic and special forms, and grading of chronic inflammation, polymorph activity, atrophy, intestinal metaplasia and *H. pylori* density into mild, moderate and marked categories were kept. This up-dated system introduced a visual analogue scale for evaluating the severity of histopathological elements (grading). It changed the routine of endoscopic biopsy sampling by the introduction of biopsy sampling from the incisura angularis and modified corpus and antrum biopsy locations from the two opposite walls to lesser and greater curvature of both parts. The Up-dated Sydney Classification received different reactions among pathologists. Most of the pathologist agreed with the need of incisural biopsy, since the most degree of atrophy and intestinal metaplasia is found in the incisural region. That would reduce the sampling error of missing premalignant lesions and improve the diagnosis of multifocal gastritis. However, later prospective studies could not really show its benefit (Stolte & Meining, 2001). Even in our conducted study higher number of intestinal metaplasia were found in antral biopsies then in the biopsies taken from the incisura angularis (Szabo et al, 2012). After the development of the visual analogue scale according to the Up-dated Sydney System, the grading of atrophy still continued to show a considerable inter-observer variability (El-Zimaity et al, 1996). The updated system categorised chronic gastritis into 'non-atrophic' and 'atrophic' forms with the latter divided into autoimmune (diffuse corpus atrophy) and multifocal. Histological reporting of gastritis should take into account the topographical pattern (antral or corpus predominant), and the final diagnostic term should ideally combine morphology and etiology to maximize the clinical value of gastric biopsy diagnosis (Dixon et al, 1997). The up-dated system beside its major benefits in further standardizing endoscopic sampling, histological assessment and formality of reporting, still showed weaknesses specially in grading atrophy as pointed out by Johan A. Offerhaus in 1999 (see ref). His proposition was to simplify the grading system to two grades (low and high).

4. Classification by Appleman

The clearest division of gastritis for clinicians was published by Appleman in 1994. He divided gastric inflammatory diseases to *acute* and *chronic* (see Table II). The most common form of gastritis that was called earlier as chronic diffuse antral gastritis, gastritis chronic type B, gastritis chronica active antralis, gastritis non-specifica or gastritis typus hypersecretions was named as *Helicobacter pylori related gastritis*. At this time lot of work proved that *H. pylori* infection causes chronic gastritis in the prepyloric region later leading to atrophy of glands and development of gastric adenocarcinoma and less frequently of lymphoma (Apelman, 1994, Kozlowski et al, 2011).

http://dx.doi.org/10.5772/52884

According to Appelman's classification the autoimmune gastritis used to be called as gastritis autoimmunogenes, gastritis chronic atrophica typus A, gastritis chronic typus A and gastritis chronic diffusa corporis, was called to *autoimmune chronic atrophic gastritis*. Appelman pointed out the presence of autoantibodies against parietal cells and intrinsic factor being important in diagnosis, enterochromaffinlike (ECL) cell hyperplasia and risk of carcinoma.

Appelman's classification of gastritis continues with the *multifocal atrophic gastritis* earlier called as environmental gastritis or type B chronic atrophic gastritis. At that time the cause of this form of gastritis was not clearly known. Beside known environmental factors responsible for geographic differences in its epidemiology, raising circumstantial evidences from an Italian study examining gastric distribution of *H. pylori*, pointed out the role of *H. pylori* in its generation (Rugge et al, 1993). Evidences suggested that *H. pylori* first infects the antrum, and later it involves the body leading to atrophic gastritis.

Appelman seeing similarity of the histological changes of patients with gastroenteric anastomosis and taking nonsteroidal anti-inflammatory (NSAID) medications, called third division of gastritis caused by bile reflux or NSAIDs to *chemical gastropathies*. Due to less inflammation these histological changes consisting foveolar hyperplasia, decrease of mucin in foveolar cells, superficial oedema, increase of smooth muscle fibres in the lamina propria were named as 'gastropathies'. Recognition of this distinction of gastritis greatly helped to simply classification, although many times elements histological changes usually found in chemical gastropathy can be noticed in other forms of gastritis as well as in other gastric disease. Finding them singular and unassociated wit other changes like atrophy, intestinal metaplasia, presence of bacteria, ulcers, polyps, should raise the possibility of chemical gastritis.

Appelman kept the name of *lymphotic gastritis* used by his frontiers for the fourth distinctive form of gastritis (Haot et al, 1988, 1990). In this form of chronic gastritis huge lymphocytic infiltration of the surface epithelium, superficial pits and lamina propria can be observed. Others used to call this as superficial gastritis, gastritis chronic erosive or gastritis varioliformis. That time in 1990, the histological changes seen in lymphocytic gastritis was already described in patients with sprues and gluten-sensitivity. Lymphocytic gastritis tends to form "varioliform gastritis" endoscopically. This includes thick folds and small bumps with central depression seen during endoscopy. But lymphocytic gastritis also can form giant folds leading clinical symptoms (Ménétrier's disease).

Appelman's division of gastritis contained a miscellaneous group of gastritis. There are many gastritis forms that do not differ significantly from similar inflammations found other organs, including those that occur in syphilis, mycobacterial and cytomegalovirus, human immunodeficiency virus infections, histoplasmosis, candidiasis, cryptosporidiosis and other opportunistic fungi. There is a family of granulomatous reactions or *granulomatous gastritis*. Some of these are part of a systemic or focal gut granulomatous disease, such as sarcoidosis or Crohn's disease, and some have been described as part of a systemic vasculitis syndrome or Whipple's disease. There are still others which are not associated with any other diseases and designated as 'isolated granulomatous gastritis'. *Allergic gastritis* is usually part of a gastrointestinal allergic disease. Appelman also categorized the recently described *collagenous gastritis* into this miscellaneous group.

Acute	Acute infectious gastritis (including Hp)	
	Erosive (caused mostly by NSAID or alcohol)	
	Necrotising and haemorrhagic (caused mostly by ischaemia)	
Chronic	**Helicobacter pylori type**	
	Atrophic	Type A: autoimmune, diffuse
		Type B: non-autoimmune, multifocal, enviromental
	Lymphocytic	Including varioliform, 'sprue-like' and Ménétrier-like
	Chemical¤	Bile reflux
		NSAIDs
		others (caused by other damaging agents and physical trauma)
	Miscellaneous	Granulomatous (part of Crohn's, Whipple's, vasculitis, sarcoidosis or isolated granulomatous gastritis)
		Allergic
		Specific infectious (HIV, mycobacterial, syphilis, Cytomegalovirus, histoplasmosis, cryptosporidiosis
		Collagenous

◦ Gastropathies

Table 2. Appleman's classification of gastritis (1994)

5. Precancerous lesions

Warren and Meissner describing intestinal metaplasia and recognising the clinical-pathological pattern of gastritis, described the bases of etiopathogenic relationship between gastric cancer and chronic gastritis (Warren & Meissner, 1944; Rugge et al, 2003). In 1980, Morson *et al.* (see ref.) defined gastric precancerous conditions as atrophic gastritis, gastric ulcer, pernicious anaemia, gastric stumps, gastric polyps, and Ménétrier's disease. They emphasized that epithelial dysplasia being a precancerous lesion is common in these conditions; dysplasia should be graded as mild, moderate and severe; and underlined the problems of differentiating inflammatory or regenerative changes from mild dysplasia, and intramucosal carcinoma from severe dysplasia (Morson et al, 1980). Japanese pathologists by studying serial sections of gastric mucosa obtained from gastric cancer patients described several border line lesions with histological and cytological changes. The premalignant significance of these was questioned for quite a long time; finally, the long-term follow-up studies closed this debate (Rugge et al, 1994, 1997). The high inter-observer inconsistency in histological assessment of premalignant lesions and new result supporting their neoplastic intraglandular nature obtained from genotyping studies highlighted the need of a broad consensus to re-

http://dx.doi.org/10.5772/52884

define precancerous lesions uniformly. International group of pathologists met in Padova, Italy in April, 1998 on an international consensus conference. The conference reached an agreement on the definitions of the spectrum of gastric premalignant lesions and on common glossary for pathologist and clinicians, and applied strict diagnostic criteria (Rugge et al, 2000) (see Table III).

<table>
<tr><td rowspan="4">Negative for dysplasia</td><td colspan="3">1.0 Normal</td></tr>
<tr><td colspan="3">1.1 Reactive foveolar hyperplasia</td></tr>
<tr><td colspan="2" rowspan="2">1.2 Intestinal metaplasia</td><td>1.2.1 Complete type</td></tr>
<tr><td>1.2.2 Incomplete type</td></tr>
<tr><td rowspan="2">Indefinite for dysplasia</td><td colspan="3">2.1 Foveolar hyperproliferation</td></tr>
<tr><td colspan="3">2.2 Hyperproliferative intestinal metaplasia</td></tr>
<tr><td rowspan="3">Non-invasive neoplasma
(flat or elevated)</td><td colspan="3">3.1 Low-grade</td></tr>
<tr><td rowspan="2">3.2 High-grade</td><td colspan="2">3.2.1 Including suspicious for carcinoma without invasion (intraglandular)</td></tr>
<tr><td colspan="2">3.2.2 Including carcinoma without invasion (intraglandular)</td></tr>
<tr><td colspan="4">Suspicious for invasive carcinoma</td></tr>
<tr><td colspan="4">Invasive carcinoma</td></tr>
</table>

Table 3. Padova Classification of gastric dysplasia and related lesions (2000)

6. Evaluation of atrophy

The Sydney System and Up-dated Sydney System attempted to incorporate etiologic, topographic, and morphologic criteria into a clinically relevant scheme to reach a broad consensus in classification of gastritis. One of the most controversial issues at the Houston Workshop was the concept of atrophy. It was pointed out that "normal" was not precisely defined; the loss of appropriate glands occurs with distinct patterns and has different functional significance in antrum and corpus; the relationship between atrophy and intestinal metaplasia remained incompletely understood; and the topographic patterns of distribution and its evolution made the atrophic gastritis to the most controversial topic of gastritis (Genta, 1996). Later long-term follow-up studies have confirmed that the extent of gastric mucosal atrophy parallels gastric cancer risk (Meining et al, 2002; Sipponen et al, 1985, 1994, 1997; Stolte et al, 2000). At the same time Sydney System did not present a reporting terminology for chronic gastritis understandable and providing prognostic and therapeutic information for clinicians. Whereas, hepatitis staging had already improved useful, simple terminology for interdisciplinary communication representing disease progression and cancer risk.

Inspired by these facts, international group of gastroenterologists and pathologists named as Operative Link on Gastritis Assessment (OLGA) developed an improved histological staging system for gastric atrophy (Rugge & Genta, 2005a, 2005b). OLGA system uses the gastric biopsy sampling protocol defined by Sydney System and the visual analogue system recommended by the Up-dated Sydney System. The gastritis staging is defined from combined extent of atrophy scored histologically with the topography of atrophy identified through biopsy mapping (see Fig. 2). Long-term follow-up studies proved that gastritis OLGA staging conveys relevant information on clinic-pathological outcome of gastritis and therefore *H. pylori* negative patients with low OLGA stages could be confidently excluded from secondary preventive surveillance invasive procedures (Rugge et al, 2010). Whereas patients with high OLGA stages (Stages III and IV) should be considered definitely candidates for endoscopic surveillance. Significant correlation was shown between OLGA stages and pepsinogen serology (marker of gastric atrophy). The ratio of pepsinogen I and II gives adequate information on the severity of atrophy, but its measurement fails to differentiate between neoplastic and non-neoplastic disease among patients with high stages of gastric mucosal atrophy (Rugge et al, 2010).

Similar to the OLGA system another system, called the Baylor system was also introduced. The Baylor system follows the Baylor biopsy protocol (which uses Sydney System biopsy sites with two additional distal corporal biopsies) and scores the atrophy of antrum and corpus independently (Graham et al, 2006). Antral atrophy stage is an average score, but corpus atrophy stage is independent of antral atrophy, independent of individual reading in each biopsy but dependent on location. As corpus atrophy starts at the incisura and extends in continuity proximally and towards the greater curve, atrophy in a distal biopsy is early and atrophy in the most proximal location is advanced. The comparison of the two atrophy grading systems is still controversial. Although there were studies performed showing the superiority of Baylor system over OLGA in indentifying cancer risk (El-Zimaity et al, 2008), the evaluation of gastric atrophy by OLGA is more widely used, further developed and more studied.

Rugge *et al*. developed the OLGIM system for more precise evaluation of cancer risk. This system basically incorporates the OLGA frame, but replaces the atrophy score with an assessment of intestinal metaplasia (IM) alone. Examining a series of more than 4500 biopsies (2007-2009) showed that OLGIM staging is less sensitive than OLGA staging in the identification of patients at high risk of gastric cancer (Rugge et al, 2011). However, replacement of atrophic gastritis by intestinal metaplasia in the staging of gastritis considerably increases inter-observer agreement. The correlation with the severity of gastritis remains at least as strong. Therefore, the OLGIM may be preferred over the OLGA for the prediction of gastric cancer risk in patients with premalignant lesions (Capelle et al, 2010).

Even though above precursor lesions were commonly known and found in everyday practice, there were no international recommendation to guide the clinicians in management of patients with such lesions. This resulted wide heterogeneity of surveillance practice and failure in diagnosing patients with early, curable stage cancer. The European Society of Gastrointestinal Endoscopy (ESGE), the European Helicobacter Study Group (EHSG), the European Society of Pathology (ESP) and the Sociedade Portuguesa de Endoscopia Digesti-

http://dx.doi.org/10.5772/52884

va (SPED) have therefore combined efforts to develop evidence-based guideline on the *management of patients with precancerous conditions and lesions in stomach* (termed *MAPS*). Panel of European gastroenterologist pathologist and other researchers met in Barcelona, Spain in 2010, agreed on methodology, set up key questions for literature search and drafted preliminary statements. The panel divided into several subgroups searched for evidence on a certain question. Finally representatives of European national societies reviewed the evidence gathered and formed statements. Later, online sessions were held for voting and further comments; finally a second meeting held in Porto, Portugal finalized the guideline. The guideline details diagnostic assessment, treatment and follow-up of individuals with atrophic gastritis or intestinal metaplasia or dysplasia of gastric mucosa (Dinis-Ribeiro et al, 2012) (see Fig. 3).

		Corpus			
	Atrophy score	No atrophy (score 0)	Mild atrophy (score 1)	Moderate atrophy (score 2)	Severe atrophy (score 3)
Antrum	No atrophy (score 0) (*including incisura angularis*)	Stage 0	Stage I	Stage II	Stage II
	Mild atrophy (score 1) (*including incisura angularis*)	Stage I	Stage I	Stage II	Stage III
	Moderate atrophy (score 2) (*including incisura angularis*)	Stage II	Stage II	Stage III	Stage IV
	Severe atrophy (score 3) (*including incisura angularis*)	Stage III	Stage III	Stage IV	Stage IV

Figure 2. Gastritis Staging by OLGA system (Rugge & Genta, 2005a, 2005b, 2007), published in Gut in 2007. Atrophy is score in a four-tiered scale (0-3) in each compartment. The atrophy stage defined from the combination of atrophic changes assessed in gastric antral and corporal biopsies.

The recommendations contain that conventional white light endoscopy cannot accurately differentiate between and diagnose pre-neoplastic gastric conditions/lesions. Thus, magnification chromoendoscopy or narrow-band imaging (NBI) endoscopy with or without magnification may be offered in these cases as it improves diagnosis of such lesions. In addition, at least four biopsies of the proximal and distal stomach, on the lesser and greater curvature, are needed for adequate assessment of premalignant gastric conditions. Systems for histopathological staging (e.g. OLGA or OLGIM assessment) may be useful for identifying subgroups of patients with different risks of progression to gastric cancer namely those with extensive lesions (i. e., atrophy and/or intestinal metaplasia in both antrum and corpus). Although only low potential applicability was reported by participants for this indicator, low serum pepsinogen levels can also predict this phenotype and, in such patients, *H. pylori* serology may also be useful for further detection of high risk individuals. Beyond a family history of gastric cancer, neither age, gender, *H. pylori* virulence factors, or host genetic variations change these clinical recommendations. Patients with extensive atrophy and/or extensive intestinal metaplasia should be offered endoscopic surveillance every 3 years. Patients with mild to moderate atrophy/intestinal metaplasia only in antrum do not need follow-up. If *H. pylori* infection is present, eradication should be offered to prevent high grade dysplasia or carcinoma. Patients with dysplasia without a visible endoscopic lesion should be closely followed up, either immediately and 6 to 12 months thereafter, or within 12 months, respectively, for those with high grade or low grade dysplasia. Those with dysplasia or cancer within an endoscopically visible lesion should undergo staging and resection (see Fig. 3.) (Dinis-Ribeiro et al, 2012).

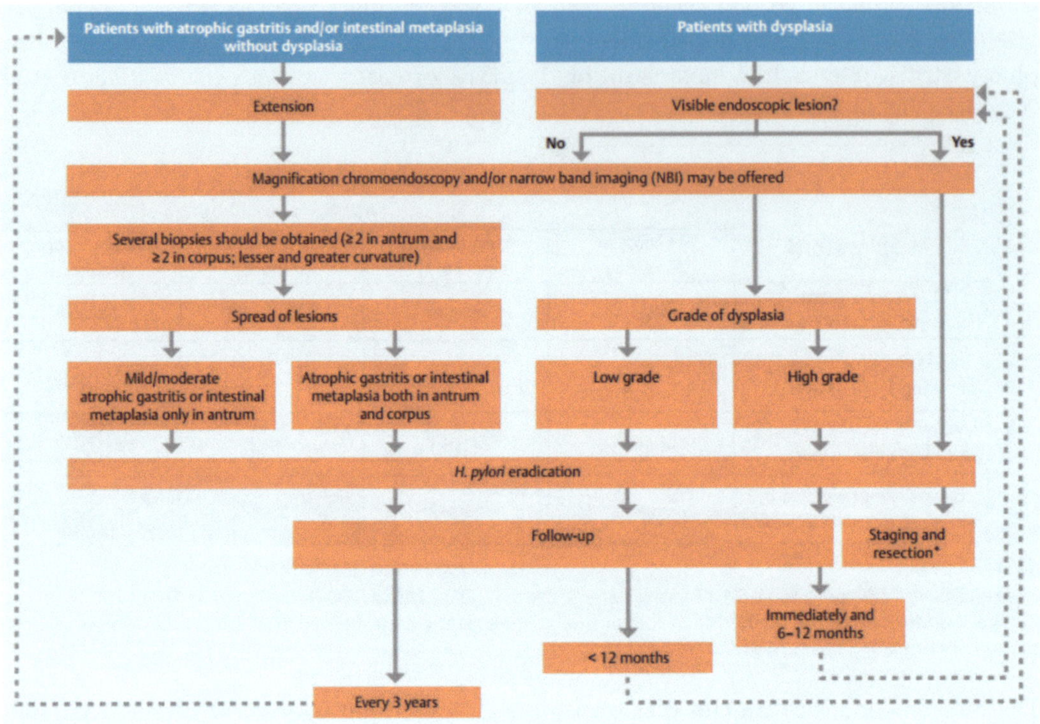

Figure 3. Summary of management for patients with atrophic gastritis, gastric intestinal metaplasia and gastric epithelial dysplasia. Published in Endoscopy, 2012 (Dinis-Ribeiro et al, 2012).

This review critically offers and emphasizes the necessity of an international consensus meeting, which will establish a more uniform classification of gastritis respecting the wider multidisciplinary aspects (morphology, clinical picture, endoscopic view, immunology, bacteriology, molecular pharmacology, general medicine, oncology and causative factors as well as social/environmental circumstances of the people) in this field.

7. Conclusion

During the about last 150 years the knowledge on "gastritides" has enlarged enormously. The discovered new forms of gastritis, the new etiopathogenic evidences have continuously

http://dx.doi.org/10.5772/52884

modified our views on gastritis classification. Recently, good agreement has been established among pathologist and clinicians to standardise the methodology of biopsy sampling, histological assessment and reporting leading to reproducible and clinically useful diagnosis. Recent recommendations for the management of bleeding, *H. pylori* infected or cancer risk patients help clinicians to endorse up-to-date therapy and follow-up. Presently there are still many unanswered questions regarding lot of segment of various forms of gastritis. Pathologist still need to issue descriptive histological report of 'chronic non-specific gastritis' to clinicians due to either lack of clinical information or knowledge of identifying gastric inflammations distinctive from known categories. For reducing the number of these cases further communication and consensus (as well as further consensus meetings) will be needed between pathologists and gastroenterologists. The growing information from research and clinical studies might show further new directions and require modification of classification. It is possible that at some day the presently known different types of gastritis will be known as various stages of the same disease, or partition of a present form could happen due to discovered futural diverse etiologic causes.

Author details

Imre Laszlo Szabo, Kata Cseko, Jozsef Czimmer and Gyula Mozsik

First Department of Medicine, University of Pécs, Hungary

References

[1] Appelman H.D. (1994). Gastritis: terminology, etiology, and clinicopathological correlations: another biased view. Hum Pathol, Vol.25, pp.1006-19.

[2] Brinton W. (1857). On the Pathology, Symptoms and Treatment of Ulcer of the Stomach, London, J. Churchill.

[3] Bock O.A. (1974). The relationship between chronic gastritis, gastric ulceration and carcinoma of the stomach. A historical review. *S Afr Med J*, Vol.48: pp.2063-6.

[4] Capelle L.G., de Vries A.C., Haringsma J., et al. (2010). The staging of gastritis with the OLGA system by using intestinal metaplasia as an accurate alternative for atrophic gastritis. *Gastrointest Endosc*, Vol.71: pp.1150-8.

[5] Cheli R., Dodero M. (1956). Sulle alterazioni ghiandolari fundiche nelle gastriti croniche. Ricerche bioetiche e correlazioni anatomo-secretorie. Min Gastroenterol, Vol.4: pp.1–6.

[6] Correa P. (1980). The epidemiology and pathogenesis of chronic gastritis; three etiologic entities. *Front Gastrointestinal Res*, Vol. 6: pp.98-108.

[7] Correa P. (1988). Chronic gastritis: a clinico-pathological classification. *Am J Gastroenterol,* Vol.83: pp.504-9.

[8] Correa P., Yardley J.H. (1992). Grading and classification of chronic gastritis: one American response to the Sydney System. *Gastroenterology,* Vol.102, pp.355-9.

[9] Crawford Q., Crawford A. (1832). Ulceration of the Brain. *The Medico-Chirurgical Review, and Journal of Practical Medicine,* Vol.16, pp.601.

[10] Dinis-Ribeiro M., Areia M., de Vries A.C., et. al. (2012). European Society of Gastrointestinal Endoscopy; European Helicobacter Study Group; European Society of Pathology; Sociedade Portuguesa de Endoscopia Digestiva. Management of precancerous conditions and lesions in the stomach (MAPS): guideline from the European Society of Gastrointestinal Endoscopy (ESGE), European Helicobacter Study Group (EHSG), European Society of Pathology (ESP), and the Sociedade Portuguesa de Endoscopia Digestiva (SPED). *Endoscopy,* Vol.44: pp.74-94.

[11] Dixon M.F. (1990). Progress in the pathology of gastritis and duodentitis. In: *Gastrointestinal Pathology,* Williams G.T. (Ed.), Springer-Verlag, Berlin, Germany, pp.1-27.

[12] Dixon M.F., Genta R.M., Yardley J.H., Correa P, Participants on the International Workshop on the Histopathology of Gastritis. (1996). Classification and grading of gastritis. The updated Sydney System. *Am J Surg Pathol,* Vol.20, pp.1161-81.

[13] Dixon M.F., Genta R.M., Yardley J.H., Correa P. (1997). Histological classification of gastritis and *Helicobacter pylori* infection: an agreement at last? The International Workshop on the Histopathology of Gastritis. *Helicobacter,* Vol.2 Suppl 1: pp.17-24.

[14] El-Zimaity H.M., Graham D.Y., al-Assi M.T., et al. (1996). Interobserver variation in the histopathological assessment of *Helicobacter pylori* gastritis. *Hum Pathol,* Vol.27: pp.35-41.

[15] El-Zimaity H. (2008). Gastritis and gastric atrophy. *Curr Opin Gastroenterol,* Vol.24: pp.682-6.

[16] Fenwick S. (1870). On atrophy of the stomach. *Lancet,* Vol. ii: pp.78-80.

[17] Genta R.M. (1996). Recognizing atrophy: another step toward a classification of gastritis. *Am J Pathol,* Vol.20 Suppl 1: pp.23-30.

[18] Glass G.B.J., Pitchumoni C.S. (1975). Atrophic gastritis. *Hum Pathol,* Vol.6: pp.219-50.

[19] Graham DY, Nurgalieva ZZ, El-Zimaity HM, et al.. (2006). Noninvasive versus histologic detection of gastric atrophy in a Hispanic population in North America. *Clin Gastroenterol Hepatol,* Vol.4: pp.306-14.

[20] Haot J., Hamichi L., Wallez L., Mainguet P. (1988). Lymphocytic gastritis: a newly described entity: a retrospective endoscopic and histological study. Gut, Vol.29: pp. 1258-64.

[21] Haot J., Jouret A., Willette M., Gossuin A., Mainguet P. (1990). Lymphocytic gastritis--prospective study of its relationship with varioliform gastritis. *Gut,* Vol.31: pp. 282-5.

[22] Kozlowski W., Jochymski C, Markiewicz T. (2011). Chronic gastritis, In: *Gastritis and Gastric Cancer – New Insights in Gastroprotection, Diagnosis and Treatments,* Tonino P. (Ed.), 76-92, In-Tech, Rijeka, Croatia.

[23] Marshall B.J., Warren J.R. (1984). Unidentified curved bacilli in the stomach of patients with gastritis and peptic ulceration. *Lancet,* Vol.1: pp.1311-5.

[24] Meining A., Riedl B., Stolte M. (2002). Features of gastritis predisposing to gastric adenoma and early gastric cancer. *J Clin Pathol,* Vol.55: pp.770-3.

[25] Misiewicz J.J., Tytgat G.N.J., Goodwin C.S., et al. (1990). The Sydney System: a new classification of gastritis. *World Congresses of Gastroenterology,* 1990 August 26–31. Sydney, pp.1-10.

[26] Morson B.C., Sobin L.H., Grundmann E., Johansen A., Nagayo T., Serck-Hanssen A. (1980). Precancerous conditions and epithelial dysplasia in the stomach. *J Clin Pathol,* Vol.33: pp.711–21.

[27] Offerhaus GJ, Price AB, Haot J, et al. (1999). Observer agreement on the grading of gastric atrophy. *Histopathology,* Vol.34: pp.320-5.

[28] Owen D.A: (1989). Stomach. In: *Diagnostic surgical Pathology and Its Clinical Implications,* Stenberg S.S. (Ed.), New York, NY, Raven Press, pp. 939-48.

[29] Palmer E.D. (1956). Clinical benmefit of routine combined oesophagogastroscopy with the help of the two trabnsoesophagoscopic gastroscope. *Bull Am Gastrosc Soc, Vol.*4: pp.7-11.

[30] Price A.B., Misiewicz J.J. (1991). Sydney classification for gastritis. *Lancet,* Vol.337:pp. 174.

[31] Price A.B. (1991). The Sydney System: Histological division. *J Gastoenterol Hepatol,* Vol.6, pp.209-22.

[32] Rugge M., Di Mario F., Cassaro M., et al. (1993). Pathology of the gastric antrum and body associated with *Helicobacter pylori* infection in non-ulcerous patients: is the bacterium a promoter of intestinal metaplasia? *Histopathology,* Vol.22: pp.9-15.

[33] Rugge M., Farinati F., Baffa R., Sonego F., Di Mario F., Leandro G., Valiante F. (1994). Gastric epithelial dysplasia in the natural history of gastric cancer: a multicenter prospective follow-up study. Interdisciplinary Group on Gastric Epithelial Dysplasia. *Gastroenterology,* Vol.107: pp.1288-96.

[34] Rugge M., Cassaro M., Farinati F., Di Mario F. (1997). Diagnosis of gastric carcinoma in Japan and western countries. *Lancet,* Vol.350: pp.448.

[35] Rugge M., Correa P., Dixon M.F., et al. (2000). Gastric dysplasia: the Padova international classification. Am J Surg Pathol, Vol.24: pp.167–76.

[36] Rugge M., Russo V.M., Guido M. (2003). Review article: what have we learnt from gastric biopsy? *Aliment Pharmacol Ther*, Vol.17 Suppl 2: pp.68-74.

[37] Rugge M., Genta R.M. (2005a). Staging and grading of chronic gastritis. Hum Pathol, Vol.36: pp.228-33.

[38] Rugge M., Genta R.M., OLGA Group. (2005b). Staging gastritis: an international proposal. *Gastroenterology*, Vol.129: pp.1807-8.

[39] Rugge M., Meggio A., Pennelli G., et al. (2007). Gastritis staging in clinical practice: the OLGA staging system. *Gut,Vol.*56: pp.631-6.

[40] Rugge M., de Boni M., Pennelli G., et al. (2010). Gastritis OLGA-staging and gastric cancer risk: a twelve-year clinico-pathological follow-up study. *Aliment Pharmacol Ther*, Vol.31: pp.1104-11.

[41] Rugge M., Fassan M., Pizzi M., et al. (2011). Operative link for gastritis assessment vs operative link on intestinal metaplasia assessment. *World J* Gastroenterol, Vol.17: pp. 4596-601.

[42] Schindler R. (1947). Gastritis. London: William Heinmann (Medical Books).

[43] Sipponen P., Kekki M., Haapakoski J., Ihamäki T., Siurala M. (1985). Gastric cancer risk in chronic atrophic gastritis: statistical calculations of cross-sectional data. *Int J Cancer*, Vol.35: pp.173-7.

[44] Sipponen P, Price A.B. (2011). The Sydney System for classification of gastritis 20 years ago. *J Gastroenterol Hepatol*, Vol.26 Suppl 1: pp.31-4.

[45] Sipponen P., Riihelä M., Hyvärinen H., Seppälä K. (1994). Chronic nonatropic ('superficial') gastritis increases the risk of gastric carcinoma. A case-control study. *Scand J Gastroenterol*, Vol.29: pp.336-40.

[46] Sipponen P., Stolte M. (1997). Clinical impact of routine biopsies of the gastric antrum and body. *Endoscopy*, Vol.29: pp.671-8.

[47] Sobala G.M., King R.F., Axon A.T., Dixon M.F. (1990). Reflux gastritis in the intact stomach. *J Clin* Pathol, Vol.43: pp.303-6.

[48] Stolte M., Meining A. (2000). *Helicobacter pylori* gastritis of the gastric carcinoma phenotype: is histology capable of identifying high-risk gastritis? *J Gastroenterol*, Vol.35 Suppl 12: pp.98-101.

[49] Stolte M., Meining A. (2001). The updated Sydney system: classification and grading of gastritis as the basis of diagnosis and treatment. *Can J Gastroenterol*, Vol.15: pp. 591-8.

[50] Strickland R.G., Mackay I.R. (1973). A reappraisal of the nature and significance of chronic atrophic gastritis. Am J Dig Dis, Vol.18: pp.426-40.

[51] Szabo I., Illes A., Godi S., et al. (2012). Gastritis staging in clinical practice by OLGA (Operative Link for Gastritis Assessment) system - Evaluation of gastric mucosal atrophy and metaplasia. *Z Gastroenterol*, Vol.50, A72.

[52] Vaughan W. (1945). Antral Gastritis: Roentgenologic and Gastroscopic Findings. Radiology, Vol.44, pp. 531-42.

[53] Warren J.R., Marshall B. (1983). Unidentified curved bacilli on gastric epithelium in active chronic gastritis. Lancet, Vol.321, pp.1273-4.

[54] Warren S., Meissner W.A. (1944). Chronic Gastritis and Carcinoma of the Stomach. *Gastroenterology*, Vol.3: pp.251-6.

[55] Whitehead R., Truelove S.C., Gear M.W. (1972). The histological diagnosis of chronic gastritis in fibreoptic gastroscope biopsy specimens. J Clin Pathol, Vol.25: pp.1–11.

[56] Wood I.J., Doig R.K., Motteram R. et al. (1949). Gastric biopsy; report on 55 biopsies using a new flexible gastric biopsy tube. Lancet, Vol.1: pp.18-21.

[57] Wyatt J.I., Dixon M.F. (1988). Chronic gastritis--a pathogenetic approach. *J Pathol*, Vol.154: pp.113-24.

[58] Yadley J.H. (1990). Pathology of chronic gastritis and duodenitis. In: *Gastrointestinal Pathology*, Ch: 3, Goldman H., Appelman H.D., Kaufman N. (Eds.), Williams & Wilkins, Baltimore, MD, pp.69-121.

Section 2

Animal Models for Study the Mechanisms of Gastritis

Chapter 2

The Role of *Helicobacter spp.* Infection in Domestic Animals

Achariya Sailasuta and Worapat Prachasilchai

Additional information is available at the end of the chapter

http://dx.doi.org/10.5772/53054

1. Introduction

1.1. Overview and pathogenesis

The discovery of the association of *Helicobacter pylori* with chronic gastritis, peptic ulcers and gastric neoplasia, mucosa-associated lymphoid tissue-type lymphoma and carcinoma, has led to fundamental changes in the understanding of gastric disease in humans. Some humans with *H. pylori* infection develop only mild, asymptomatic gastritis. Whether more severe disease develops thought to be influenced by individual host factors and pathogenicity of the bacteria involved. The odd of developing symptomatic *H. pylori* infection varies by geographic location and age. Different strains of *H. pylori* have recently been identified. Therefore, *H. pylori* should be considered a population of closely related but genetically heterogenous bacteria of different genotypes and virulence.

A gastric spiral bacteria of superkingdom bacteria, phylum proteobacteria, subphylum delta/epsilon subdivisions, class epsilonproteobacteria, order campylobacter, family helicobacteraceae, genus *Helicobacter spp.* is gram-negative, spiral-shaped bacteria. At least 13 species have been reported, and most are suspected or proven gastric or hepatic pathogens. *Helicobacter spp.* have been reported in humans: mainly *H. pylori*, nonhuman primates: *H. nemestrinae*, cats and dogs various species, including *H. pylori, H. felis, H. salomonis, H. rappini, H. heilmannii*, and *H. bizzozeronii*, pigs: *H. heilmannii*, ferrets: *H. mustelae*, and cheetahs: *H. acinonys*. More recently we have learned that nearly all mammmals harbor their own species of *Helicobacter* infection. Some are suggesting now that infection might be benign or even beneficial by protecting againts development of esophageal reflux and cancer of the esophagus.

Risk factors for *H. pylori* infection in humans include age and socioeconomic status, with children and those with low socioeconomic status at greater risk. The role of *Helicobacter spp.* in gastrointestinal disease in dogs and cats is uncertain. It has been known for years that gastric *Helicobacter*-like organisms (HLO) are commonly present in stomach of dogs but the relationship of these organisms and gastric disease is unresolved. *H. pylori* transmission is proposed to be fecal-oral, oral-oral, and gastro-oral (via vomited fluids). The exact details of transmission are still unclear. A higher incidence of *H. pylori* infection has been reported by gastroenterologists, suggesting that transmission from patient to physician is possible. It has been suggested that *Helicobacter spp.* infection might be zoonotic by contact with dogs and cats and has been correlated with human *H. heilmannii* infection. There is no correlation between pet ownership and human *H. pylori* infection.

H. pylori is one of the major causes of chronic gastritis and plays an important role in the pathogenesis of peptic ulcer, gastric carcinoma, gastric adenocarcinoma, and primary B-cell gastric lymphoma. *H. pylori* is the second most common cause of cancer morbidity and mortality worldwide, and the development of gastric non-Hodgkin's lymphoma. Histological gastritis is essentially universal among *H. pylori*-infected individuals, but only a few develop a clinically significant outcome, such as peptic ulcer disease or gastric cancer. The clinical significance of this bacterium has recently been emphasized by a National Institutes of Health consensus panel and thus recommending antibiotic therapy for the large majority of peptic ulcer patients who are infected with *H. pylori* and by classification of *H. pylori* as a classification of *H. pylori* as a class I (definite) carcinogen by the World Health Organization. The bacteria were often seen in malignant or ulcerated gastric tissue, and the possibility of an infectious cause of peptic ulcer was considered. *H. pylori* often estabishes life-long infections of the gastric mucosa. These bacteria produce a powerful urease that is regulated in response to acid. So the ammonia and carbonate produced by this enzyme most likely create an alkaline microenvironment. This mechanism is unprecedented. Further study shows that the high density of colonization by *H. pylori* occurs in the antrum (lower portion of the stomach) where conditions are less acidic. As the infection becomes more pronounced or under conditions where the antrum becomes more alkaline, the motile bacteria migrate up into the cardia (body) of the stomach. Infection with *H. pylori* bacteria is basically located in three dimensions, as these bacteria not only can move north and south in the mucosa in response to acid levels, but they are able to move freely up and down in the mucus layer that coats the gastric mucosa and provides a protective barrier against the diffusion of strong acid onto the epithelium. The notion of being "off shore" and therefore out of reach of the macrophages and cells of host immune defense may also play an important role in survival of these bacteria. Finally, the mounting evidence suggests that *H. pylori* may control the immune response and selective release of inflammatory factors. The balance between increase of inflammation and immune suppression is a key to the persistence and an area where novel therapeutics, perhaps in combination with vaccine strategies, could be directed.

The discovery of *Helicobacter spp.*, a relative of *Campylobacter spp.* (bacterial pathogens of the lower GI tract), fortunately coincided with the beginning of the genomics era, and is the beneficiary of two completely sequenced genomes of *H. pylori*. The results reveal a small genome (1.67 megabases) containing some 1553 genes encoding around 1,300 proteins. Despite possessing a limited number of genes, *H. pylori* displays auxotropy for only a few amino acids and appears to possess most catabolic and anabolic pathways found in bacteria with larger genomes. Recent studies examining essentiality testing on a genome scale suggested that there are few redundancies and backups in metabolic pathways and thus the percentage of *H. pylori* genes found essential may be greater than expected for organisms with larger genomes perhaps opening a door for development of *Helicobacter* selective therapeutics.

Helicobacter-like bacteria have been identified in the stomachs of all mammalian species examined to date. Many epidemiological studies have shown a strong association between chronic *H. pylori* infection and subsequent development of gastric carcinoma in humans. Studies of *H. pylori* and gastric carcinoma from the view point of animal model showed that persistent *H. pylori* infection has recently been achieved in the Japanese monkeys and Mongolian gerbil models, with results demonstrating that the sequential histopathological changes in the gastric mucosa are closely mimic the gastric mucosal changes caused by *H. pylori* infection in humans. Gastric mucosa infected with *H. pylori* exhibited significantly higher gastritis score, reduction in glandular height, increase in the number of Ki-67 positive cells and over expression of p53 protein and p53 gene mutation in the Japanese monkey model. In the Mongolian gerbil model, *H. pylori* infection enhances gastric and also demonstrated that *H. pylori* infection alone can result in the development of gastric carcinoma

In gnotobiotic dogs were used as experimental hosts for *H. pylori* infection. All dogs tested were successfully colonized with *H. pylori*. In addition, two inoculated dogs co-housed with experimental dogs also became colonized which indicating transmission of infection. The subsequent use of dogs as *H. pylori* models has been limited. One recent study showed that conventionally housed dogs are also susceptible to experimental infection. In addition to experimental studies, efforts have been made to determine the presence of natural gastric *Helicobacter* spp. infections in dogs. Surveys of pet dogs have repeatedly failed to show natural infection with *H. pylori*. However, natural infection with other gastric *Helicobacters* commonly occurs. *H. felis, H. bilis, H. bizzozeronii, H. salomonis, H. heilmannii* and *Flexispira rappini* have all been identified in surveys of gastric infections in dogs. A significant association between their presence and the occurrence of gastritis has never been demonstrated. There have been many studies confirm other studies which suggested the presence of *Helicobacter spp.* is naturally found in dogs. It has been reported that the gastric biopsies found *Helicobacter*-like organism infection and dogs were postulated to be infected with several species of *Helicobacter spp.* While, it is said to be the most commonly occurring of *Helicobacter*-like organisms in dogs and cats. The role of *Helicobacter spp.* infection in gastrointestinal disease in dogs and cats is uncertain. It has been known for years that gastric *Helicobacter*-like organisms (HLO) are commonly presented in stomach of dogs but the relationship of these organisms and gastric disease is unresolved. Infection with HLO is highly prevalent in dogs. It is seen the clinical sign of vomiting and also clinically healthy pet dogs. *Gastrospirillum hominis*, another *Helicobacter*-like organism, has so far not been cultivated.

H. pylori transmission is proposed to be fecal-oral, oral-oral, and gastro-oral (via vomited fluids). The exact details of transmission are still unclear. A higher incidence of *H. pylori* infection has been reported by gastroenterologists, suggesting that transmission from patient to physician is possible. It has been suggested that *Helicobacter spp.* infection might be zoonotic by contact with dogs and cats and has been correlated with human *H. heilmannii* infection. There is no correlation between pet ownership and human *H. pylori* infection.

Helicobacter spp. produce urease, which breaks down urea into ammonia and bicarbonate ions. In stomach, ammonia has a buffering effect that may help *Helicobacter spp.* colonize on mucosa in the acidic gastric environment. In addition, ammonia is directly toxic to gastric epithelial cells. *H. pylori* infection is associated with increased gastric acid secretion (hyperacidity), which causes inflammation of the gastric antrum (antral gastritis) and duodenal ulceration. It has been proposed that hyperacidity is caused by hypergastrinemia resulting from the inhibition of somatostatin-secreting cells (somatostatin inhibits gastrin release). Hypergastrinemia also increases parietal cell mass through a trophic effect on gastric mucosa. *H. pylori* infection can also be associated with lack of gastric acid (achlorhydria). This is thought to occur when *H. pylori* causes mucosal atrophy in the gastric fundus and body or inhibits functioning of the parietal cells. Chronic gastric inflammation may progress to chronic atrophic gastritis and intestinal metaplasia, which are precancerous conditions. It appears that *Helicobacter spp.* infection significantly alter gastric acid secretion in dogs.

The pathological significance of these organisms in the dog is currently unknown. Study of naturally infected dogs and cats has shown that *Helicobacter spp.* predominantly colonizes the gastric fundus and cardia and is associated with mild to moderate mononuclear cell inflammation in appearance of chronic gastritis. In an experimental study of beagles which infected with *H. felis and H. bizzozeronii-like* organisms, it has been concluded that acid secretion was not markedly disturbed by infection and that treatment had been temporarily suppressed. Infected dogs showed no clinical signs and had mild gastritis histologically before and after treatment. No correlation was identified between the severity of inflammation and degree of bacterial colonization. It has been suggested that successful treatment of *Helicobacter spp.* in pet dogs did not change gastric histology and that mild chronic gastritis still persisted.

1.2. Helicobacter diagnosis

Non-invasive test methods for detecting *Helicobacter spp.* (e.g., urea breath testing, antibody testing, stool antigen testing) are not routinely available for dogs and cats. Urease testing from breath and blood, has been investigated in dogs but is not widely available. Antibody testing is potentially used but more difficulty apply than in human because of the variety of *Helicobacter spp.* infecting dogs and cats. Nevertheless, antibody testing is being investigated, and infected animals are known to develop antibodies. Theoretically, stool antigen testing could be useful in *H. pylori*-infected cats or in animals infected with *Helicobacter spp.* that have antigenic homology. Thus cross-reactivity with *H. pylori* should be concerned. This has not yet been investigated. The confirmation of the presence of *Helicobacter spp.* in dogs and cats, the invasive methods has already been discussed. Endoscopically obtained gastric mu-

http://dx.doi.org/10.5772/53054

cosal biopsies are commonly used, and direct observation of organisms by histology or cytology and rapid urease testing are common methods. Because of *Helicobacter spp.* distribution in the stomach may be in locally site, evaluation of multiple biopsies and anatomic location (i.e., cardia, fundus, and antrum) is also recommended. Gastric *Helicobacter spp.* was found in the cardia, fundus, body, and pylorus. It has been reported that the most prevalent location of stomach were in cardia, fundus, body and pylorus respectively. In addition, naturally infected dogs has shown that *Helicobacter spp.* predominantly colonizes in the gastric cardia and fundus. *Helicobacter spp.* was demonstrated considerable affinity for parietal cells and is found in their intracellular canaliculi as well as in the cytoplasm. They had been observed in large numbers in the mucus covering the surface epithelium, the gastric pits and the glandular lumina. It appears that *Helicobacter spp.* infection does not significantly alter gastric acid secretion in dogs. Study of naturally infected dogs has shown that Helicobacter predominantly colonizes the gastric cardia and fundus. However, the predilection site of infection is recommended as fundic area of the stomach.

Direct observation of *Helicobacter spp.* organisms in biopsy specimens and necropsied dogs usually requires special stains. It has been reported that there was no statistically different significant between the locations of histopathological lesion and *Helicobacter spp.* infection using H&E. The presence of lymphoid follicles in the gastric mucosa has traditionally been considered a common, nonspecific finding in the gastric mucosa of dogs. Most dogs had many bacteria and only mild gastritis. It is suggested that in dogs, the bacteria did not induce histological evident of certain diseases. In naturally infected with *Helicobacter spp.*, the lymphoid follicles are frequently found in subglandular areas and sometimes extended between the glands. Moreover, it was reported that, gnotobiotic dogs which experimentally infected with *Helicobacter spp.* developed large numbers of lymphoid follicles throughout the gastric mucosa, while the dogs had no follicles. The occurrence of lymphoid follicles were indicated the *Helicobacter spp.* infection from gastrointestinal specimens which depend on the sites. In comparable to the *H. pylori* infection in children which frequently results in marked gastric lymphoid hyperplasia, have led to the hypothesis that lymphoid follicles in the human gastric mucosa can result from chronic *H. pylori* antigenic stimulation and, therefore, represent a specific immune response directed against the organisms. Also, by inducing lymphoid tissue formation in the gastric mucosa, *H. pylori* may be a necessary precursor for the development of primary gastric MALT lymphoma. It should be noted that the histopathological changes in the dogs was much less severe than those seen in *H. pylori* gastritis in human which could be due to species variation. It will be of interest to study dogs which have been subjected to different environmental conditions or dietary changes to ascertain if differences in the gastritis profile occur with manipulation of these variables.

The Histopathology diagnosis, *Helicobacter spp.* can be visualized at the high magnification with conventional Hematoxylin & eosin (H&E) stained sections. Bacteria are located in the mucus adherent to the surface epithelium and are often found deep within the crypts. However, H&E staining may be unclear when few bacteria are also presented. In addition, luminal debris on the surface of the epithelium can be mistaken for *Helicobacter spp.* in H&E stained sections. Although these organisms with certain morphology 2.5-5.0 μm length, 0.5- 1.0 μm width and had five to nine helical turns could be notified. But the other organisms such as *Bacillus* organisms were difficult to histology evaluation. Because of the presented things were presented quite similar to *Helicobacter spp.* in color by H&E staining in histology evaluation (Fig. 1). Using special stains such as Warthin Starry stain (WSS) facilitates histological identification of bacteria. *Helicobacter spp.* was obviously presented in dark-brown color on yellow background. These bacteria were located mainly in the gastric pits and the upper portions of gastric glands, where they were often in intimate association with the epithelial cell surface (Fig. 2). These bacteria were located within the gland lumens, sometimes attached to the epithelial cell surface, and within the cytoplasm of parietal cells. WSS sections of stomach part revealed tightly coiled helical bacteria that were generally 2.5- 5.0 μm length. It is suggested that WSS is high occurence than H&E. It is likely that the additional of WSS is offset by a reduction in time required for slide evaluation and improvement of identification of *Helicobacter spp.* infection. A sensitive staining technique consisting of a combination of H&E and WSS has been developed. WSS could be used for detecting *Helicobacter spp.* in gastric tissues short period of time, cheap and easy to use. The WSS examination of large numbers of sections in a relatively short period of time. However, the special staining procedure can be technically difficult, and require experiences. Its meaning acceptance among gastrointestinal pathologists has not been proved yet. Other factors that could influence gastric pathology include the number of organisms present, the host species and genotype, environmental factors such as diet, and concurrent infection with undetected organisms. However, it is suggested the significantly different correlations for *Helicobacter spp.* detection between H&E and WSS. Therefore, the diagnostic method of choice for diagnosis of *Helicobacter spp.* infection in canine stomach is depended on the purpose and appropriate site of specimen collection.

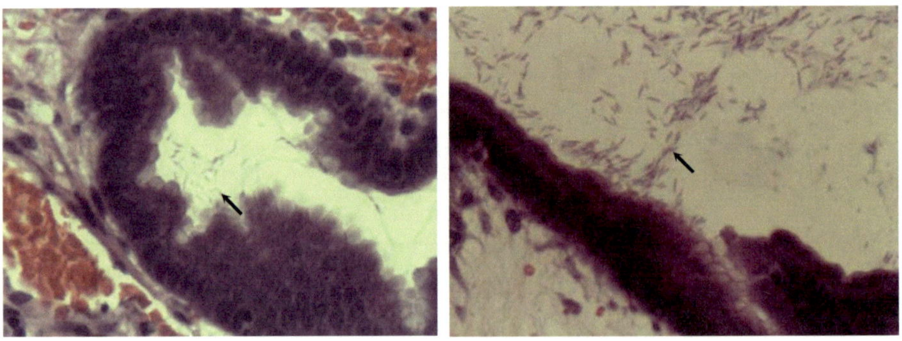

A B

Figure 1. The numerous spiral shape organisms: *Helicobacter spp.* was presented in the surface of gastric mucosa in fundus part of stomach in dog (Arrow) (A) (H&E, Bar = 10 μm) *Helicobacter spp.* was demonstrated on the gastric epithelium in higher magnification. (B) (H&E, Bar = 5 μm)

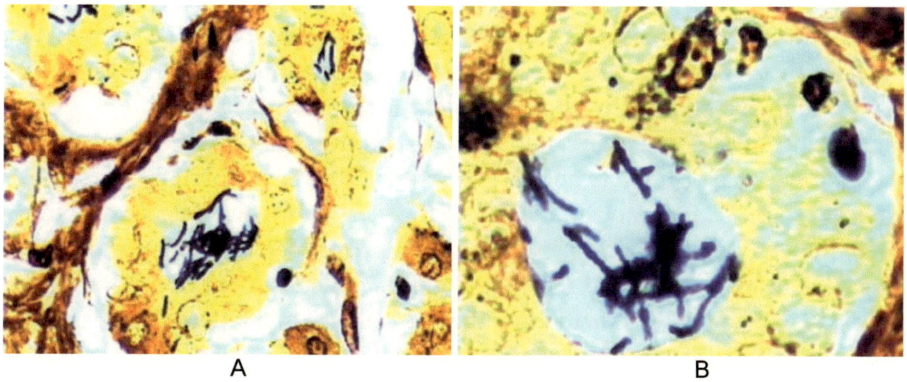

Figure 2. Spiral-shape *Helicobacter spp.* was positive in dark brown color was showning 3.0 - 5.0 μm in length and 0.5 – 1.0 μm in width in the gastric pit in fundus. In higher magnification of spiral-shape with dark brown color of *Helicobacter spp.* (WSS, A : Bar = 10 μm, B : Bar = 5 μm)

In case of Immunohistochemical staining, IHC was much more sensitive for detecting infection than the routinely used H&E and WSS. IHC staining also have been developed to detect *Helicobacter spp.* antigen. The IHC using monoclonal anti-*H. pylori* antibody is the best diagnostic tool for formalin-fixed samples (Fig. 3). And IHC is very high specificity. But IHC is rather expensive, long period of time and good experience. Such IHC are usually not necessary but may prove worthwhile in cases where stains are difficult to evaluate for confirmations.

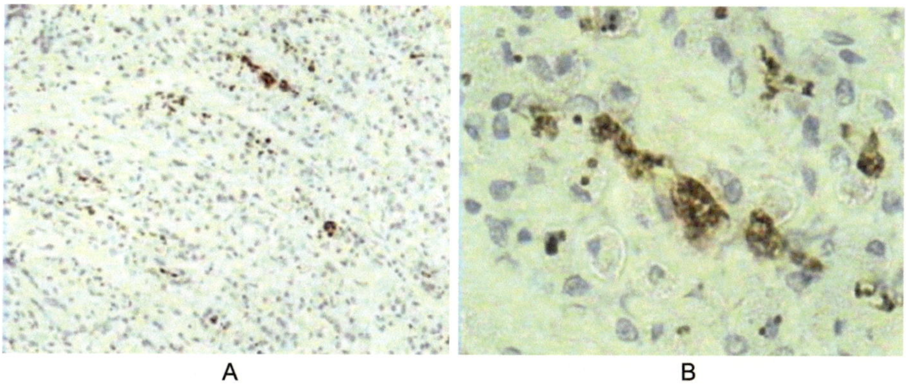

Figure 3. *Helicobacter spp.* demonstrated brown color in positive sites by Immunohistochemistry using rabbit polyclonal anti-*H. pylori* antibody in lumen of gastric gland in fundus part of stomach. Meyer's Hematoxylin counterstained, ABC, DAB (A Bar =20 μm, B Bar =10 μm)

For PCR offers great promise as a highly sensitive and specific technique for the detection of *Helicobacter spp.* and *H. pylori.* PCR technique for the detection of *H. pylori* in gastric biopsy specimens has been described by a number of laboratories although the accuracy of such technique varies widely. The identification of *Helicobacter spp.* in biopsies from dogs using

PCR has been reported and applied for detection of identification to species of *Helicobacter spp.* in dogs with naturally occurring gastric helicobacteriosis. Several observations shown that PCR was sensitive and specific which is in agreement with studies in mice infected with *H. felis* and in humans and cats infected *H. pylori,* which showed that PCR was more sensitive than histology, bacterial culture, and urease mapping. Factors affecting test accuracy of PCR include the choice of primers and target DNA, specimen preparation, bacterial density and technical issues. PCR demonstrated excellent accuracy for the detection of *H. pylori* infection in a limited number of samples. PCR technique for the detection of *H. pylori* is still in its infancy. It is unlikely that such technique will have widespread use in the initial detection of *H. pylori.* However, PCR method hold great promise in the detection of genetic differences between *H. pylori* strains for research and epidemiological studies. Repeat endoscopy or biopsy is required, which is expensive and unappealing to many pet owners. However, an advantage of follow up endoscopy in noninvasive testing is the opportunity to reassess gastric morphologic changes.

2. Treatment

Treatment of the *Helicobacter spp.* infection in dogs is controversial. Whether treatment is needed in all cases and which drugs are preferred. Efficacy of treatment and whether drug resistance is a problem in veterinary patients and should be awared. Recent studies suggested that treatment might only suppress infection but not eradicate it. More reports of post treatment follow-up assessing bacterial status and gastrointestinal (GI) changes are needed for naturally acquired clinical signs in a dog should be considered. A profile of investigations to rule out underlying GI disease (e.g., food inflammatory bowel disease, neoplasia) should be undertaken before treating *Helicobacter spp.* infection. Even with such a work set up, it may be difficult to know whether all GI inflammation is caused by *Helicobacter spp.* infection alone or whether underlying with other inflammatory diseases. This is especially true for patients in which inflammation persists following treatment and apparent *Helicobacter* spp. prevention and control.

The treatment protocols in dogs and cats have been adapted from human medicine and included various combination of antibiotic and antisecretory therapy. Traditional veterinary triple therapy consists of metronidazole, amoxicillin, and bismuth subsalicylate and has been used as initial treatment for *Helicobacter spp.* infection in dogs and cats. Other antimicrobial drugs that have been used in animals in which traditional triple therapy fails include tetracycline and clarithromycin. Antisecretory drugs that have been used include H2-receptor antagonists and proton-pump inhibitors. Treatment is typically administered for 2 to 4 weeks, but the optimal duration of treatment is unknown. The clinical gastritis resolve following 4 weeks of treatment with traditional veterinary triple therapy (in dogs) or a combination of amoxicillin, metronidazole, and famotidine (in dogs and cats). These therapeutic protocol has been practically used.

Author details

Achariya Sailasuta[1*] and Worapat Prachasilchai[2]

*Address all correspondence to: achariya.sa@chula.ac.th

1 STAR, Molecular Biology Research on Animal Oncology, Department of Pathology, Faculty of Veterinary Science, Chulalongkorn University, Bangkok, Thailand

2 Department of Small animal clinic, Department of Companion animals and wildlife clinic, Faculty of Veterinary Medicine, Chiangmai University, Chiangmai, Thailand

References

[1] Ashton-Key, M., Diss, T.C. and Isaacson. 1996. Detection of Helicobacter pylori in gastric biopsy and resection specimens. J. Clin. Pathol. 49: 107-111.

[2] Barber, M. and Franklin, R.H. 1946. Bacteriology and duodenum in cases of peptic ulcer and gastric carcinoma. Br. Med. J. 1: 951-953.

[3] Berg, D.E., Hoffman, P.S., Appelmelk, B.J., Kusters, J.G. 1997. The Helicobacter pylori genome sequence: genetic factors for long life in the gastric mucosa. Trends Microbiol. 5(12): 468-474.

[4] Blanchard, J.F. and Czinn, S.J. 2001. Helicobacter pylori acquisition and transmission: Where does it all begin ? [editorial]. Gastroenterology.121: 483-490

[5] Buczolits, S., Hirt, R., Rosengarten, R. and Busse, H.J. 2003. PCR-based genetic evidence for occurrence of Helicobacter pylori and novel Helicobacter species in the canine gastric mucosa. Vet. Microbio. 95: 259-270.

[6] Cattoli, G., van Vugt, R., Zanoni, R.G., Sanguinetti, V., Chiocchetti, R., Gualtieri, M., Vandenbroucke-Graals W. and Kusters, J.G. 1999. Occurrence and characterization of gastric Helicobacter spp. in naturally-infected dogs. Vet. Microbiol. 70: 239.

[7] Deltenre, M. and de Koster, E. 2000. How come I've got it ? (A review of Helicobacter pylori transmission). Eur. J. Gastroenterol. Hepatol. 12: 479-482.

[8] Dewhirst, F.E., Fox, J.G. and On, S.L. 2000. Recommended minimal standards for describing new species of the genus Helicobacter. Int. J. Syst. Evol. Microbiol. 50 (6): 2231-2237.

[9] Dunn, B.E., Cohen, H. and Blaser, M.J. 1997. Helicobacter pylori. Clin. Microbiol. Rev. 10: 720-741.

[10] Eaton, K.A. 1999. Man bites dog : Helicobacter in the new millennium [editorial]. J. Vet. Intern. Med. 13: 505-506.

[11] Eaton, K.A., Dewhirst, F.E., Paster, B.J., Tzellas, N., Coleman, B.E., Paola, J. and Sherding, R. 1996. Prevalence and varieties of Helicobacter species in dogs from random sources and pet dogs: animal and public health implications. J. Clin. Microbiol. 34: 3165-3170.

[12] Eaton, K.A., Dewhirst, F.E., Paster, B.J., Tzellas, N., Coleman, B.E., Paola, J. and Sherding, R. 1996. Prevalence and varieties of Helicobacter species in dogs from random sources and pet dogs: animal and public health implications. J. Clin. Microbiol. 34: 3165-3170.

[13] Esteves, M.I., Schrenzel, M.D., Marini, R.P., Taylor, N.S., Xu, S., Hagen, S., Feng, Y., Shen, Z. and Fox, J.G. 2000. Helicobacter pylori gastritis in cats with long-term natural infection as a model of human disease. Am. J. Pathol. 156(2): 709-721.

[14] Flatland, B. 2002. Helicobacter Infection in Humans and Animals. Compendium. 24(9): 688-696.

[15] Fox, J.G. and Lee, A. 1997. The role of Helicobacter species in newly recognized gastrointestinal disease of animals. Lab. Anim. Sci. 47: 222-255.

[16] Fox, J.G. 1998. Gastric helicobacters, in Greence CE (ed.): Infectious Diseases of the Dog and Cat. Philadelphia, W.B. Saunders Co. 229-233.

[17] Fox, J.G., Correa, P., Taylor, N.S., Lee, A., Otto, G., Murphy, J.C. and Rose, R. 1990. Helicobacter mustelae-associated gastritis in ferrets. An animal model of Helicobacter pylori gastritis in humans. Gastroenterology. 99: 352-361.

[18] Fox, J.G. and Lee, A. 1997. The role of Helicobacter species in newly recognized gastrointestinal disease of animals. Lab. Anim. Sci. 47: 222-255.

[19] Freedberg, A.S. and Barron, L.E. 1940. The presence of spirochactes in human gastric mucosa. Am. J. Dig. Dis. 38: 443-445.

[20] Fujioka, T., Murakami, K., Kodama, M., Kagawa, J., Okimoto, T. and Sato, R. 2002. Helicobacter pylori and gastric carcinoma from the view point of animal model. Keio. J. Med. 51(suppl. 2): 69-73.

[21] Geyer, C., Colbatzky, F., Lechner, J. and Hermanns, W. 1993. Occurrence of spiral-shaped bacteria in gastric biopsies of dogs and cats. Vet.Rec. 133: 18-19.

[22] Graham, D.Y. 1997. Helicobacter pylori infection in the pathogenesis duodenal ulcer and gastric cancer: a model. Gastroenterology. 113:1943-1911.

[23] Graham, D.Y. and Yamaoka, Y. 1998. Helicobacter pylori and CagA: relationships with gastric cancer, duodenal ulcer and reflux esophagitis and its complications. Helicobacter. 3:145-151.

[24] Hall, J.A. 2000. Diseases of the stomach, in Ettinger, S.J., Feldman, E.C.(eds): Textbook of Veterinary Internal Medicine. Philadephia. W.B. Saunders: 1154-1181.

[25] Handt, L.K., Fox J.G., Stalis, I.H., Rufo, R., LEE., G., Linn, J., Li., X. and Kleanthous, H. 1995. Characterization of feline Helicobacter pylori strains and associated gastritis in a colony of domestic cats. J. Clincl. Microbiol. 33(9): 2280-2289.

[26] Happonen, I., Saari, S., Castren, L., Tyni, O., Hanninen, M.L. and Westermarck, E. 1996. Occurrence and topographical mapping of gastric Helicobacter-like organisms and their association with histopathological changes in apparently healthy dogs and cats. J. Vet. Med. A. 43: 305-315.

[27] Happonen, I., Linden, J., Saari, S., Karjalainen, M.L., JALAVA, K. and Weastermarck, E. 1998. Detection and effects of helicobacters in healthy dogs and dogs with signs of gastritis. J. Am. Vet. Med. Assoc. 213: 1767.

[28] Henry, G.A., Long, P.H., Burns, J.L. and Charbonneau, D.L. 1987. Gastric spirillosis in Beagles. Am. J. Vet. Res. 48: 831-836.

[29] Herbrink, P. and van Doorn, L.J. 2000. Serological methods for diagnosis of Helicobacter pylori infection and monitoring of eradication therapy. Eur. J. Clin. Microbiol. Infect. Dis. 19: 164-173.

[30] Hermanns, W., Kregel, K., Breuer, W. and Lechner, J. 1995. Helicobacter-like organisms: histopathological examination of gastric biopsies from dogs and cats. J. Comp. Pathol. 112: 307-318.

[31] Huang, J.Q., Sridhar, S., Chen, Y. and Hunt, R.H. 1998. Meta-analysis of the relationship between Helicobacter pylori seropositivity and gastric cancer. Gastroenterology. 114: 1169-1179.

[32] Issacson, P.G. and Spencer, J. 1993. Is gastric lymphoma an infection disease? Hum. Pathol. 24:569-570.

[33] Laine, L., Lewin , D.N., Naritoku, W. and Cohen, H. 1997. Prospective comparison of H&E, Giemsa and Genta stains for the diagnosis of Helicobacter pylori. Gastrointest. Endosc. 45: 463-467.

[34] Lee, A., Krakowka, S., Fox, J.G., Otto, G., Eaton, K.A. and Murphy, J.C. 1992. Role of Helicobacter felis in chronic canine gastritis. Vet. Pathol. 29: 487-494.

[35] Lee, A., Krakowka, S., Fox, J.G., Otto, G., Eaton, K.A. and Murphy, J.C. 1992. Role of Helicobacter felis in chronic canine gastritis. Vet. Pathol. 29: 487-494.

[36] Lee, A., Fox, J.C. and Hazell, S. 1993. Pathogenicity of Helicobacter pylori: a perspective. Infect. Immun. 61: 1601-1610.

[37] Lee, A. and O'Rourke, J.1993. Gastric bacteria other than Helicobacter pylori. Gastroenterol. Clin. North. Am. 22(1): 21-42.

[38] Lin, S.K., Lambert, J.R. and Schembri, M.A. 1994. Helicobacter pylori prevalence in endoscopy and medical staff. J. Gastroenterol. Hepato. 9: 319-324.

[39] Marais, A., Mendz, G.L., Hazell, S.L., Megraud, F. 1999. Metabolism and genetics of Helicobacter pylori: the genome era. Microbiol. Mol. Biol. Rev. 63(3): 642-674.

[40] Marini, R.P., Labato, M.A., Taylor, N.S., Schrenzel, M.D., Xu, S., Speilman, B., Shen, Z., Yan, L., Feng, L. and Fox, J.G. 2000. Failure to detect Helicobacter pylori in gastric endoscopic biopsies from dogs and cats. Contemp. Topics Lab. Anim. Sci. 39: 52.

[41] Montiero, L., de Mascarel, A. and Sarrasqueta, A.M. 2001. Diagnosis of Helicobacter pylori infection: Noninvasive methods compared to invasive methods and evaluation of two new tests. Am. J. Gastroenterol. 96: 353-357.

[42] Moss, S.F., Legon, S. and Bishop, A.E. 1992. Effect of Helicobacter pylori on gastric somatostatin in duodenal ulcer disease. Lancet 340(8825): 930-932.

[43] Nakajima, S., Graham, D.Y., Hattori, T. and Bamba, T. 2000. Strategy for treatment of Helicobacter pylori infection in adults. Updated indications for test and eradication therapy suggested in 2000. Curr. Pharm. Design. 6(15): 1503-1514.

[44] Nomura, A., Stemmerman, G.N., Chyou, P.H., Kato, I.,Perez-Perez, G.I. and Blaser, M.J. 1991. Helicobacter pylori infection and gastric carcinoma among Japanese Americans in Hawaii. N. Engl. J. Med. 325: 1132-1136.

[45] Parsonnet, J., Friedman, G.D., Vandersteen, D.P., Chang, Vogelman, J.H., Orentreich, N. and Sibley, R.K. 1991. Helicobacter pylori infection and the risk of gastric carcinoma. N. Engl. J. Med. 325: 1127-1136.

[46] Peyrol, S., Lecoindre, P., Berger, I., Deleforge, J. and Chevallier, M. 1998. Differential pathogenic effect of two Helicobacter-like organisms in dog gastric mucosa. J. Submicrosc. Cytol. Pathol. 30: 425.

[47] Pirarat, N., Makbunsri, T., Sukkamon, S., Amornchailertrat, S., Rungsipipat, A., Sunyasootcharee, B. 2003. The relationship between pathological gastric changes and Helicobacter spp. in dog. Thai J. Vet. Med. 33(3): 73-80.

[48] Prachasilpchai, W., Prachasilpchai W., Nuanualsuwan S., Chatsuwan T., Techangamsuwan S., Wangnaitham S., Sailasuta A. 2007. Diagnosis of Helicobacter spp.infection in canine stomach. J. Vet. Sci. 8(2): 139-145.

[49] Queiroz, D.M.M., Rocha, G.A., Mendes, E.N., Moura, S.B., Oliveira, A.M.R. and Miranda, D. 1996. Association between Helicobacter and gastric ulcer disease of the pars esophagea in swine. Gastroenterology. 111: 19-27.

[50] Radin, M.J., Eaton, K.A., Krakowka, S., Morgan, D.R., Lee, A., Otto, G. and Fox, J. 1990. Helicobacter pylori gastric infection in gnotobiotic beagle dogs. Infect. Immun. 58(8): 2606-2612.

[51] Rossi, G., Rossi, M., Vitali, C.G., Fortuna, D., Burroni, D., Pancotto, L., Capecchi, S., Sozzi, S., Renzoni, G., Braca, G., Del Giudice, G., Rappuoli, R., Ghiara, P. and Taccini, E. 1999. A conventional beagle dog model for acute and chronic infection with Helicobacter pylori. Infect. Immun. 67: 3112.

[52] Scott, D., Weeks, D., Melchers, K., Sachs, G. 2000. UreI-mediated urea transport in Helicobacter pylori: an open and shut case? Trends Microbiol. 8(8): 348-349.

[53] Simpson, K.W., McDonough, P.L., Strauss- Ayali, Chang, Y.F., Harpending, P. and Valentine, B.A. 1999 (a). Helicobacter pylori infection in dogs: effect on gastric structure and function. Vet. Pathol. 36: 237-248.

[54] Simpson, K.W.,Strauss- Ayali, D., McDonough, P.L., Chang, Y.F. and Valentine, B.A. 1999 (b). Gastric function in dogs with naturally acquired gastric Helicobacter spp. infection. J. Vet. Intern. Med. 13: 507-515.

[55] Smoot, D.T. and Hamilton, F.A. 1995. Summary of the national institutes of health consensus development conference on Helicobacter pylori. Gastrointest. Dis. Today. 4: 1-10.

[56] Solnick, J.V., O'Rourke, J., Lee, A., Paster, B.J., Dewhirst, F.E., Tompkins, L.S. 1993. An uncultured gastric spiral organism is a newly identified Helicobacter in humans. J. Infect. Dis. 168(2): 379-385.

[57] Solte, M., Bayerdorffer, E. and Morgner, A. 2002. Helicobacter and gastric MALT lymphoma. Gut 50(Suppl3): 19-24.

[58] Tomb, J.F., White, O., Kerlavage, A.R., Clayton, R.A., Sutton, G.G., Fleischmann, R.D., Ketchum, K.A., Klenk, H.P., Gill, S., Dougherty, B.A., Nelson, K., Quackenbush, J., Zhou, L., Kirkness, E.F., Peterson, S., Loftus, B., Richardson, D., Dodson, R., Khalak, H.G., Glodek, A., McKenney, K., Fitzegerald, L.M., Lee, N., Adams, M.D., Venter, J.C. 1997. The complete genome sequence of the gastric pathogen Helicobacter pylori. Nature. 388(6642): 539-547.

[59] Tompkins, L.S. and Falkow, S. 1995. The new path to preventing ulcers. Science. 267: 1621-1622.

[60] Vaira, D., Holton, J. and Menegatti, M. 2000. Review article: Invasive and noninvasive tests for Helicobacter pylori infection. Aliment. Pnarmacol. Ther. 14(Suppl. 3); 13-22.

[61] Yamasaki, K., Suematsu, H. and Takahashi, T. 1998. Comparison of gastric lesions in dogs and cats with and without gastric spiral organisms. J. Am. Vet. Med. Assoc. 212: 529-533.

[62] Zucca, E., Bertoni, F., Rogerreo, E., Bosshard, G., Cazzaniga, G.,Pedrinis, E., Biondi, A. and Cavalli, V. 1998. Molecular analysis of the progression from Helicobacter pylori-associated chronic gastritis to mucosa-associated lymphoid tissue lymphoma of the stomach. N. Eng. J. Med. 338: 804-810.

Section 3

Epidemiology of Gastritis

Chapter 3

Helicobacter Pylori Infection and Its Relevant to Chronic Gastritis

Mohamed M. Elseweidy

Additional information is available at the end of the chapter

http://dx.doi.org/10.5772/46056

1. Introduction

Gastric inflammation is highly complex biochemical protective response to the cellular tissue injury. Chronic gastritis is associated with the inflammatory cellular infiltrate predominantly consisting of lymphocyte and plasma cells in gastric mucosa. Many evidences suggest that Helicobacter pylori (H. pylori) infection and non steroidal anti- inflammatory drug (NSAID) ingestion are major causative factors. Both are highly implicated in the pathogenesis of gastric mucosal oxidative injury in humans.

Chronic gastritis is mainly divided into two main categories namely non-atrophic and atrophic gastritis (*Rugge et al, 2011*). In the gastric mucosa, atrophy is defined as the loss of appropriate glands. Atrophic gastritis, resulting mainly from long standing H. pylori infection and is a major risk factor for the onset of gastric cancer.

Two main types of atrophic gastritis can be recognized, one characterized by the loss of glands, accompanied by fibrosis or fibromuscular proliferation in the lamina propria and the other characterized by the replacement of normal mucosa into an intestinal type of mucosa i.e intestinal metaplasia (Rugge et al, 2007).

Helicobacter pylori is spiral –shaped, flagellated, Gram-negative bacterium. It colonizes the stomach of about 50 percent of the world population, especially in the developing countries (Marshall BJ and Warren, 1983, Bruce and Maaroos, 2008). It is directly implicated in the dyspepsia, acute and chronic gastritis, peptic ulceration, MALT lymphoma and it is an independent risk factor for gastric adenocarcinoma (Atherton, 2006). It may also be a risk factor for pancreatic including cancer (Trikudanathan et al, 2011). H. pylori has been also associated to some extra-gastric diseases including several autoimmune diseases.

2. Geographical distribution of the prevalence of H. pyloriinfection

The prevalence of H. pylori infection varies from country to country with large differences between developed and developing countries (Neunert et al, 2011) The epidemiology of H. pylori infection in developing countries is characterized by a rapid rate of acquisition of the infection such that approximately 80 percent of the population is infected by the age of 20 (Robinson et al, 2007) because the disease is most often acquired in childhood or when young children are present in the household. The prevalence of H. pylori is inversely related to socioeconomic status (Sobala et al, 1991, Blaser and Atherton, 2004).The major variable being the status childhood, the period of highest risk. Attempts to understand the different infection rates in defined groups have focusedon differences in socioeconomic states defined by occupation, family income level and living conditions. Each of these variables measures a different component of the socioeconomic complex.

3. Routs of transmission

H. pylori is a true opportunistic bacterium that will use any method available for gaining access to the human stomach. Gastro-oral (e.g. exposure to vomit) and fecal-oral routs are believed to be the primary means of transmission. The bacterium can also be transmitted through exposure to contaminated food or water. The majority of the data support the notion that transmission is mainly within families. Thus close contact and the level of house hold sanitation appear to be the most important variables. These findings may support the concept that the most likely sources of transmission are person-to-person and /or exposure to a common source of infection.

H. pylori from the Hispanic families living in certain place was examined for relatedness based on the geno types using the cag A, vac A and ice A genes. H. pylori isolated from the children and their mothers had the same genotype and were different from the associated with children's fathers or brothers-in-law (Graham et al, 2004). The high rate of transmission to spouses also suggests that genetic factors are less critical than living conditions for transmission of the bacterium.

4. Relationship between H. pylori infection and associated diseases

AS reported before H. pylori infection causes chronic gastritis, peptic ulcer disease, primary gastric B-cell lymphoma, (indirectly) gastric adenocarcinoma and patients with infection develop gastric damage (Harford et al, 2000, Nomura et al, 2002). Approximately 17 percent of infected patients develop peptic ulcer and one quarter of such patients experience an ulcer complication (Crabtree et al, 1991, Censini et al, 1996). Numerous trials have shown that ulcer relapse is prevented following infection cure (Yamaoka et al, 1998, Yamaoka et al, 1999). Histological and serologic studies have also shown that the infection preceded the ulcer and

H. pylori infection is now accepted as one of the major causes of peptic ulcers (the other being use of non-steroidal anti-inflammatory drugs) (Higashi et al, 2002).Accordingly development of the disease depends on bacterial, host and environmental factors.

The risk of ulceration is higher with more virulent strains. The best described virulence determinants are expression of active forms of a vacuolating cytotoxine (Vac A)(Crabtree et al, 1995) and possession of a protein secretory apparatus called cag (cytotoxin-associated gene products) that stimulates the host inflammatory response (Ando et al, 2002). Cag+ strains interact more closely with epithelial cells and induce release of pro-inflammatory cytokines, thereby increasing inflammation.

However it is unclear whether it is this or the direct translocation of a bacterial protein (Cag A) into gastric epithelial cells that is the primary cause of the disease, including gastric adenocarcinoma.

Host genetic susceptibility and environmental factors also affect disease risk; for example, smoking is strongly associated with peptic ulceration in H. pylori –infected individuals. H. pylori induced duodenal ulceration arises in people with antral predominant gastritis (Backert et al, 2004, Majumdar et al, 2010). Antral inflammation leads to reduced somatostatin production and, because somatostatin has a negative feedback effect on gastrin production, this results in hypergastrinaemia. Gastrin stimulates enterochromaffin-like cells to release histamine, which acts on parietal cells, resulting in stimulated acid production, increased duodenal acid load and the formation of protective gastric metaplasia in the duodenum. Helicobacter pylori cannot colonize the normal duodenum, but can colonize gastric metaplasia, causing inflammation and ulceration (Majumdar et al, 2010). Hypergastrinemia on the other hand and inconsequence to antral inflammation may leads to an increase of acid production from the acid secreting areas of the stomach in response to food and other stimuli. The resulting increased acid load in the duodenum is one factor encouraging duodenal ulceration. Gastric ulceration occurs on a background of pangastritis often arising at the highly inflamed transitional zone between antrum and corpus, particularly on the lesser curve.

5. Clinical features

Chronic H. pylori –associated gastritis per se is asymptomatic but the initial acquisition of the infection cause acute gastritis with hypochlorhydria which may cause abdominal pain, nausea and vomiting that resolve within a few days (Fischer et al, 2001). Uncomplicated peptic ulcers typically cause epigastric pain and less commonly, nausea, vomiting and weight loss, whereas some ulcers (particularly NSAID ulcers) are asymptomatic. The classically described pain of duodenal ulcer is felt as a growing or burning sensation, often with a relation to meals; occurring 1-3 hours after meals and /or at night and relieved by food. Gastric ulcer pain is instead often precipitated by food. However symptoms are actually very poorly discriminatory for ulceration site and even for whether or not an ulcer is present. Examination usually reveals epigastric tenderness but may be normal.

6. Complications

H. pylori ulcers usually heal and relapse spontaneously but ulcers of any cause, and particularly NSAID –induced ulcers, may cause serious complications.

Acutely bleeding ulcers cause anemia, perforation results in peritonism and gastric outlet obstruction causes persistent vomiting. The discovery of H. pylori therefore has revolutionized the management of peptic ulcers; its eradication heals H. pylori –induced ulcers and prevents their relapse.

7. Dyspepsia in the community

Older patients presenting for the first time and those with alarm symptoms or signs (weight loss, dysphagia, persistent vomiting, gastrointestinal bleeding, unexplained anemia, epigastric mass, previous gastric ulcer or gastric surgery) should be referred for upper gastrointestinal endoscopy and /or other investigations, both to exclude malignancy and to make a positive diagnosis. Other patients (with simple dyspepsia) should normally be treated without endoscopy or specialist referral. These patients should have one of two initial approaches. In populations where H. pylori prevalence is high (≥ 20-25 percent), patients should be tested for H. pylori non-invasively, and given treatment to eradicate H. pylori if positive.

In populations with lower H. pylori prevalence another approach may be followed (inhibitors). In either case, if the first approach fails, the second can be tried (Wirth et al, 1998, Mason et al, 2005, Delaney et al, 2008).

8. Upper gastrointestinal endoscopy

Upper gastrointestinal endoscopy is the investigation of choice in older patients with dyspepsia and those with alarm symptoms because it enables diagnosis of ulceration and of other macroscopic abnormalities such as malignancy and Oesophagitis. Histological examination of gastric mucosal biopsy specimens is useful in confirming the nature of any abnormalities seen, and in identifying whether gastritis is present and its cause. However it is seldom necessary if macroscopic appearances are normal. Treatment with acid –suppressing drugs before endoscopy may heal ulcers, rendering endoscopic findings misleading since proton pump inhibitors, bismuth compounds and antibiotics may cause false-negative H. pylori tests. If possible, acid suppressing agents should be avoided for at least two weeks and preferably 4, bismuth compounds and antibiotics may be avoided for at least 4 weeks before endoscopy.

http://dx.doi.org/10.5772/46056

9. H. pylori infection and oxidative stress expression

Oxidative stress is associated with many diseases (Yamaoka et al, 2000), including gastric disorders like chronic gastritis, peptic ulcers, gastric cancer and mucosa-associated lymphoid tissue (MALT) lymphoma (Majumdar et al, 2010). These gastric diseases can be the result of infection with Helicobacter pylori, which is believed to be the major etiological age (Chen et al, 2005). Several studies have been carried out focusing bacterial factors in gastric diseases and it has been assumed that H. pylori strains having Cag A+ /VacAs1 genotype are more virulent than other genotypes.

Some studies have reported that Vac As1 strain is usually toxigenic and tends to be CagA+ (Moss et al, 1992).

H. pylori infection induces an inflammatory response that is also oxidative. The gastric epithelium and the bacteria induce production of interleukin-8 (IL-8) that contributes to the generation of great amounts of toxic reactive oxygen species (ROS), with marked infiltration of inflammatory cells and can elicit induction of interleukin-1β (IL-1β), interleukin -6 (IL-6), IL-8, IL-12, tumor necrosis factor-α (TNF-α) and interferon-γ (INF-γ) (Marshall et al, 1985). The inflammatory response induced during H. pylori infection does not appear to confer protective immunity and the resulting oxidative burst caused by phagocytic cells can damage gastric tissues (Graham et al, 2004). Increased pathogen- inducible nitric oxide synthase (iNos) has also been observed in the gastric mucosa of the patients with duodenal ulcer (2010), gastric cancer (Mason et al, 2005), gastritis (Delaney et al, 2008) caused by H. pylori infection. iNos is induced by a variety of stimuli, including bacterial Lipopolysaccharide, cytokines and products from the bacterial wall (Janssen et al, 1992) and its expression contributes to oxidative stress.

Another oxidative enzyme induced by H. pylori in gastric disease is Nox1 (NADH oxidase 1) (Blaser and Atherton, 2004). It constitutively produces both superoxide anion and Hydrogen peroxide (H_20_2). Increased expression of Nox1 mRNA moderately increases superoxide generation, which leads to a reduction in aconitase activity, making Nox1 a good marker of oxidative stress (Tandon et al, 2004).H. pylori also induces ROS production by gastric epithelial cels, contributing to increased damage in the mucosa (Naito and Yoshikawa, 2002) and H. pylori itself generates great amounts of superoxide anions to inhibit bactericidal action of nitric oxide (N0) produced by inflammatory cells (Atherton, 1997).

Another source of ROS that contributes to oxidative stress is the H202 generated by TNF-α and other cytokines that are essential for their activity (Atherton et al, 1995) since H202 in the presence of ferrous or cuperous ions can catalyzes the generation of the highly reactive hydroxyl radical by Fenton reaction (Noach et al, 1994), an increase in H202 concentration induced by cytokines makes also TNF-α expression a good oxidative stress marker.

TNF-α is produced by a wide variety of cell types and it is positively regulated under stress and pathological conditions (Meyer et al, 2000). Protection of cells against ROS is accomplished through the activation of oxygen-scavenging enzymes such as superoxide dismutase (SOD), glutathione peroxidase (GPX) and catalase (CAT).

However it is not well known how H. pylori bacteria products and inflammation affect the ability of gastric cells to protect themselves from damage caused by ROS. The virulence of the strain acts primarily as an accelerator in the disease process and not as a predictor of outcome.

10. The immune response to H. pylori

H. pylori is an active stimulator of both the innate and acquired immune responses. Local innate recognition of H. pylori by epithelial cells is thought to be an important disease determinant. There are also strong local and systemic antibody and cell-mediated immune response

11. The innate immune response

H. pylori colonization of the gastric mucosa triggers innate host defense mechanism thus stimulating the expression of pro-inflammatory and anti-bacterial factors by gastric epithelial cells (Antos et al, 2001). The first line of defence results in gastritis and H. pylori also stimulates innate immune responses from these infiltrating cells (Kawahara et al, 2001) which may subsequently influence bacterial colonization density (Arnold et al, 2001), the inflammation level and also the generation of adaptive response may represent a central determinant of disease severity and participation is thought to be a major mediator in gastric carcinogenesis.

12. Antimicrobial peptides

Secreted antimicrobial peptides, including defensins are produced as part of the innate immune response to H. pylori. Elevated levels of human β defensin (hBD2) and the neutrophil-derived alpha defensins 1,2 and 3 are present in the gastric juice of H. pylori –infected patients (Nagata et al, 1998) and increased expression of hBD2 (Beutler and Cerami, 1986),hBD3 (Meneghini, 1998), adrenomedullin (Jung et al, 1997), angiogenin (George et al, 2003) and the human cationic antimicrobial peptide 18 (Gobert et al, 2004) LL-37 (Harris et al, 1998) has been shown in infected human gastric epithelial cells.

13. The acquired immune response

H. pylori infection provokes a vigorous humoral and cellular immune response in humans, but the organism is rarely eliminated from the gastric mucosa and infection persists lifelong in the absence of treatment (Blaser and Atherton, 2004). One possibility is

http://dx.doi.org/10.5772/46056

that H. pylori itself influences the immune response to avoid its own clearance by the host and to down-regulate excessive host damage thus promoting a relatively peaceful co-existence. However, there is good evidence that the acquired immune response itself contributes to gastro-duodenal disease processes (Zevering et al, 1999). Mouse models have shown that the cellular immune response is a central regulator of H. pylori-induced gastric inflammation and pathology. Mice deficient in IL-10 mount a vigorous inflammatory response to H. pylori, successfully and rapidly clear H. pylori infections (Chen et al, 2001).

14. Humoral immunity

H. pylori stimulates the production of mucosal and systemic IgA and IgG s, but the effect of antibody upon bacterial colonization remains controveial. One report showed that the intragastric administration of specific monoclonal IgA mediated protection against H.fellis infection in mice (George et al, 2003). In contrast, others have shown that specific IgA and IgG in mice actually promote bacterial colonization and reinhibit protective immune mechanisms (Akhiani et al, 2004, Akhiani et al, 2005). H. pylori is susceptible to the compliment-mediated bactericidal activity of serum (Gonzalez-Valencia et al, 1996) but it is possible to successfully immunize B-cell deficient mice (Ermak et al, 1998, Sutton et al, 2000), indicating that antibodies are not essential for protection. The B-cell response plays an important role in pathogenesis through participating in an H. pylori –precipitated autoimmune process (D'Elios et al, 2004). In this, antibodies cross-react with host antigens such as those on gastric epithelial cells and the parietal cell H+,K+_ATPase(Amedei et al, 2003), potentially inducing local- inflammation and damage.

15. The T-cell response

In humans, the T-cell response to H. pylori is dominated (Fan et al, 1994, Bamford et al, 1998). Th1 cells produce IFNγ and this type of response is associated with pro-inflammatory cytokine expression, for example TNFα, IL-12 and IL-18. When macrophages are activated in the presence of such type I cytokines, the resulting " angry " macrophages secrete pro-inflammatory factors and have enhanced bactericidal activity compared to those activated in the presence of Th2 cytokines (Ma et al, 2003). The number of IFNγ-secreting cells in the infected human gastric mucosa correlates with the severity of gastritis (Lehmann et al, 2002). IFNγ itself appears to be a key mediator, as infusion into mice, even in the absence of H. pylori infection, induces pre-cancerous gastric atrophy, metaplasia and dysplasia (GeaCui, 2003). Some strains of mice, such as C57BL/6, which mount a strong Th1 response to H. pylori, have more severe gastritis but reduced colonization densities (Gerhart et al, 2000)

16. Tests for H. pylori

16.1. Tests not requiring endoscopy

Serology:serological tests involve detection of IgG antibodies against H. pylori and the best are very accurate. However, accuracy depends critically on the precise serological test used. Serology may remain positive for years after successful eradication of H. pylori and therefore is not used for checking the treatment success, it is cheap (Majumdar et al, 2010)

Urea breath test (UBT): the UBT is a simple, non invasive test based on H. pylori urease. It is particularly useful for checking the success of treatment. It is also more accurate than serology and often used as a first-line diagnostic test in places where it is readily available. It must be performed at least 4 weeks after any bismuth compounds, antibiotics or proton pump inhibitors have been stopped. If not, false-negative results are common. It is inexpensive and readily available to general practioners in most countries.

Stool antigen test:It is more developed as alternative to the urea breath test (Gisbert et al, 2006). Like the latter it assesses active infection and so can be used for assessing treatment success since it is less expensive than the UBT.

16.2. Test requiring endoscopy

Biopsy UREASE TEST: The biopsy is placed in a urea solution or gel with a PH indicator. When H. pylori is present, the urea is hydrolysed by its urease, resulting in a color change. Some positive results may be available within minutes, although initially negative tests must be kept for 24 hours to avoid occasional false-negative results. Blood in the upper GIT may also sometimes cause a false-negative test. The biopsy urease test is cheap and widely available

Histology: H. pylori infection can be diagnosed accurately by histology if special stains are used. The distribution of gastritis may give information on disease risk if biopsies are taken from antrum and corpus (Figure 1)

Histology can also give further information, for example on whether gastric atrophy or intestinal metaplasia- markers of increased risk of gastric adenocarcinoma- are present. Histology is relatively expensive, particularly if special stains are used (Figure 2)

Culture: Endoscopic mucosal biopsy specimens can be cultured for H. pylori. Although some studies referred to it as being not useful as a purely diagnostic test as H. pylori is not straightforward to grow, and culture is often falsely negative. However success rates are high in others, isolates obtained from biopsy of certain individuals having positive IgM serologically were used for induction of gastritis in experimental rats (Elseweidy et al, 2010).

The serum concentrations of pepsinogen 1 and 11 (Pg1, Pg11), gastrin (G17) and HP antibodies of IgG class have been used to assess the risk of atrophic gastritis and to differentiate between HP-related and non HP- related gastritis (Elseweidy et al, 2010).

http://dx.doi.org/10.5772/46056

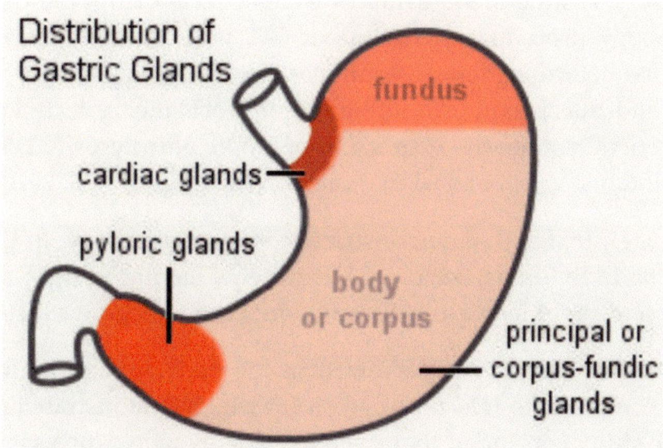

Figure 1. Zones of antrum and corpus-fudic glands of the stomach

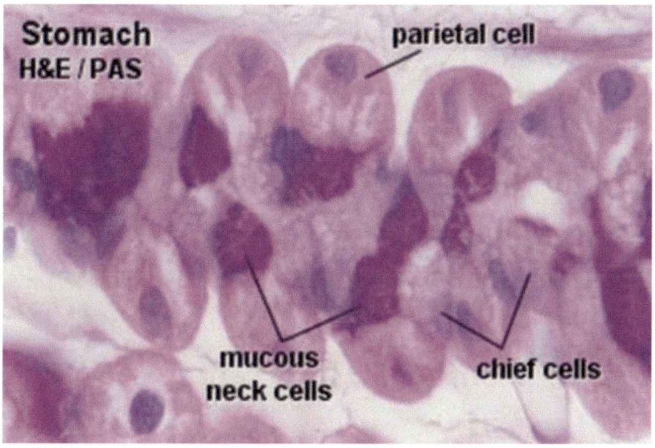

Figure 2. Distribution of parietal and chief cells of normal tissues (H&E stain)

To verify such concept, certain clinical study was designed mainly to identify the pattern of chronic gastritis and the potential effect of HP infection. Certain biomarkers, histological and immunochemical tests were used for assessment.

Fifty eight patients, clinically diagnosed as having chronic gastritis (median age 45 y; range 38-52 y, 9 females, 49 males) were participated in the present study. They were categorized into two groups.

The first one 31 percent demonstrated positive reaction to IgM- Ab of HP (≥ 40 u/ml) and the second group 69 percent demonstrated negative reaction. All the patients had signs of chronic gastritis which vary between them like abdominal pain, heartburn, vomiting or nausea, flatulence or chronic dyspepsia, epigastric pain or nausea, constipation and anorexia

(Robinson et al, 2007). Fasting blood samples were collected from the patients before their direction to endoscopy procedure of the upper GIT with gastric biopsies. Blood samples were directed for the determination of serum gastrin (G-17), Pepsinogens (Pg1,Pg11), Prostaglandin (PGE2) and Interleukin 6(IL -6).Immunohistochemistry technique was also done in antral biopsy to demonstrate the expression of INOS, Nitrotyrosin, DNA fragmentation, myeloperoxidase and histopathological examination (Elseweidy et al, 2010)(Figures 3,4).

Serum gastrin, Pg1, 11, PGE2, IL-6 demonstrated significant increase in gastritis patients as compared to normal individuals. Sector of HP patients having +veIgM showed significant increase of Pg1, 11 and slight increase of IL-6 as compared to negative sector

Immunostaining tests in antral biopsy showed strong positive reaction for the above mentioned markers as compared to IgM negative group which demonstrated mild positive reactions (Figure 5)The study concluded that gastritis patients who express positive IgM for HP infection showed higher gastrinaemia and more pronounced atrophic, inflammatory and apoptotic damage than those not expressing IgM- Ab(Elseweidy et al, 2010).

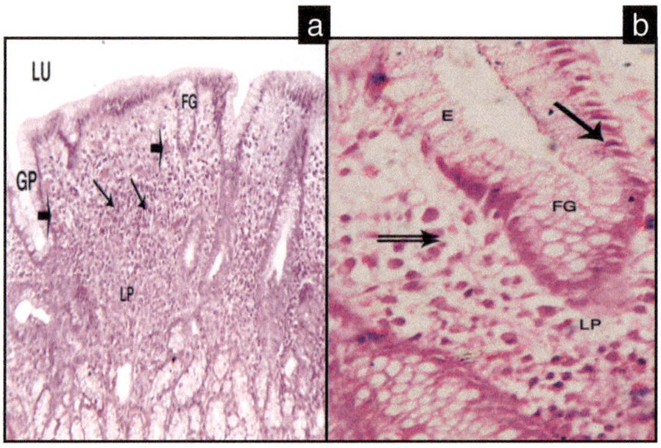

Figure 3. Histological section of human fundic gland of patient suffering from gastritis with anti H. pylori IgM positive group showing (a) x100 irregular short fundic gland (FG), wide gastric pit (GP), multiple inflammatory cells (arrows) and blood vessels (double arrows) filling lamina propria (LP), (b) x400 showing irregular simple columnar epithelium (E), small pyknotic nuclei (arrows) of cells lyningfundic gland (FG) and multiple inflammatory cells (double arrows) filling lamina propria (LP)(Elseweidy et al, 2010).

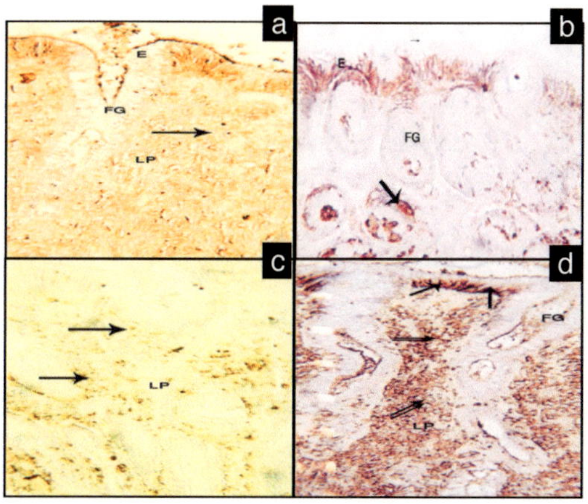

Figure 4. Immunostaining section of Gastritis patients IgM(+) category for (a) nitrotyrosine showing strong positive reaction in the epithelial (E) lining fundic gland (FG) and inflammatory cells (arrows) filling lamina propria (LP), (b) myeloperoxidase showing strong positive reaction in the surface columnar epithelial cells (E) and other cells (arrows) lining fundic gland (FG) (c) iNOS showing strong positive reaction in the inflammatory cells rows) filling lamina propria (LP), (d) DNA fragmentation factor (DFF) showing strong positive reaction in the epithelial (arrows) lining fundic gland (FG) and inflammatory cells (double arrows) fill lamina propria (LP) (x200)(Elseweidy et al, 2010).

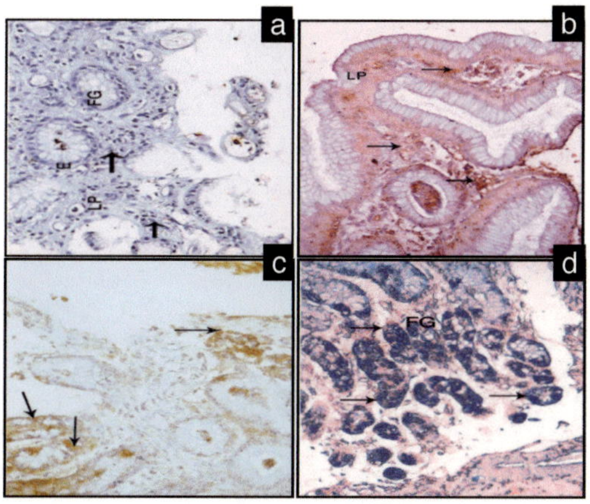

Figure 5. Immunostaining section of human fundic gland from gastritis patients, with anti-H. pylori IgM(-) showing for (a) nitrotyrosine negative reaction in the epithelial (E) lining fundic gland (FG) and inflammatory cells (arrows) filling lamina propria (LP), (b) myeloperoxidase showing strong positive reaction in the inflammatory cells (arrows) infiltrating lamina propria (LP) (c) iNOS showing moderate positive reaction in the cells of the fundic gland (arrows), (d) DNA fragmentation factor (DFF) showing mild positive reaction in the epithelial cell (arrows) lining fundic gland (FG) (x20) (Elseweidy et al, 2010).

17. Eradication of Helicobacter pylori

First –line treatment is usually a 1 or 2-week triple combination therapy comprising twice-daily use of omeprazole, clarithromycin plus metronidazole or amoxicillin. It is successful in 80-90 percent of cases (Marshall et al, 1985). The most common reasons for failure are antibiotic resistance and poor compliance with treatment. Resistance to clarithromycin is increasing and is a crucial determining factor in treatment success. Patients with previous exposure to clarithromycin should not receive this drug for H. pylori treatment unless antibiotic susceptibility testing shows that they have a sensitive strain. Metronidazole resistance is also very common, in particular amongst those having previous exposure to the drug.

So new research has been developed in natural products with anti HP activity.

When Nigella sativa L. (Ranunculaceae) seeds were given to patients with dyspeptic symptoms and found positive for HP infection in a dose of 2g/d along with 40 mg/d omeprazole, it possessed clinically useful anti HP activity (O'Mahony et al, 2005). Solamumlyratum-Thunp (SLE, Solanaceae) showed a moderate ability in inhibiting growth of HP and its association with host cells (Enomoto et al, 2010)

Curcumin from turmeric (Curcuma longa, longa, Zingiberaceae) has been lastly shown to arrest HP growth. Its potential was highly effective in eradication of HP from infected mice and to restore gastric damage, induced by chemicals like iodoacetamide(Elseweidy et al, 2008, Chowdhury and Mukhopadhyay, 2009). Crude essential oil obtained from the dried aerial parts of Thymus Caramanicusjalas (Lamiaceae) at a concentration of 0.33 ul/ml was tested in vitro against clinical isolates and proved to be highly effective.

Aqueous extract of Glucyrrhiza –globra L (Fabaceae) 1mg /ml significantly inhibited the adhesion of HP to human stomach tissue. The effect was related to the polysaccarIdes isolated from the extract (Eftekhar et al, 2009)

18. Prospects for future vaccines

The prevalence of antibiotic resistance amongst H. pylori isolates is increasing, and there are reports of over 50 percent of isolates being resistant to metronidazole in parts of Asia and Africa (Lwai-Lume et al, 2005, Kim et al, 2006).Such antibiotic resistance is a problem for many pathogenic bacterial infections, and large scale control of such infections is probably best achieved through vaccination programmes. Although vaccination appears the logical approach to control H. pylori, however vaccine research has not been straightforward and may need extensive efforts to achieve significant results.

Author details

Mohamed M. Elseweidy

Faculty of Pharmacy, Zagazig University, Zagazig, Egypt

References

[1] WWW.nice.org.uk/nicemedia/pdf /GG017 nice guideline.pdf (accessedMay (2010).

[2] Akhiani, A. A., Schon, K., Franzen, L. E., Pappo, J., Lycke, N., & (2004, . (2004). Helicobacter pylori-specific antibodies impair the development of gastritis, facilitate bacterial colonization, and counteract resistance against infection. J Immunol, 172, 5024-5033.

[3] Akhiani, A. A., Stensson, A., Schon, K., Lycke, N. Y., (2005, , & Ig, . (2005). IgA antibodies impair resistance against Helicobacter pylori infection: studies on immune evasion in IL-10-deficient mice. J Immunol, 174, 8144-8153.

[4] Amedei, A., Bergman, M. P., Appelmelk, B. J., Azzurri, A., Benagiano, M., Tamburini, C., van der Zee, R., Telford, J. L., Vandenbroucke-Grauls, C. M., D'Elios, M. M., & Del Prete, G. (2003). Molecular mimicry between Helicobacter pylori antigens and H +, K+--adenosine triphosphatase in human gastric autoimmunity. J Exp Med, 198, 1147-1156.

[5] Ando, T., Peek, R. M., Jr Lee, Y. C., Krishna, U., Kusugami, K., Blaser, M. J., & (2002, . (2002). Host cell responses to genotypically similar Helicobacter pylori isolates from United States and Japan. Clin Diagn Lab Immunol, 9, 167-175.

[6] Antos, D., Enders, G., Rieder, G., Stolte, M., Bayerdorffer, E., & Hatz, R. A. (2001). Inducible nitric oxide synthase expression before and after eradication of Helicobacter pylori in different forms of gastritis. FEMS Immunol Med Microbiol, 30, 127-131.

[7] Arnold, R. S., Shi, J., Murad, E., Whalen, A. M., Sun, C. Q., Polavarapu, R., Parthasarathy, S., Petros, J. A., & Lambeth, J. D. (2001). Hydrogen peroxide mediates the cell growth and transformation caused by the mitogenic oxidase Nox1. Proc Natl Acad Sci U S A, 98, 5550-5555.

[8] Atherton J C(1997). The clinical relevance of strain types of Helicobacter pylori. Gut, 40, 701-703.

[9] Atherton J C(2006). The pathogenesis of Helicobacter pylori-induced gastro-duodenal diseases. Annu Rev Pathol, 1, 63-96.

[10] Atherton, J. C., Cao, P., Peek, R. M., Jr Tummuru, M. K., Blaser, M. J., & Cover, T. L. (1995). Mosaicism in vacuolating cytotoxin alleles of Helicobacter pylori. Association

of specific vacA types with cytotoxin production and peptic ulceration. J Biol Chem, 270, 17771-17777.

[11] Backert, S., Schwarz, T., Miehlke, S., Kirsch, C., Sommer, C., Kwok, T., Gerhard, M., Goebel, U. B., & , . (2004). Functional analysis of the cag pathogenicity island in Helicobacter pylori isolates from patients with gastritis, peptic ulcer, and gastric cancer. Infect Immun72: 1043-1056.

[12] Bamford, K. B., Fan, X., Crowe, S. E., Leary, J. F., Gourley, W. K., Luthra, G. K., Brooks, E. G., Graham, D. Y., Reyes, V. E., & Ernst, P. B. (1998). Lymphocytes in the human gastric mucosa during Helicobacter pylori have a T helper cell 1 phenotype. Gastroenterology, 114, 482-492.

[13] Beutler, B., & Cerami, A. (1986). Cachectin/tumor necrosis factor: an endogenous mediator of shock and inflammation. Immunol Res, 5, 281-293.

[14] Blaser, M. J., & Atherton, J. C. (2004). Helicobacter pylori persistence: biology and disease. J Clin Invest, 113, 321-333.

[15] Bruce, M. G., & Maaroos, H. I. (2008). Epidemiology of Helicobacter pylori infection. Helicobacter13Suppl , 1, 1-6.

[16] Censini, S., Lange, C., Xiang, Z., Crabtree, J. E., Ghiara, P., Borodovsky, M., Rappuoli, R., & Covacci, A. (1996). cag, a pathogenicity island of Helicobacter pylori, encodes type I-specific and disease-associated virulence factors. Proc Natl Acad Sci U S A, 93, 14648-14653.

[17] Chen, T. S., Lee, Y. C., Li, F. Y., Chang, F. Y., & (2005, . (2005). Smoking and hyperpepsinogenemia are associated with increased risk for duodenal ulcer in Helicobacter pylori-infected patients. J Clin Gastroenterol, 39, 699-703.

[18] Chen, W., Shu, D., Chadwick, V. S., & (2001, . (2001). Helicobacter pylori infection: mechanism of colonization and functional dyspepsia Reduced colonization of gastric mucosa by Helicobacter pylori in mice deficient in interleukin-10. J Gastroenterol Hepatol, 16, 377-383.

[19] Chowdhury, A., & Mukhopadhyay, A. (2009). Curcumin exhibits anti-bacterial activity against HP infection. Green-Med Info summary Antimicrob agents Chemother , 53, 1592-1597.

[20] Crabtree, J. E., Shallcross, T. M., Heatley, R. V., Wyatt, J. I., & (1991, . (1991). Mucosal tumour necrosis factor alpha and interleukin-6 in patients with Helicobacter pylori associated gastritis. Gut, 32, 1473-1477.

[21] Crabtree, J. E., Xiang, Z., Lindley, I. J., Tompkins, D. S., Rappuoli, R., Covacci, A., & (1995, . (1995). Induction of interleukin-8 secretion from gastric epithelial cells by a cagA negative isogenic mutant of Helicobacter pylori. J Clin Pathol, 48, 967-969.

[22] D'Elios, M. M., Appelmelk, B. J., Amedei, A., Bergman, M. P., Del Prete, G., & (2004, . (2004). Gastric autoimmunity: the role of Helicobacter pylori and molecular mimicry. Trends Mol Med, 10, 316-323.

[23] Delaney, B. C., Qume, M., Moayyedi, P., Logan, R. F., Ford, A. C., Elliott, C., Mc Nulty, C., Wilson, S., & Hobbs, F. D. (2008). Helicobacter pylori test and treat versus proton pump inhibitor in initial management of dyspepsia in primary care: multicentre randomised controlled trial (MRC-CUBE trial). Bmj, 336, 651-654.

[24] Eftekhar, F., Nariman, F., Yousefzadi, M., Hadiand, J., Ebrahimi, S. N., (2009, , & Anti, . (2009). Anti-Helicobacter pylori activity and essential oil composition of Thymus caramanicus from Iran. Nat Prod Commun, 4, 1139-1142.

[25] Elseweidy, M., Taha, M. M., & , N. N. Y. (2010). pattern of Gastritis as manipulated by current state of H. pylori infection Int J of Biology and biomedical engineering , 4, 1998-4510.

[26] Elseweidy, M. M., Taha, M. M., Younis, N. N., Ibrahim, K. S., Hamouda, H. A., Eldosouky, M. A., & Soliman, H. (2010). Gastritis induced by Helicobacter pylori infection in experimental rats. Dig Dis Sci, 55, 2770-2777.

[27] Elseweidy, M. M., Younis, N. N., Amin, R. S., Abdallah, F. R., Fathy, A. M., & Yousif, Z. A. (2008). Effect of some natural products either alone or in combination on gastritis induced in experimental rats. Dig Dis Sci, 53, 1774-1784.

[28] Enomoto, S., Yanaoka, K., Utsunomiya, H., Niwa, T., Inada, K., Deguchi, H., Ueda, K., Mukoubayashi, C., Inoue, I., Maekita, T., Nakazawa, K., Iguchi, M., Arii, K., Tamai, H., Yoshimura, N., Fujishiro, M., Oka, M., & Ichinose, M. (2010). Inhibitory effects of Japanese apricot (Prunus mume Siebold et Zucc.; Ume) on Helicobacter pylori-related chronic gastritis. Eur J Clin Nutr, 64, 714-719.

[29] Ermak, T. H., Giannasca, P. J., Nichols, R., Myers, G. A., Nedrud, J., Weltzin, R., Lee, C. K., Kleanthous, H., & Monath, T. P. (1998). Immunization of mice with urease vaccine affords protection against Helicobacter pylori infection in the absence of antibodies and is mediated by MHC class II-restricted responses. J Exp Med, 188, 2277-2288.

[30] Fan, X. J., Chua, A., Shahi, C. N., Mc Devitt, J., Keeling, P. W., & Kelleher, D. (1994). Gastric T lymphocyte responses to Helicobacter pylori in patients with H pylori colonisation. Gut, 35, 1379-1384.

[31] Fischer, W., Puls, J., Buhrdorf, R., Gebert, B., Odenbreit, S., Haas, R., & (2001, . (2001). Systematic mutagenesis of the Helicobacter pylori cag pathogenicity island: essential genes for CagA translocation in host cells and induction of interleukin-8. Mol Microbiol, 42, 1337-1348.

[32] GeaCui(2003). IFN-gamma infusion induces gastric atrophy, metaplasia and dysplasia in the absence of H. pylori infection : a role for the immune response in Helicobacter disease. Gastroenterology124.

[33] George, J. T., Boughan, P. K., Karageorgiou, H., Bajaj-Elliott, M., & (2003, . (2003). Host anti-microbial response to Helicobacter pylori infection. Mol Immunol, 40, 451-456.

[34] Gisbert, J. P., de la Morena, F., Abraira, V., & (2006, . (2006). Accuracy of monoclonal stool antigen test for the diagnosis of H. pylori infection: a systematic review and meta-analysis. Am J Gastroenterol, 101, 1921-1930.

[35] Gobert, A. P., Bambou, J. C., Werts, C., Balloy, V., Chignard, M., Moran, A. P., & Ferrero, R. L. (2004). Helicobacter pylori heat shock protein 60 mediates interleukin-6 production by macrophages via a toll-like receptor (TLR)-2-, TLR-4-, and myeloid differentiation factor 88-independent mechanism. J Biol Chem, 279, 245-250.

[36] Gonzalez-Valencia, G., Perez-Perez, G. I., Washburn, R. G., Blaser, M. J., & (1996, . (1996). Susceptibility of Helicobacter pylori to the bactericidal activity of human serum. *Helicobacter*, 28-33.

[37] Graham, D. Y., Opekun, A. R., Osato, M. S., El -Zimaity, H. M., Lee, C. K., Yamaoka, Y., Qureshi, W. A., Cadoz, M., & Monath, T. P. (2004). Challenge model for Helicobacter pylori infection in human volunteers. Gut, 53, 1235-1243.

[38] Harford, W. V., Barnett, C., Lee, E., Perez-Perez, G., Blaser, M. J., & Peterson, W. L. (2000). Acute gastritis with hypochlorhydria: report of 35 cases with long term follow up. Gut, 47, 467-472.

[39] Harris, P. R., Ernst, P. B., Kawabata, S., Kiyono, H., Graham, M. F., & Smith, P. D. (1998). Recombinant Helicobacter pylori urease activates primary mucosal macrophages. J Infect Dis, 178, 1516-1520.

[40] Higashi, H., Tsutsumi, R., Muto, S., Sugiyama, T., Azuma, T., Asaka, M., & Hatakeyama, M. (2002). SHP-2 tyrosine phosphatase as an intracellular target of Helicobacter pylori CagA protein. Science, 295, 683-686.

[41] Janssen, Y., Van Houten, B., Bormp, J., & , B. T. M. (1992). Cell and tissue responses to oxidative damage. Lab Invest, 69, 261-274.

[42] Jung, H. C., Kim, J. M., Song, I. S., Kim, C. Y., & (1997, . (1997). Helicobacter pylori induces an array of pro-inflammatory cytokines in human gastric epithelial cells: quantification of mRNA for interleukin-8,-1 alpha/beta, granulocyte-macrophage colony-stimulating factor, monocyte chemoattractant protein-1 and tumour necrosis factor-alpha. J Gastroenterol Hepatol, 12, 473-480.

[43] Kawahara, T., Teshima, S., Oka, A., Sugiyama, T., Kishi, K., Rokutan, K., & (2001, . (2001). Type I Helicobacter pylori lipopolysaccharide stimulates toll-like receptor 4 and activates mitogen oxidase 1 in gastric pit cells. Infect Immun, 69, 4382-4389.

[44] Kim, J. M., Kim, J. S., Kim, N., Kim, S. G., Jung, H. C., & Song, I. S. (2006). Comparison of primary and secondary antimicrobial minimum inhibitory concentrations for Helicobacter pylori isolated from Korean patients. Int J Antimicrob Agents, 28, 6-13.

[45] Lehmann, F. S., Terracciano, L., Carena, I., Baeriswyl, C., Drewe, J., Tornillo, L., De Libero, G., & Beglinger, C. (2002). In situ correlation of cytokine secretion and apoptosis in Helicobacter pylori-associated gastritis. Am J Physiol Gastrointest Liver Physiol283: G, 481-488.

[46] Lwai-Lume, L., Ogutu, E. O., Amayo, E. O., Kariuki, S., & (2005, . (2005). Drug susceptibility pattern of Helicobacter pylori in patients with dyspepsia at the Kenyatta National Hospital, Nairobi. East Afr Med J, 82, 603-608.

[47] Chen, J., Mandelin, T., Ceponis, J., Miller, A., Hukkanen, N. E., , M. G. F., & Konttinen, Y. T. (2003). Regulation of macrophage activation. Cell Mol Life Sci, 60, 2334-2346.

[48] Majumdar, D., Bebb, J., & (2010, J. A. (2010). H. pylori infection and peptic ulcers.Medicine, 39, 154-161.

[49] Marshall, B. J., Armstrong, J. A., Mc Gechie, D. B., Glancy, R. J., & (1985, . (1985). Attempt to fulfil Koch's postulates for pyloric Campylobacter. Med J Aust, 142, 436-439.

[50] Marshall, B. J., & warren, R. (1983). Unidentified curved bacilli on gastric epithelium in active chronic gastritis. Lancet, 1, 1273-1275.

[51] Mason, J. M., Delaney, B., Moayyedi, P., Thomas, M., Walt, R., & (2005, . (2005). Managing dyspepsia without alarm signs in primary care: new national guidance for England and Wales. Aliment Pharmacol Ther, 21, 1135-1143.

[52] Meneghini, R. (1998). Genotoxicity of active oxygen species in mammalian cells Mutat Res , 195, 215-230.

[53] Meyer, F., Wilson, K. T., James, S. P., & (2000, . (2000). Modulation of innate cytokine responses by products of Helicobacter pylori. Infect Immun, 68, 6265-6272.

[54] Moss, S. F., Legon, S., Bishop, A. E., Polak, J. M., & Calam, J. (1992). Effect of Helicobacter pylori on gastric somatostatin in duodenal ulcer disease. Lancet, 340, 930-932.

[55] Nagata, K., Yu, H., Nishikawa, M., Kashiba, M., Nakamura, A., Sato, E. F., Tamura, T., & Inoue, M. (1998). Helicobacter pylori generates superoxide radicals and modulates nitric oxide metabolism. J Biol Chem, 273, 14071-14073.

[56] Naito, Y., & Yoshikawa, T. (2002). Molecular and cellular mechanisms involved in Helicobacter pylori-induced inflammation and oxidative stress. Free Radic Biol Med, 33, 323-336.

[57] Neunert, C., Lim, W., Crowther, M., Cohen, A., Solberg, L., Jr , , & Crowther, M. A. (2011). The American Society of Hematology 2011 evidence-based practice guideline for immune thrombocytopenia. Blood, 117, 4190-4207.

[58] Noach, L. A., Bosma, N. B., Jansen, J., Hoek, F. J., van Deventer, S. J., & Tytgat, G. N. (1994). Mucosal tumor necrosis factor-alpha, interleukin-1 beta, and interleukin-8 production in patients with Helicobacter pylori infection. Scand J Gastroenterol, 29, 425-429.

[59] Nomura, A. M., Perez-Perez, G. I., Lee, J., Stemmermann, G., Blaser, M. J., & (2002, . (2002). Relation between Helicobacter pylori cagA status and risk of peptic ulcer disease. Am J Epidemiol, 155, 1054-1059.

[60] O'Mahony, R., Al-Khtheeri, H., Weerasekera, D., Fernando, N., Vaira, D., Holton, J., & Basset, C. (2005). Bactericidal and anti-adhesive properties of culinary and medicinal plants against Helicobacter pylori. World J Gastroenterol, 11, 7499-7507.

[61] Robinson, K., Argent, R. H., Atherton, J. C., & (2007, . (2007). The inflammatory and immune response to Helicobacter pylori infection. Best Pract Res Clin Gastroenterol, 21, 237-259.

[62] Rugge, M., Fassan, M., Pizzi, M., Pennelli, G., Nitti, D., & Farinati, F. (2011). Operative Link for Gastritis Assessment gastritis staging incorporates intestinal metaplasia subtyping. Hum Pathol, 42, 1539-1544.

[63] Rugge, M., Meggio, A., Pennelli, G., Piscioli, F., Giacomelli, L., De Pretis, G., & Graham, D. Y. (2007). Gastritis staging in clinical practice: the OLGA staging system. Gut, 56, 631-636.

[64] Sobala, G. M., Crabtree, J. E., Dixon, M. F., Schorah, C. J., Taylor, J. D., Rathbone, B. J., Heatley, R. V., & Axon, A. T. (1991). Acute Helicobacter pylori infection: clinical features, local and systemic immune response, gastric mucosal histology, and gastric juice ascorbic acid concentrations. Gut, 32, 1415-1418.

[65] Sutton, P., Wilson, J., Kosaka, T., Wolowczuk, I., Lee, A., & (2000, . (2000). Therapeutic immunization against Helicobacter pylori infection in the absence of antibodies. Immunol Cell Biol, 78, 28-30.

[66] Tandon, R., Khanna, H. D., Dorababu, M., Goel, R. K., & (2004, . (2004). Oxidative stress and antioxidants status in peptic ulcer and gastric carcinoma. Indian J Physiol Pharmacol, 48, 115-118.

[67] Trikudanathan, G., Philip, A., Dasanu, C. A., Baker, W. L., & (2011, . (2011). Association between Helicobacter pylori infection and pancreatic cancer. A cumulative meta-analysis. Jop, 12, 26-31.

[68] Wirth, H. P., Beins, M. H., Yang, M., Tham, K. T., & Blaser, M. J. (1998). Experimental infection of Mongolian gerbils with wild-type and mutant Helicobacter pylori strains. Infect Immun, 66, 4856-4866.

[69] Yamaoka, Y., El -Zimaity, H. M., Gutierrez, O., Figura, N., Kim, J. G., Kodama, T., Kashima, K., & Graham, D. Y. (1999). Relationship between the cagA 3' repeat region of Helicobacter pylori, gastric histology, and susceptibility to low pH. Gastroenterology, 117, 342-349.

[70] Yamaoka, Y., Kodama, T., Kashima, K., Graham, D. Y., & Sepulveda, A. R. (1998). Variants of the 3' region of the cagA gene in Helicobacter pylori isolates from patients with different H. pylori-associated diseases. J Clin Microbiol, 36, 2258-2263.

[71] Yamaoka, Y., Kwon, D. H., Graham, D. Y., & (2000, . (2000). A M(r) 34,000 proinflammatory outer membrane protein (oipA) of Helicobacter pylori. Proc Natl Acad Sci. U S A, 97, 7533-7538.

[72] Zevering, Y., Jacob, L., Meyer, T. F., & (1999, . (1999). Naturally acquired human immune responses against Helicobacter pylori and implications for vaccine development. Gut, 45, 465-474.

Section 4

Afferent Vagal Neural Pathway in the Development and Healing of Chronic Gastritis in Patients

Chapter 4

Capsaicin-Sensitive Afferentation Represents a New Mucosal Defensive Neural Pathway System in the Gastric Mucosa in Patients with Chronic Gastritis

Jozsef Czimmer, Imre Laszló Szabo,
Janos Szolcsanyi and Gyula Mozsik

Additional information is available at the end of the chapter

http://dx.doi.org/10.5772/52883

1. Introduction

The name of capsaicin is generally used in the medical research, however this material does not contain a uniform chemical entity. Capsaicinoids covers 5 analogues and 2 homologues components (Mozsik et al. 2009) (Fig. 1).

It has been established that capsaicinoids interact with capsainin-sensitive afferent nerves representing a novel regulatory pathway of gastrointestinal funcions (Jancsó et al. 1967, 1968, 1970). Capsaicin-sensitive afferent nerves contain a temperature-gated ion channel called capsaicin receptor or transient receptor potencil vanilloid 1 (TRPV1) which is expressed by a subgroup of primary afferent nociceptive neurons (Szolcsanyi, 2004). The capsaicin receptor has been cloned (Caterina et al., 1997) and has been found to be linked to a cation channel. It is gated by capsaicin and other capsaicinoids (some vanilloids) by various treatments including low pH, noxius heat and various pain-producing endogenous an exogenous chemicals. Thus, those sensory nerve endings possessing these ion channels are susceptible to being stimulated in the gastric mucosa. Upon stimulation with capsaicin, these afferent fibers develop four response stages (excitation, sensory-blocking, long-term selective neurotoxic impairment, and irreversible cell destruction), depending on the dose and duration of exposure of the component (Mózsik et al. 2001). A low dose of capsaicin (nanograms to micrograms per kilogram) causes excitation of the nerve endings, and neuropeptides (substance P [SP], calcitonin gene-related peptide [CGRP], and somatostatin) are released (Holzer et al. 1998, 1999) (Szolcsányi 2004). These mediators can increase mucosal blood flow by vasodilatation (Holzer et al. 1991), can activate mast cells and immunocells in the mucosa (Stead 1992), and are involved in drug effects (Mózsik et al. 2004, 2005), and somatostatin can elicit systemic anti-inflammatory and analgetic "sensory functions." The immunodistribution of neuropeptides (SP, VIP, NPY, SOM, GAL, and TH) released from the sensory neurons and their neuroimmune function are known in *H. pylori*-positive gastritis (Sipos et al. 2006). Notwithstanding studies supported that this gastric mucosal protective mechanism provided by capsaicin-sensitive afferent nerves exists in patients with chronic gastritis, and its extent does not depend on the presence or absence of *H. pylori* infection. In other words, the gastric mucosal protection produced by capsaicin-sensitive afferent nerves is one of the general defense mechanisms against the different noxious agents that induce chronic gastritis (Dömötör et al. 2006).

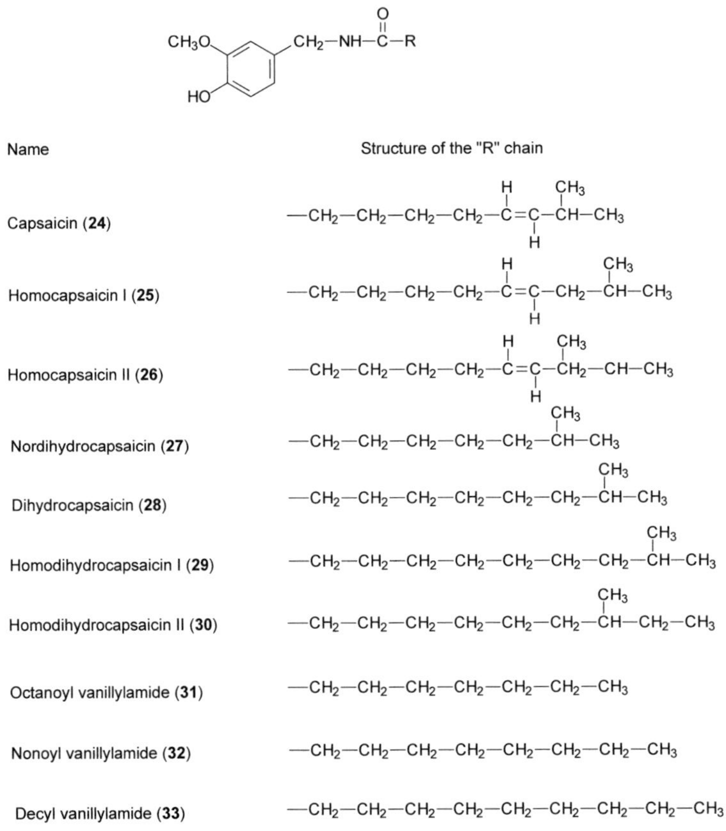

Figure 1. Names and chemical structures of capsaicin homologs and analogs (with knowledge and allowance of Mozsik et al. 2009).

The vagal nerve has a key-role in the development of gastrointestinal mucosal damage and prevention (Mozsik et al., 1982). The key-role of vagal nerve has been emphasized dominantly in the aggressive processes to gastrointestinal (GI) mucosa (such as in peptic ulcer disease, gastric mucosal damage, etc.) as evidenced from GI investigations in animal models and as well as in human clinical practice. The application of capsaicin in the animal experimentswas used as a specific tool to investigate those primary afferent nociceptive neurones (Szolcsanyi, 2004; Buck and Burks, 1986; Holzer, 1988; 1991; Szállasi and Blumberg, 1999) involved in the different physiological, pathological processes.

Szolcsanyi and Bartho (1981) were the first authors, who clearly identified the beneficial and harmful effect of capsaicin in experimental peptic ulcer in rats, following varying doses of capsaicin. Later, Holzer undertook extensive investigations on the mode of action of capsaicin on GI functions (Holzer, 1998; 1999; Buck and Burks, 1986; Szállasi and Blumberg, 1999). We also contributed during the 1980's to GI capsaicin research from studies in animal models (Mózsik et al., 1997c). Recently the new drug, lafutidine, was introduced in the medical treatment of GI mucosal damage (Ajioka et al., 2000; 2002; Onodera et al., 1995; 1999; Takeuchi, 2006). Lafutidine is a histamine histamine type 2 receptor (H2R) blocking compound which uniquely has typical capsaicin actions on the target organ.

Capsaicin-sensitive vagal neural afferentation is one of the defensive mechanisms. These nerves have been shown to play a role in gastric mucosal protection by preventing drug - induced mucosal injury in animals (Abdel-Salam et al. 1999; Mózsik et al. 1997a; Reinshagen at al. 1996) and by decreasing the amount of indomethacin (IND)-induced gastric microbleeding in healthy human subjects (Kang JY et al. 1995; Mózsik et al. 2004b; Mózsik et al. 2005). These mechanisms are well known to be important in protection against gastritis caused by various harmful effects. The TRVP 1 receptors were also detected in the area postrema and in the nucleus tractus solitary, where the afferent fibres of the vagus nerve taper, and have key role in regulation of gastric functions i.e. secretion, motiity and protestion mechanisms.

The vagus nerve consists of 10% efferent nerves, 90% afferents. About 10% of these afferent nerves are capsaicin-sensitive. The amount of efferent nerves and the capsaicin-sensitive afferent nerves is roughly equal in the vagus nerve. Capsaicin exposure exerts various responses in these afferent nerves depending on dose and exposure duration (excitation, sensory-blocking, long-term selective neurotoxic impairment and irreversible cell destruction) (Vincze et al. 2004). During exposure to small doses of capsaicin (from ng/kg to μg/kg body weight) neurotransmitters, such as: substance P (SP), calcitonin gene-related peptide (CGRP) and somatostatin, are released from the nerve endings (Caterina et al. 1997; Mózsik et al. 2001; Holzer 1998). These mediators are responsible for increasing mucosal blood flow by vasodilatation (Holzer 1999), activation of mast cells and other immune cells in the mucosa (Szolcsányi 2004; Holzer et al. 1991) and defense of gastrointestinal mucosa.

Capsaicin has been used in human studies, looks to be a suitable treatment tool in several fields of medicine that can be seen from several running and completes multicentric controlled studies worldwide. The United States Pharmacopeia (USP) describes the list of capsaicins and their definition, identification, melting range, and content of capsaicin, dihydrocapsaicin and other capsaicinoids as follows (USP30-NF25. 2006 Edition, pp.1609): capsaicin contains not less than 90.0 % and more than 110.0 % of the labelled percentage of total capsaicinoids. The content of capsaicin is not less than 55 %, and the sum of the contents of capsaicin and dihydrocapsaicin should not be less than 75 %. The content of other capsaicinoids should not be more than 15 %, all calculated on the dried basis. The circumstances of plant cultivation, preparation, storage and other facts are summarized in the drug master file (DMF). The DMF of capsaicin originated from India was signed by Food and Drug Administration (FDA) in the United States as existing registration, which allows the usage of capsaicin as basic source for capsaicin-containing drugs. This type of capsaicinoids (briefly capsaicin) was used in our previous studies (Mozsik et al. 2009a, 2009b, 2011).

Gastritis is a pathomorphological appearance of inflammation in the gastric mucosa. Acute and chronic gastritis can be differentiated on the basis of the development and process of the disease. Chronic gastritis may be caused by different factors such as *Helicobacter pylori* infection, bacterial overgrowt in a hypochlorhydric stomach, autoimmune mechanisms, or chemical agents such as long-term nonsteroidal anti-inflammatory drug (NSAID) treatment, and bile reflux (Owen 2003; Appelman 1994, Szabo et al. 2012), for details about mechanisms we refere to the other chapters of this book. Nowdays, the importance of *Helicobacter pylori* infection is increasing as the main causative factor in gastric diseases in humans. This bacterium is highly prevalent in many countries (Parsonnet 1995) and it increases the risk for development of gastric and duodenal ulcer disease, gastric cancer, and gastric mucosa-associated lymphoid tissue lymphoma (Janulaityte-Gunther et al. 2005; Mitani et al. 2004; Peng et al. 1998; Salih et al. 2005; Zhang et al. 2005a, 2005b). Dysfunction of gastrointestinal mucosal defense mechanisms is also involved in the development of gastric diseases. Capsaicin-sensitive afferent nerves take part in gastric mucosal protection in animals (Mózsik et al. 1997a; Reinshagen et al 1996) and in healthy human subjects (Kang et al. 1995; Mózsik et al. 2004a, 2005a), and the presence of these fibers is proved to play a role in the development of human gastrointestinal disorders including gastritis, peptic ulcer, polyp without and with dysplasia, tumor, and inflammatory bowel diseases (Dömötör et al. 2005; Vincze et al. 2004). The immunodistribution of neuropeptides (SP, VIP, NPY, SOM, GAL, and TH) released from the sensory neurons and their neuroimmune function are known in *H. pylori*-positive gastritis (Sipos et al. 2006).

2. Recent results in human studies

Presentation of capsaicin-sensitive afferentation in the *H. pylori* positive and *H. pylori* negative chronic gastritis in patients has been studied by Mózsik et al. (2011): The symptoms of patients sufferring from chronic gastritis with or without *H. pylori* infection (*H. pylori* positive, n=21, age 39-68 years, screened with [^{14}C] urea breath test, rapid urease test, Warthin-Starry silver staining and specific histological examinations; *H. pylori* negative, n=30, age 39-68 years) were nonspecific including gastric dyscomfort sensation, nausea, loss of apetite and vomiting. The gastric tissue samples from the stomach and antrum were examined by an independent histopathologist and classified of chronic gastritis according to the Sydney's System (Price et al. 1991). The immunohistological studies were carried out on formalin fixed, parafin embedded tissue samples of gastric mucosa using the peroxidase-labeled polymer method (Lab Vision Co., Fremont, USA). SP was detected by the NC1/34HL rat monoclonal antibody, the TRPV1 receptor and CGRP were labeled using polyclonal rabbit antisera (all from Alcam Ltd., UK, Cambridge) (Dömötör et al. 2006) (Figs. 2-4).

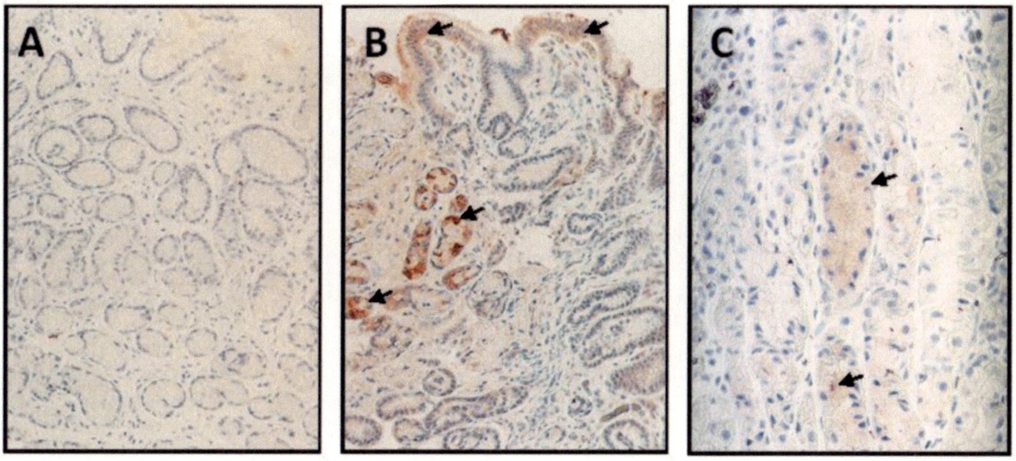

Figure 2. Immunohistochemical distribution of capsaicin receptor (transitoric receptor potential vanilloid) (TRPV1 in the gastric mucosa of a healthy (A) and of patient with *H. pylori* negative (B) and *H. pylori* positive (C) chronic gastritis. Arrows indicate the immunosigns in the epithelial layer of the gastric mucosa (original magnification: 100x). From the ref. (Mózsik et al. 2011), with permission.

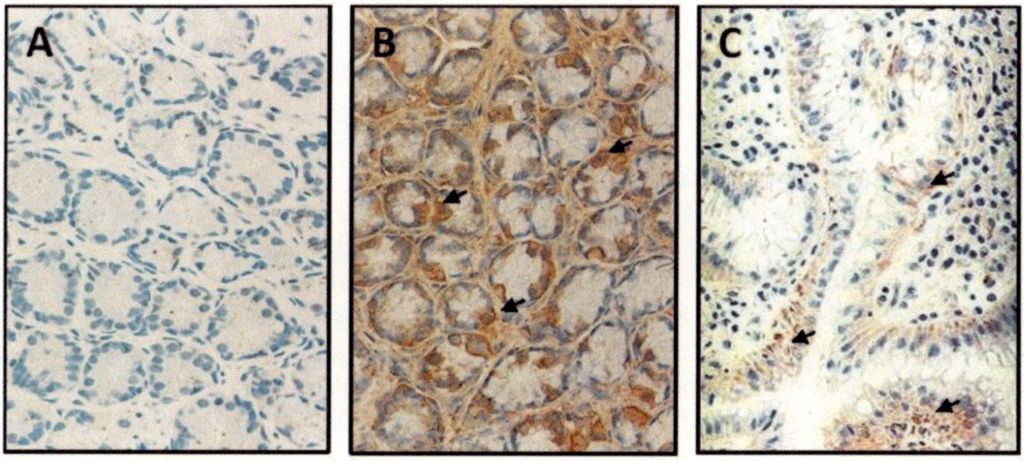

Figure 3. Immunoshistochemical distribution of calcitonin gene-related peptide (CGRP) in the gastric mucosa of healthy subject (A), of patient with *H. pylori* negative (B) and *H. pylori* positive (C) chronic gastritis. Arrows demosntrate the immunosign in the epithelial layer of the gastric mucosa (original magnification: 100x). From the ref. (Mózsik et al. 2011), with permission.

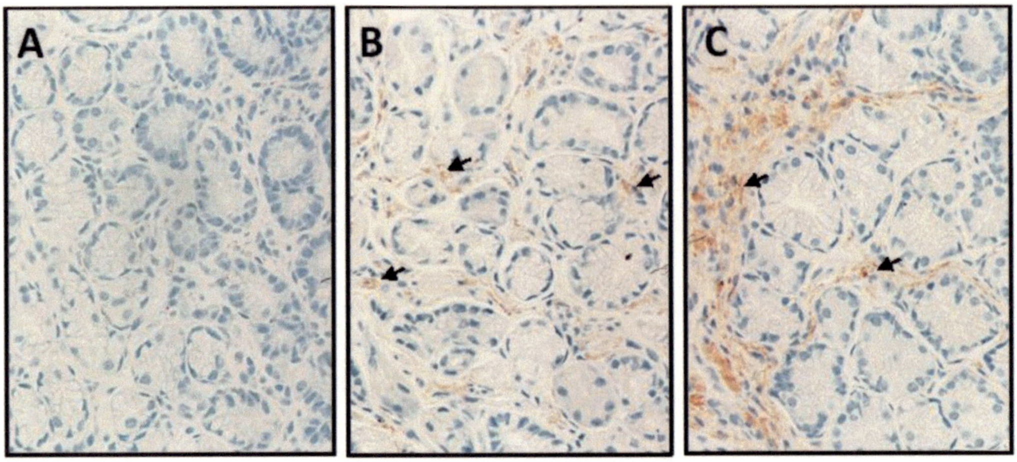

Figure 4. Immonohsitochemical distribution of subastane P (SP) in gastric mucosa of healthy subject (A), of pateints with *H. pylori* negative (B) and positive (C) chronic gastritis. Arrows show the immunosigns in the epithelial layer of the gastric mucosa (original magnification: 100x). From the Ref. (Mózsik et al 2011), with permission.

Presentation of capsaicin-sensitive afferention of vagal nerve in patients with *H. pylori* positve chronic gastritis of patients, before after after eradication treatment (Mózsik et al 2011):Very recently the same clinical and immunohistochemical examinations were carried out as those mentioned above in patients with *H. pylori* positive chronic gastritis before and after eradication treatment. These observations were carried out in 38 persons, including 20 healthy subjects and 18 patients with *H. pylori* positive gastritis. The age of persons with histologically intact gastric mucosa (controls) were between 41 and 67 years (mean=52.2 years). The age of patients (6 males, 12 females) was 39 to 68 years (mean = 56.4 years).

The time period between the first and control gastroscopy was 6 weeks. The biopsies were taken from the corpus and antrum of patients with chronic gastritis, before and after eradidation treatment, and from healthy persons. *H. pylori* positive patients underwent 7 days eradication treatment with combination of double dose PPI (pantoprazole 2x40 mg/day), amoxicillin (1000 mg twice daily) and clarithromycin (500 mg twice daily) according to current European guidelines (Malferteiner et al. 2007). After this one week combination treatment, patients continued to take normal dose of PPI for another week. The *H. pylori* infection was detected before and after by [^{14} C] urea breath test, rapid urease test, Warthing-Starry silver staining and specific histological and immmunohistological examinations. The results of eradication treatment was succesfull in 89%, the gastric histology indicated normal picture in 22% of cases, and in 78 per cent patient the mucosa showed moderate gastritis (Lakner et al. 2011).

Expression of TRPV1 receptor, CGRP and SP in the gastric mucosa of patients with *H. pylori* negative and positive chronic gastritis, and before and after successful eradication treatment (Mózsik et al 2011): The expression of TRPV1 and CGRP increased in the gastric mucosa of patients with chronic gastritis, however, it was an unexpected that the increase expresson of

TRPV1 and CGRP did not depend on the presence of *H. pylori* infection. The changes in expression of SP were not significant between these groups of patients.

Another surprising result was obtained in patients with *H. pylori* positive chronic gastritis before and after sucessfull eradication treatment. The extent of expression of TRPV1, CGRP remained at the same level after eradication. No significant changes were obtained in the expression of SP in the gastric mucosa in these patients (Fig. 4) (Mózsik et al 2011).

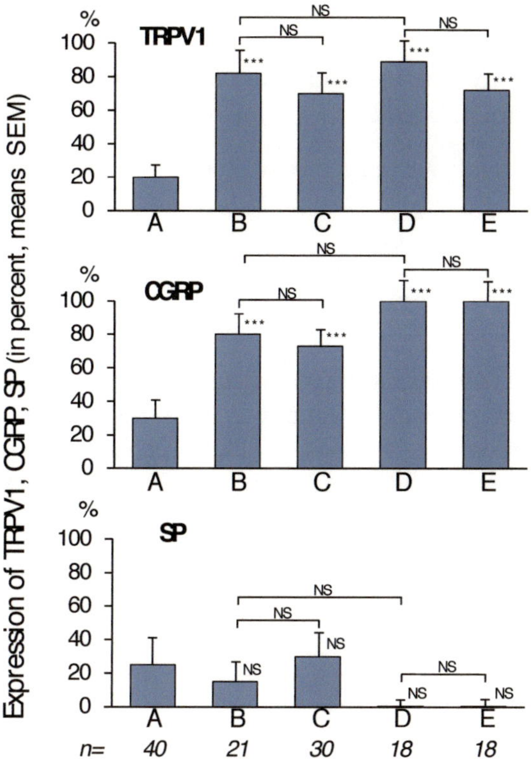

Figure 5. Chamges in the expression of capsaicin receptor (TRPV1), calcitonin gene-ralated peptide (CGRP) and substabtance P (SP) in the human gastric mucosa of healthy voluntaries(histologically intact) (A), *H. pylori* positive (B), *H. pylori* negative (C) and *H. pylori* positive before (D) and after eradication (pantoprazole 40, amoxicillin 1000 and clarithromycin 500 mg, all two times per day, for seven days) (n=number of patients) (Mózsik et al 2012).

These findings suggest potential role of capsaicin-sensitive afferent vagal nerve in the development of chronic gastritis and the eradication treatment (Mózsik et al 2011): From the experimental observations it could be concluded that actions of capsaicin are dose-dependent (Mozsik et al. 2001, 2005a, 2009b). The types of gastric mucosal injuries could be prevented by application of small doses (200 to 800µg/person) of capsaicin (Mózsik et al. 2001). Results of these observations suggest mucosal protecting effect of capsaicin (acting via the stimulation of capsaicin-sensitive afferent fibres of vagal nerve) in healthy human subjects. These observations showed that the expression of TRPV1 and CGRP increased siginicantly in inflamated chronic gastritis, and no significant change was obtained in SP levels. However, these immunohistochemical results did not differ in patients with *H. pylori* positive and negative chronic gastritis. Capsaicin-sensitive afferention did not differ before and after (6 weeks) successfull eradication treatment in patients with chronic *H. pylori* positive gastritis (meanwhile the control biopsy was normal in 22% and in 78% indicated in moderated histological picture of gastritis) (Lakner et al. 2011).

Explantaion of study group of the for the unchanged immunohistochemical distribution of TRPV1, CGRP and SP of gastric *H. pylori* positive chronic gastritis before vs. after eradication treatment were as follows (Mozsik et al. 2011):

1. Six week time period (including the eradication treatment) is not enough time for the complete healing of chronic gastritis.
2. The six-week time period (after eradication treatment) is probably not enought time for complete histologically recovery of chronic *H. pylori* positive infection in patients in term of histology and immunohistology.
3. The *H. pylori* bacteria as etiological factors might represent only one of the factors causing chronic gastritis (in term of histology);
4. The immunohistological distribution (expression rate) of TRPV1, CGRP and SP are independent ont the chronic gastritis produced by different physical, chemical, bacterological or immunological agents. However, the increased expression of TRPV1, CGRP is involved in the gastric mucosal damage and the normalization of these changes can be obtained by other way as the classical eradication treatment (Lakner et al. 2011).

Kozlowski et al. (2011) conluded from their study on chronic gastritis: 1. Chronic supeficial gastritis coexists with significantly higher proliferative activity of gastric mucosal glandular epithelium, particulary in relation to the prepyloric area and 2. Changes of proliferative activity of gastric mucosal glandular epithelium are independent of age, histotopography and of *H. pylori* colonization.

Recent investigations showed that the expression of TRPV1 and CGRP increased significantly inthe epithelial layer of the gastric mucosa in patients with *H. pylori* - positive and -negative chronic gastritis. The significant etiological role of *H. pylori* in the development of chronic gastritis has received great attention in the pertinent literature; for this reason, we compared the differences in TRPV1,CGRP, and SP expression in *H. pylori* positive or -negative chronic gastritis, suggesting their etiological role in the development of chronic gastritis. No significant differences were obtained between *H. pylori*-positive and *H. pylori*-negative patients, but values of both groups with chronic gastritis differed significantly from those of histological intact mucosa of healthy human subjects. Results also indicated that chronic gastric inflammation is one of the general tissue reactions to different noxious agents, and *H. pylori* is only one of these in patients. It must be emphasized that clinicians are able to specifically demonstrate the presence of *H. pylori* (by UBT, rapid urease test, and specific histological staining), however, we have no specific methods for well demonstration of other (suggested) etiological factors.

In animal experiments, different noxious agents produce the same (or basically similar) pathological, biochemical (oxygen free radicals), etc., events in the development of gastrointestinal mucosal injury and its prevention (Mózsik et al. 1992). Gastric mucosal damage can be produced by direct application of ethanol and indomethacin and it can be dose dependently prevented by the topical application of capsaicin in healthy volunteers (Mózsik et al., 2005a). Endogenous (increased production of gastric HCl in 4-hr pylorus-ligated rats) and exogenous (indomethacin given s.c. in a 4-hr experiment, without pylorus ligation) factors produced changes in functional status and damaged the gastric mucosa in rats. The immunohistochemical distribution of TRPV1, CGRP, and SP decreased significantly during this time; the levels of TRPV1 and CGRP returned to those of healthy controls dose dependently by application of omeprazole and omeprazole-like compounds, and no significant change was detected in the immunodistribution of SP (Mózsik et al. 1997b). There is no real explanation for the different expression rates of TRPV1 and mediators released from the sensory nerves. Similar differences in TRPV1, CGRP, and SP have been observed in many other conditions (in acute animal models and in patients with chronic gastrointestinal disorders). The following explanations have been suggested for these differences in expression of TRPV1 and mediators released from sensory nerves (Dömötör et al., 2007): (1) the regulation of SP differs from that of TRPV1 and CGRP regarding the development of chronic gastritis and (2) the sensitivity of SP regulation is lower than in the cases of TRPV1 and CGRP. The increased level of TRPV1 and CGRP is accepted as a signal of an increased defense mechanism produced by capsaicin-sensitive afferent nerves in animal experiments (Mózsik et al. 2005a), and the topical application of capsaicin dose-dependently prevented the mucosal injury produced by intragastrically applied ethanol and indomethacin in healthy human subjects (Mózsik et al. 2005b). These findings suggest that increased expression of TRPV1 and CGRP is associated with increased gastric mucosal protection. This gastric mucosal protective mechanism provided by capsaicin-sensitive afferent nerves exists in patients with chronic gastritis, and its extent does not depend on the presence or absence of *H. pylori* infection. In other words, the gastric mucosal protection produced by capsaicin-sensitive afferent nerves is one of the general defensive mechanisms against the different noxious agents that induce chronic gastritis.

3. Conclusions

The results of above mentioned animal and human observations indicated clearly the following considerations:

1. Both acute and chronic gastritis can be induced by different reasons, like chemicals (drugs) or bacteria (most emphysized one H. Pylori). Both H. pylori positive and negative gastritis can be acute or chroinic. In case of patients with H.plyori negative gastritis, the therapeutic approach follows the traditional medical treatment, while H.pylori positive patients with gastritis are suggested a rational eradtication treatment only (accepted by many international consensus meetings).

Mózsik et al. and Lakner et al. (2011) have demonstrated that while chronic H. pylori pozitive gastritis heals entirely after a sucessful eradication therapy (which represents an important step to prevent development of gastric cancer), the extents of TRVP1, CGRP remained in increased level (in comparison to the normal gastric mucosa). This indicates that there is at least one other important defensive mechanism than antibiotic eradiction treatment, the capsaicin-sensivite afferention of vagal nerve (results clearly indicated that independent from H. pylori status and independent from eradication).

Generally it can be concluded that: 1. there can be different mucosal defensive mechanisms playing key role in treatment of H. plyori positive chronic gastritis: a. eradication treatment and b. stimulation of capsaicin sensitive afferentation; 2. eradication treatment is independent from capsaicin-sensitive afferention (defensive) mechanism; 3. it should be considered to amend treatment protocols of H. pylori positive chronic gastritis (conventional eradication therapy and success control) with modification of functional state of capsaicin-sensitive afferentation. Medical effect of capsaicin for modification of capsacin-sensitive afferent nerves depends on its dosages, more clinical findngs are needed in the field, that observations are in progress (Mozsik et al. 2009b, 2011).

Acknowledgements

This chapter was supported by MEDICZIM Kft, Hungary and ALAPITVANY AZ EGESZSEG UGYEBEN DOLGOZOKERT, Hungary.

Author details

Jozsef Czimmer[1*], Imre Laszló Szabo[1], Janos Szolcsanyi[2] and Gyula Mozsik[1]

*Address all correspondence to: jozsef.czimmer@aok.pte.hu

1 First Department of Medicine, University of Pécs, Hungary

2 Department of Pharmacology and Pharmacotherapy, University of Pécs, Hungary

References

[1] Abdel-Salam, O. M. E., Debreceni, A., & Mózsik, Gy. (1999). Capsaicinsensitive afferent sensory nerves in modulating gastric mucosal defense against noxious agents. J Physiol Paris , 93, 443-454.

[2] Aijoka, H., Miyake, H., & Matsuura, N. (2000). Effect of FRG-8813, a new-type histamine H2-receptor antagonist, on the recurrence of gastric ulcer healing by drug treatment. Pharmacology. , 61, 83-90.

[3] Aijoka, H., Matsuura, N., & Miyake, H. (2002). High quality of ulcer healing in rats by lafutidine and new-tipe histamine H2-receptor antagonist: involvement of capsaicin of sensitive sensory neurons. Inflammopharmacology , 10, 483-493.

[4] Appelman HD(1994). Gastritis: terminology, etiology, and clinicopathological correlations: another biased view. Hum Pathol , 25, 1006-1019.

[5] Buck SH, Burks TF.(1986). The Neuropharmacology of capsaicin: review of some recent observation. Pharmacol Rev. , 38, 179-226.

[6] Caterina, Chumacher., Tominaga, M., Rosen, T. A., & Levine, Julius. D. (1997). The capsaicin receptor: a heat-activated ion channel in the pain pathway. *Nature,* 389, 816-824.

[7] Dixon, M. F., Genta, R. M., Yardley, J. H., & Correa, P. (1996). Classification and grading of gastritis: the updated Sydney system. Am J Surg Pathol , 20, 1161-1181.

[8] Dömötör, A., Peidl, Zs., Vincze, Á., Hunyady, B., Szolcsányi, J., Kereskay, L., Szekeres, Gy., & Mózsik, Gy. (2005). Immunohistochemical distribution of vanilloid receptor (TRPV1), calcitonin generelated peptide (CGRP) and substance-P (SP) in the gastrointestinal mucosa of patients with different gastrointestinal disorders. Inflammopharmacology , 13, 161-177.

[9] Dömötör, A., Kereskay, L., Szekeres, Gy., Hunyady, B., Szolcsányi, J., & Mózsik, Gy. (2006). Participation of capsaicin sensitive afferent nerves in the gastric mucosa of patients with helicobacter pyloripositive or-negative chronic gastritis. Dig Dis Sci. , 52, 411-417.

[10] Holzer, P., & Lippe, I. T. (1988). Stimulation of afferent nerve endings by intragastric capsaicin protects against ethanol-induced damage of gastric mucosa. *Neuroscience,* 27, 981-7.

[11] Holzer, P., Livingston, E. H., Saria, A., & Guth, P. H. (1991). Sensory neurons mediate protective vasodilatation in rat gastric mucosa. Am J Physiol , 260, 363-370.

[12] Holzer, P. Afferent nerve-mediated control of gastric mucosal blood flow and protection. In: Costa M, Surrenti C, Gorini S, Maggi CA, Meli A, Eds. Sensory nerve and neuropeptides in gastroenterology. From basic science to clinical perspective. New York: Plenum Press; (1991). , 97-108.

[13] Holzer, P. (1998). Neural emergency system in the stomach. *Gastroenterology,* 114, 823-830.

[14] Holzer, P. (1999). Capsaicin cellular targets, mechanisms of action and selectivity for thin sensory neurons. Pharmacol Rev , 43, 143-201.

[15] Jancsó, N., Jancsó-Gábor, A., & Szolcsányi, J. (1967). Direct evidence for neurogenic inflammation and its prevention by denervation and by pretreatment with capsaicin. Br J Pharmacol , 31, 138-51.

[16] Jancsó, N., Jancsó-Gábor, A., & Szolcsányi, J. (1968). The role of sensory nerves endings in the neurogen inflammation induced in human skin and in the eye and paw of the rat. Br J Pharmacol , 33, 32-41.

[17] Jancsó-Gábor, A., Szolcsányi, J., & Jancsó, N. (1970). Irreversible impairment of the irregulation induced by capsaicin and similar pungent substances in rat and guinea-pigs. J Physiol (London). , 206, 495-507.

[18] Janulaityte-Gunther, D., Kucinskiene, R., Kupcinskas, L., Pavilonis, A., Labanauskas, L., Cizauskas, A., Schmidt, U., Wadstrom, T., & Andersen, L. P. (2005). The humoral immune response to Helicobacter pylori infection in children with gastrointestinal symptoms. FEMS Immunol Med Microbiol , 44, 205-212.

[19] Kang, J. Y., Yeoh, K. G., Chia, H. P., Lee, H. P., Chia, Y. W., Guan, R., & Yap, I. (1995). Chili-Protective factor against peptic ulcer? Dig Dis Sci , 40, 576-579.

[20] Kozlowski, W., Jochymski, C., Markiewiocz, T., Chronic, gastritis., In, Tonino. P., & Ed, . Gastritis and Gastric Cancer- New Insights in Gastroportection, Diagnosis and Treatment. Publisher by inTech, Rijeka, Croatia. (2011). , 75-92.

[21] Lakner, L., Dömötör, A., Tóth, Cs., Szabo, I. L., Mecker, Á., Hajós, R., Kereskai, L., Szekeres, Gy., Döbrönte, Z., & Mózsik, Gy. (2011). Capsaicin-sensitive afferentation represents an indifferent defensive patway from eradication in patients with H.pylori positve gastritis. World J Gastrointest Pharmacol Ther , 2, 36-41.

[22] Malfertheiner, P., Megraud, F., O'Morain, C., Bazzoli, F., El -Omar, E., Graham, D., Hunt, R., Rokkas, T., Vakiel, N., & Kuipers, E. J. Current concepts in the management of Helicobacter pylori infection. The Maastricht III. Consensus Repor. t. Gut (2007). , 56, 772-81.

[23] Mitani, K., Tatsuta, M., Iishi, H., Yano, H., Uedo, N., Iseki, K., & Narahara, H. (2004). Helicobacter pylori infection as a risk factor for gastric ulceration. Hepato-Gastroenterology , 51, 309-312.

[24] Mózsik, Gy., Moron, F., & Jávor, T. (1982). Cellular mechanisms of the development of gastric mucosal damage and of gastroprotection induced by prostacyclin in rats. A pharmacological study, Prostagland. Leukot. Med. , 9, 71-84.

[25] Mózsik, Gy., Király, Á., Sütő, G., & Vincze, Á. (1992). ATP breakdown in the development of gastrointestinal mucosal damage and its prevention in animals and human (An overview of 25 years ulcer research studies). Acta Physiol Hung , 80, 39-80.

[26] Mózsik, Gy., Nagy, L., & Király, Á. (1997a). Eds. Twenty-five Years of Peptic Ulcer Research in Hungary. from Basic Science to Clinical Practice 1971-1995. Budapest: Akademiai Kiadó; , 1-448.

[27] Mózsik, Gy., Nagy, L., Pár, A., & Rainsford, . (1997b). Eds. Cell Injury and Protection in the Gastrointestinal Tract: from Basic Science to Clinical Perspectives. Dordrecht: Kluwer Academic Publisher.

[28] Mózsik, Gy., Abdel-Salam, O. M. E., & Szolcsányi, J. (1997c). Capsaicin-Sensitive Afferent Nerves in Gastric Mucosal Damage and Protection. Budapest: Akadémiai Kiadó; 1997c.

[29] Mózsik, Gy., Vincze, Á., & Szolcsányi, J. (2001). Four response stages of capsaicin-sensitive primary afferent neurons to capsaicin and its analog: gastric acid secretion, gastric mucosal damage and protection. J Gastroenterol Hepatol , 16, 1093-1097.

[30] Mózsik, Gy., Belágyi, J., Szolcsányi, J., Pár, G., Pár, A., Rumi, Gy., & Rácz, I. (2004a). Capsaicin-sensitive afferent nerves and gastric mucosal protection in the human healthy subjects. A critical overview. In: Takeuchi K, Mózsik Gy (Eds) Mediators in Gastrointestinal Protection and Repair. Research Signpost, Kerala, , 43-62.

[31] Mózsik, Gy., Pár, A., Pár, G., Juricskay, I., Figler, M., & Szolcsányi, J. (2004b). Insight into the molecular pharmacology to drugs acting on the afferent and efferent fibers of the vagal nerve in the gastric mucosal protection. In: Sikiric P, Seiwerth P, Mózsik Gy, Arakawa T, Takeuchi K (Eds) Ulcer Research. Proceedings of the 11th International Conference. Monduzzi, Bologna, , 163-168.

[32] Mózsik Gy, Peidl Zs, Szolcsányi J, Dömötör A, Hideg K, Szekeres Gy, Karádi O, Hunyady B (2005a). Participation of vanilloid/ capsaicin receptors, calcitonin gene-related peptide and substance P in gastric protection of omeprazole and omeprazole-like compounds. Inflammopharmacology 13:139–159.

[33] Mózsik Gy., Rácz I., Szolcsányi J. (2005b). Gastroprotection induced by capsaicin in human healthy subjects. World J Gastroenterol 11:5180–5184.

[34] Mózsik, Gy., Dömötör, A., Past, T., Vas, V., Perjési, P., Kuzma, M., Blazics, Gy., & Szolcsányi, J. (2009a). Capsaicinoids: From the Plant Cultivation to the Production of the Human Medical Drug. Akadémiai Kiadó, Budapest

[35] Mózsik, Gy., Past, T., Abdel-Salam, O. M. E., Kuzma, M., & Perjési, P. (2009b). Interdisciplinary review for correlation between the plant origin capsaicinoids, non-steroidal antiinflammatory drugs, gastrointestinal mucosal damage and prevention in animals and human beings. *Inflammopharmacology*, 17, 113-150.

[36] Mózsik, Gy., Past, T., Dömötör, A., Kuzma, M., & Perjési, P. (2010). Production oforally applicable new drug or drug combinations from natural origin capsaicinoids for human medical therapy. Curr Pharm Des , 16, 1197-1208.

[37] Mózsik, Gy., Szabó, I. L., & Dömötör, A. (2011). Approach to role of capsaicin-sensitive afferent nerves in the development and healing in patients with chronic gastritis. In: Tonino P (ed). Gastritis and New Gastric Cancer- New Insights in Gastroprotection, Diagnosis and Treatments. 2011 Publisher by in Tech. Rijeka, Croatia 2011. , 25-46.

[38] Mózsik, Gy., Szabó, I. L., & Czimmer, J. (2012). Vulnerable points of the Helicobacter pylori story- based on animal and human observations (1975-2012). Buzás G (Ed.): Helicobacter pylori: 2012. Bentham Science Publishers (in press).

[39] Onodera, S., Shibata, M., Tanaka, et., & al, . (1999). Gastroprotective mechanisms of lafutidine, a novel anti-ulcer drug with histamine H2-receptor antagonist activity,. Artneim Forsch. Drug Res. , 49, 519-26.

[40] Owen DAMB(2003). Gastritis and carditis. Mod Pathol , 16, 325-341.

[41] Parsonnet, J. (1995). The incidence of Helicobacter pylori infection. Aliment Pharmacol Ther , 2, 45-51.

[42] Peng, H., Ranaldi, R., Diss, T. C., Isaacson, P. G., Bearzi, I., & Pan, L. (1998). High frequency of CagA+ Helicobacter pylori infection in high-grade gastric MALT B-cell lymphomas. J Pathol , 185, 409-412.

[43] Price AB, Misiewicz JJ. (1991). Sydney classification for gastritis. *Lancet*, 174 EOF.

[44] Reinshagen, M., Patel, A., Sottili, M., French, S., Sternini, C., & Eysselein, V. E. (1996). Action of sensory neurons in an experimental rat colitis model of injury and repair. Am J Physiol , 270, 79-86.

[45] Salih, Abasiyanik. M. F., Saribasak, H., Huten, O., & Sander, E. (2005). A follow-up study on the effect of Helicobacter pylori radication on the severity of gastric histology. Dig Dis Sci , 50, 1517-1522.

[46] Sipos, G., Altdorfer, K., Pongor, E., Chen, L. P., & Fehér, E. (2006). Neuroimmune link in the mucosa of chronic gastritis with Helicobacter pylori infection. Dig Dis Sci. 2006; , 51, 1810-7.

[47] Stead RH(1992). Innervation of mucosal immune cells in the gastrointestinal tract. Reg Immunol , 4, 91-99.

[48] Szabó, I. L., Cseko, K., Czimmer, J., & Mózsik, Gy. (2012). Diagnosis of Gastritis- Review from Early Pathological Evaluation to Present Day Management. In: Mózsik Gy (Ed). "Gastritis" Publisher by In Tech. Rijeka, Croatia (in press).

[49] Szállasi, A., & Blumberg, M. (1999). Vanilloid (capsaicin) receptors and mechanisms. Pharmacol Rev. , 51, 159-211.

[50] Szolcsányi, J., & Barthó, L. (1981). Impaired defense mechanisms to peptic ulcer in the capsaicin-desensitized rat. In: Mózsik Gy, Hanninen O, Jávor T, Eds. Advances in Physiological Sciences, Gastrointestinal Defense Mechanisms. Oxford and Budapest: Pergamon Press and Akadémiai Kiadó; , 29, 39-51.

[51] Szolcsányi, J. (2004). Forty years in capsaicin research for sensory pharmacology and physiology. Neuropeptide. , 38, 377-84.

[52] Takeuchi, K. (2006). Unique profile of lafutidine: a novel histamine Hreceptor antagonist: mucosal protection throughout GI mucosal mediated by capsaicin-sensitive afferent nerves. Acta Pharmacol Sinica Suppl. 27-35., 2.

[53] Vincze, Á., Szekeres, Gy., Király, Á., Bódis, B., & Mózsik, Gy. (2004). The immunohistochemical distribution of capsaicin receptor, CGRP and SP in the human gastric mucosa in patients with different gastric disorders. In: Sikiric P, Seiwerth S, Mózsik Gy, Arakawa T, Takeuchi K (Eds) Ulcer Research. Proceedings of 11th International Congress of Ulcer Research. Monduzzi, Bologna, , 149-153.

[54] Zhang, C., Yamada, N., Wu, Y. L., Wen, M., Matsuhisa, T., & Matsukura, N. (2005a). Comparison of Helicobacter pylori infection and gastric mucosal histological features of gastric ulcer patients with chronic gastritis patients. World J Gastroenterol , 11, 976-981.

[55] Zhang, C., Yamada, N., Wu, Y. L., Wen, M., Matsuhisa, T., & Matsukura, N. (2005b). Helicobacter pylori infection, glandular atrophy and intestinal metaplasia in superficial gastritis, gastric erosion, erosive gastritis, gastric ulcer and early gastric cancer. World J Gastroenterol , 11, 791-796.

Section 5

Diagnostic Backgrounds

Chapter 5

The Genetic and Epigenetic Bases of Gastritis

Alejandro H. Corvalan, Gonzalo Carrasco and
Kathleen Saavedra

Additional information is available at the end of the chapter

http://dx.doi.org/10.5772/53131

1. Introduction

Gastritis, the inflammation of the mucosal layer of the stomach, is a major clinical entity due to its association with gastric cancer and peptic ulcer disease. The primary cause of gastritis is the infection with the microaerofilic gram negative Helicobacter pylori that during the early phases elicits an acute inflammatory response which eventually evolves to a long-standing chronic gastritis (Ruggiero 2012). In the case of gastric cancer development, chronic gastritis is the first step of the so-called multistep cascade of gastric cancer. This sequence includes the non-atrophic chronic gastritis, multifocal atrophic gastritis, intestinal metaplasia, dysplasia and invasive carcinoma as were described in detail by Correa as the "human model of gastric carcinogenesis" (Fig. 1) (Correa et al. 2007). This multistep model hypothesizes that the sequence of these lesions reflects a dynamic process from a naive inflammation caused by H. pylori infection to a fully malignant neoplasm of the stomach (Correa et al. 1976; Cuello et al. 1976; Haenszel et al. 1976; Correa et al. 1990). Independent epidemiological studies have confirmed that non-atrophic, atrophic, intestinal metaplasia and dysplasia are all linked through a sequential cause-effect relationship, thus supporting the concept of a human model for gastric carcinogenesis (Ohata et al. 2004). However, the risk of malignant transformation of these lesions is poorly defined. Long-term follow-up studies have shown a risk from 10% to 17% in the case of dysplasia (Saraga et al. 1987; Coma del Corral et al. 1990; Koch et al. 1990; Whiting et al. 2002; Rugge et al. 2003). For intestinal metaplasia, the risk assessment has conflicting results and therefore a limited clinical value (Ramesar et al. 1987; Silva et al. 1990; Rokkas et al. 1991; Conchillo et al. 2001; Vannella et al. 2012). The recently developed Operative Link for Gastritis Assessment (OLGA) staging system (Rugge et al. 2007), through the evaluation of the extension and site of the atrophic changes, is an attempt to evaluate the risk of chronic gastritis to progress to intestinal metaplasia and gastric cancer (Rugge et al. 2008; Capelle et al. 2010; Rugge et al. 2010). In this scenario, the identification of molecular bases in the multistep process of gastric carcinogenesis is highly relevant since it will contribute greatly to the risk assessments of the precursor lesions of gastric cancer. In this chapter we will primarily attempt to summarize and integrate our current knowledge of the genetic as well as epigenetic bases of the dynamic process of chronic gastritis, as well as the other entities of the so-called multistep cascade of gastric cancer.

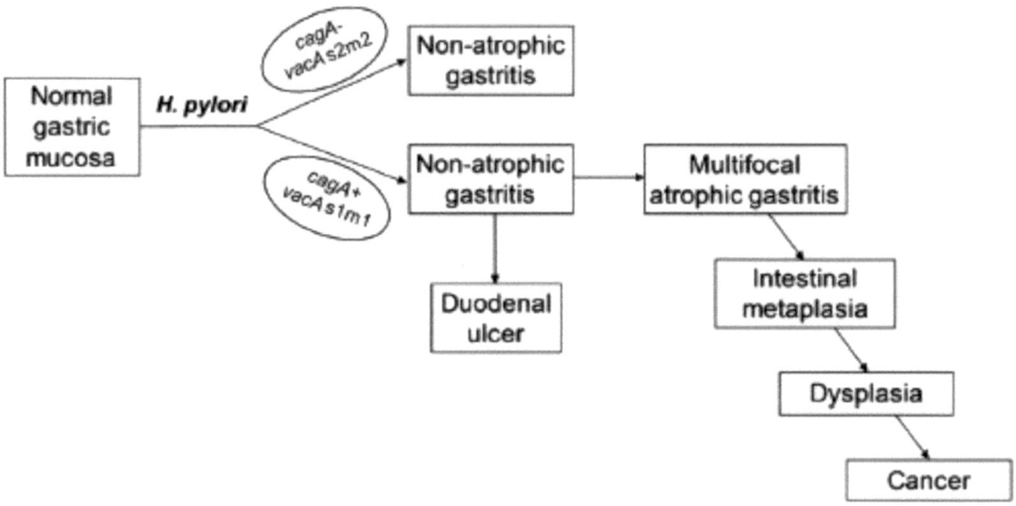

Figure 1. Multistep cascade of gastric cancer. This sequence begins with the infection of H.pylori to sequential steps of the precancerous cascades. Taken from Correa & Piazuelo J Dig Dis. 2012;13:2–9.

2. The genetic bases of gastritis

Human allelic variations at single nucleotide polymorphisms (SNP) are involved at different stages of gastric carcinogenesis. Accordingly, the dynamics of chronic gastritis might be associated with specific allelic variants. These variants, recognized as polymorphisms when occur with a frequency of >1% in the normal population, affects mostly genes of the inflammatory response genes, detoxification enzymes, and cancer-related procesess (Gonzalez et al. 2002).

Polymorphisms in inflammatory response genes

Two clear examples of polymorphisms associated with inflammatory response are interleukin-1 gene cluster and Toll-like receptors (TLRs). As shown in Table 1, Interleukin-1-beta (IL-1B) -31 T genotype and interleukin-1-receptor antagonist (IL1RN) IVS 86 bp VNTR, 2/2 genotype enhance the production of IL-1B, which is associated with an increased risk of hypochlorhydria induced by H. pylori. Because IL-1B is an important pro-inflammatory cytokine and a powerful inhibitor of gastric acid secretion, it might explain the higher risk of development of gastric cancer in chronic gastritis - H. pylori infected patients (El-Omar et al. 2000; Hwang et al. 2002; Yuzhalin 2011). The presence of polymorphisms in the non-coding but regulatory regions may also alter the levels of gene transcription and therefore the susceptibility to gastric cancer. In this sense, single A/T SNP at position -251 from the transcription start site in the promoter region of the IL-8 gene is one of the best examples. The presence of the -251A allele tended to be associated with an increase in IL-8 production and has been reported that this allele is associated with an increased risk for gastric cancer at cardia location (Hull et al. 2000; Xue et al. 2012). It could be extrapolated that IL-8 -251A allele may increase the risk of developing cancer through the elevation of its IL-8 expression. Mediators of the innate immune response, which provide first line of host defense against harmful pathogens are also involved in the dynamics of chronic gastritis. A good example for this type of inflammatory response are the Toll-like receptors (TLRs) (El-Omar et al. 2008). It has been reported that both, the 22-bp nucleotide deletion (-196 to –174 del) in the promoter region of the TLR-2 gene and the +896A/G and +1196C/T polymorphisms (Asp299Gly and Thr399Ile) in the coding region of the TLR-4 gene, promotes a rapidly progressive chronic gastritis (de Oliveira et al. 2012). Since it is well known that not all H. pylori are equally associated with the risk of development of gastric cancer, the combination of bacterial and inflammatory host genotypes have been explored. Figueiredo et al (2002) have shown that the infection with aggressive cagA-positive strains of H. pylori were associated with an increased risk of gastric cancer. In addition, the homozygous IL-1B-511*T carriers (IL-1B-511*T/*T or IL-1B-511*T/*C) and the short allele of IL-1RN (IL-1RN*2/*2) also had an increased susceptibility. However, for each combination of bacterial/host genotype, the odds of having gastric cancer were greatest in those with both bacterial and host high-risk genotypes.

Polymorphisms in genes associated with detoxification enzymes

Members of the cytochrome P-450 superfamily belong to the detoxification enzymes. One of the members of this family is the CYP2E1, a naturally ethanol-inducible enzyme involved in the metabolic activation of low molecular weight compounds such as N-nitrosamines (Boccia et al. 2007). Functional CYP2E1 polymorphisms in the 50-flanking region (PstI, RsaI) alter the transcriptional activity of the gene. A meta-analysis by Boccia et al (2007) suggests that the CYP2E1 PstI/RsaI polymorphism may be a risk factor for gastric cancer in asiatic populations and a synergic relation with tobacco-related detoxification Glutathione S-transferase (GST) genes (see below) may account for a proportion of these cases. GSTs and the polymorphic arylamine N-acetyltransferases (NAT1 and NAT2) are another type of detoxification enzymes that metabolize tobacco-related carcinogens. Zendehdel et al (2009) reported a weak linkage between the GSTP1 Ile105Val polymorphism and the risk for gastric cancer at cardia location (OR = 1.4; 95% CI 0.9-2.1). On the other hand, Katoh et al (2000) found that the NAT1*10 allele should be considered a risk factor among heavy smokers with well-differentiated tumors (Table 1).

Polymorphisms of cancer-related genes

In cancer-related processes, polymorphisms have been reported in the promoter region of the MET gene, a crucial gene to multiple oncogenic pathways and metastatic behavior (Gherardi et al. 2012). Sequencing of the promoter region of MET revealed some alterations scattered in a proportion of clinical samples of gastric cancer. The most common substitutions were -304C>A and 206C>G. The presence of these SNPs altered the junction sites for putative transcription factors such as Sp1 and AP-1/AP-2. As a consequence, the transcription of MET was constantly being activated (Trzyna et al. 2012). Another example is the polymorphism -160 A at the promoter region of the E-cadherin gene (CDH1), which has been associated with the DNA hypermethylation (see below) of the promoter region (Borges Bdo et al. 2010). In a Japanase study, 117 cases of gastric cancer with H. pylori-induced chronic gastritis were compared with 116 cancer-free yet H. pylori-induced chronic gastritis controls. It was found that the Pro/Pro allele of CDH-1 was associated with an increased risk of developing diffuse-type of gastric cancer compared to the Arg/Arg (Hiyama et al. 2002; Zhou et al. 2007). Finally, other polymorphims of cancer-related genes were reported to show significant associations with gastric cancer risk including EGFR, VEGF and p53 (Tahara et al. 2009). Taken together, data presented here suggest that allelic variations at regulatory or coding regions will affect gene expression patterns and modify the balance towards a more rapid progression of chronic gastritis and other preneoplastic lesions of the multistep cascade of gastric cancer (Fig. 2).

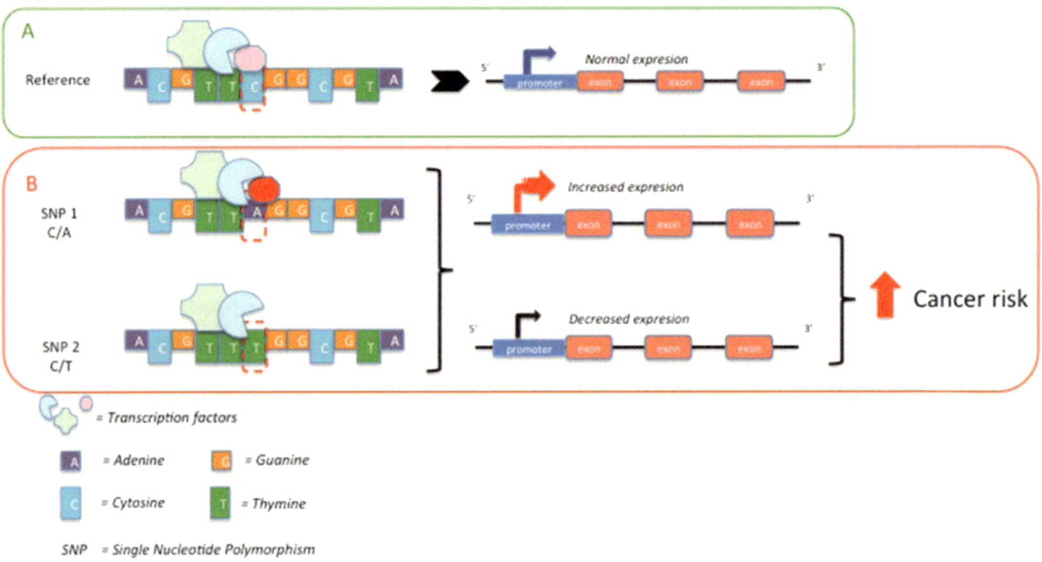

Figure 2. Allelic variations at regulatory regions will affect gene expression patterns. (A) Single nucleotide polymorphisms (SNP) in promoter region can alter the binding of transcription factors required for the expression of a gene. (B) These variations may increase or decrease the expression of the affected gene, which eventually can increase the risk of developing cancer.

http://dx.doi.org/10.5772/53131

Gene	Variation Allelic	SNP	rs number	Effect	Reference
IL1B	SNP	-31 T/C	rs1143627	Increased IL-1beta production and inhibit gastric acid secretion.	(Yuzhalin et al., 2011)
IL-8	SNP	-251 A/T	rs4073	Increased IL-8 production.	(Xue et al., 2012)
IL-10	SNP	-1082 A/G	rs1800896	Reported associated with the pathologically intestinal-type gastric cancer or anatomically cardia-type gastric cancer.	(Ni et al., 2012)
TLR2	Deletion	-196 to -174del	not applicable	Susceptibility to gastric cancer in the Southeastern Brazilian population.	(de Oliveira et al, 2012)
TLR4	SNP	+ 896 A/G	rs4986790		
CYP2E1	RFLP	CYP2E1 c2 allele homozygote	not applicable	Risk for gastric cancer among Asians	(Boccia et al., 2006)
GSTP1	SNP	+562 A/G	rs1695	Increased risk of esophageal squamous cell carcinoma and tended to be weakly, positively linked to cardia cancer	(Zendehdel et al., 2009)
NAT	RFLP	NAT1*10 allele	not applicable	Risk factor among the well-differentiated type of tumors of gastric cancer	(Katoh et al., 2000)
MET	SNP	-304C> A	undefined	Activate the transcription.	(Trzyna et al., 2012)
	SNP	206 C>G	undefined		
CDH1	SNP	-160 C/A	rs16260	Associated with DNA methylation linking genetic and epigenetics fields in the pathogenesis of gastritis.	(Borges Bdo et al., 2010)

Table 1. Selected single nucleotide polymorphisms (SNP) in inflammatory response genes, detoxification enzymes, and cancer-related processes associated to increase susceptibility of gastric cancer. The sign (-) indicates that the SNP is located in the direction of the promoter region, the sign (+) indicates that the SNP is located in the direction of the coding region, the number indicates the nucleotide positionfrom TSS and the first nucleotide is substituted (/) by the second.

3. Epigenetic bases of gastritis

Epigenetic processes control the packaging and function of the human genome, and contribute to normal development and disease (Callinan et al. 2006). Epigenetic mechanisms such as DNA methylation, histone modifications and microRNAs are important events toward regulating gene expression for the biology and disease of the gastrointestinal tract. In particular, DNA methylation, a process in which cytosines acquire a methyl group in the 5' position only if they are followed by a guanine (Corvalán et al. 2010), virtually affects all of the pathways in the cellular network, such as DNA repair, cell cycle, and apoptosis (Esteller et al. 2002). Furthermore, a growing body of evidence has shown that aberrant DNA methylation (DNA hypermethylation or DNA hypomethlation) is an early event in carcinogenesis (Jones et al. 2002; Herman et al. 2003; Kopelovich et al. 2003). In addition, aberrant DNA methylation has been recently considered to be an excellent candidate to explain how certain environmental factors may increase the risk of developing cancer (Chan et al. 2006). Accordingly, an emerging catalog of cancer-related genes inactivated by DNA hypermethylation in gastric cancer has been established (Hamilton et al. 2006; Wu et al. 2006; Bernal et al. 2008). However, there are limited reports on DNA hypermethylation analysis in precursor lesions of gastric cancer. Kang et al. (2001) tested five genes (p16, hMLH1, DAP-kinase, THBS1, and TIMP-3) in precancerous conditions to identify three different classes of hypermethylated genes. Hypermethylation of DAP-kinase was found in all premalignant conditions, whereas hMLH1 and p16 were preferentially methylated in intestinal metaplasia (6.3% and 2.1%, respectively), adenomas (9.8% and 11.5%, respectively) and gastric cancer (20.3% and 42.2%, respectively). THBS-1 and TIMP-3 were also hypermethylated at a similar frequency in all premalignant conditions, but showed a marked increase from chronic gastritis to intestinal metaplasia (10.1% & 34.7% and 14.5% & 36.7%, respectively; $P < 0.05$), as well as from adenomas to carcinomas (28.3% & 48.4% and 26.7% & 57.4% respectively). Another study including 11 genes (COX-2, DAP-kinase, E-cadherin, GSTP1, MGMT, hMLH1, p14, p16, THBS1, TIMP3, and RASSF1A) and 268 premalignant conditions (Kang et al. 2003) identified specific patterns of aberrant DNA methylation associated to aging. Specifically five genes (DAP-kinase, E-cadherin, p14, THBS1, and TIMP-3) showed a progressive increase in aberrant methylation frequency as a function of aging, whereas the other genes (COX-2, GSTP1, MGMT, hMLH1, p16, and RASSF1A) were rarely methylated. Male patients showed higher numbers of hypermethylated genes than females (3.2 vs. 2.1, respectively, $P = 0.002$) and cases with severe intestinal metaplasia also showed a higher frequency of aberrantly methylated genes. Taken together, these findings suggest that hypermethylation occurs early in the multistep gastric carcinogenesis and that accumulate during this process. In addition, age and gender are closely associated with increased frequency of aberrant DNA methylation. A further study demonstrated that DNA methylation of E-cadherin was associated with H. pylori infection ($p=0.002$) in an independent way of age and/or gastritis (Chan et al. 2003). Similarly, Maekita et al. (2006) carried out a more detailed analysis of the effect of H. pylori infection in the progression of aberrant DNA methylation in chronic gastritis. These authors collected gastric mucosa samples from 154 healthy volunteers (56 H. pylori negative and 98 H. pylori positive) and from 72 cases with gastric cancers (29 H. pylori negative and 43 H. pylori positive). Among the healthy volunteers, methylation levels were 5.4- to 303-fold higher in H. pylori positive subjects than in H. pylori negative ones ($P < 0.0001$). Particularly, methylation levels of the LOX, HAND1 and THBD at their promoter regions were identified in H. pylori-positive individuals. Among H. pylori-negative individuals, methylation levels were 2.2- to 32-fold higher in gastric cancer cases than in age-matched healthy volunteers. These findings suggest that H. pylori infection potently induces aberrant DNA methylation of several genes beyond E-cadherin, and that methylation levels of specific genes seemed to reflect the risk of gastric cancer in H. pylori-negative subjects. A recent quantitative analysis of the promoter region of a novel gene Reprimo (RPRM), per-

http://dx.doi.org/10.5772/53131

formed in Colombian residents from areas with high and low incidence of gastric cancer, demonstrated an association with virulent factors such as cagA and vacA s1/m1 regions of H. pylori strains. This data suggests that certain strains of H. pylori are associated with aberrant DNA methylation on specific genes (Schneider et al. 2010). Interestingly, we have shown that Reprimo is not only found in gastric mucosa but also in the plasma of gastric cancer patients (Bernal et al. 2008). Thus, hypermethylated circulating DNA offers the opportunity for non-invasive detection of gastric cancer and premalignant gastritis (Corvalán et al. 2010; Sapari et al. 2012). As mentioned before, an aberrant of DNA methylation could be considered as a candidate to explain how environmental factors increase the susceptibility of gastric cancer. One approach to explain this phenomena could be through the evaluation of the effect of the eradication of H. pylori in the pattern of DNA methylation of the gastric mucosa. Chen et al (2003) evaluate the presence of DNA methylation of E-cadherin promoter regions before the erradication of H. pylori and after 6 weeks of treatment. DNA methylation of E-cadherin was detected in 46% (19/41) and 17% (7/41) of both untreated and treated patients, respectively. Mucosal biopsy showed chronic inactive gastritis in 35 patients, intestinal metaplasia in one patient and normal mucosa in five patients after the treatment. This data suggests that H. pylori eradication therapy could reverse aberrant DNA methylation in patients with chronic gastritis. Similar results were reported by Leung et al. (2006), although they evaluated mucosal biopsies from the antrum and corpus of H. pylori-infected subjects at the baseline, and after one year of successful H. pylori eradication. In addition, these authors identified a significant reduction in the methylated density of the promoter region of the E-cadherin gene (Leung et al. 2006). Taken together, both reports are clear examples of how the environment affects DNA methylation and shows that the eradication of H. pylori infection reverses E-cadherin promoter hypermethylation. Although less explored, DNA hypomethylation can also be involved in the risk of developing cancer. The concept of DNA hypomethylation, although identified 30 years ago (Christman et al. 1977), was overlooked in preference to DNA hypermethylation. Recently, gene activation by promoter hypomethylation has been rediscovered (Ichinose et al. 1988; Cravo et al. 1996; Fang et al. 1996; Akiyama et al. 2003; Cho et al. 2003; Mesquita et al. 2003; Oshimo et al. 2003; Chalitchagorn et al. 2004; Honda et al. 2004; Kaneda et al. 2004; Yanagawa et al. 2004; Jung et al. 2005; Nishigaki et al. 2005). Emerging data suggests that global DNA hypomethylation is thought to occur during the early stages of gastric carcinogenesis (Goelz et al. 1985; Cravo et al. 1996; Narayan et al. 1998; Lin et al. 2001; Bariol et al. 2003) but hypomethylation of individual genes, such as MAGE, synuclein-alpha, MUC2, maspin, CAGE and family A melanoma antigen (Akiyama et al. 2003; Cho et al. 2003; Mesquita et al. 2003; Honda et al. 2004; Yanagawa et al. 2004; Jung et al. 2005) is thought to occur during the advanced stages. Interestingly, overexpression of well known oncogenes, such as MYC, HRAS1 and cyclin D2 has been linked to hypomethylation in their promoter region, suggesting an inverse correlation between methylation and gene expression (Fang et al. 1996; Oshimo et al. 2003). Taken together, this data suggests that promoter hypomethylation is an underlying mechanism of gene activation that should be explored in gastric carcinogenesis. In these sense, recent work from Daskalos et al (2011) has shown that the overexpression of p73, a well stablish cancer-related gene associated with apoptosis and DNA repair (Zaika et al. 2011), might be associated with hypomethylation of the P2 promoter region that controls the DeltaNup73 isoform. Although this work was not performed in a gastric cancer model, our preliminary findings suggests similar results in gastric cancer cases (Corvalán et al. 2008). Based on both data, we decide to analysed the protein overexpression of p73 as well as other seven well stablished cancer-related genes activated by hypomethylation (BRCA1, HSP90, STAT1, FHIT, EGFR, p73, p53, p16INK4a) (Tanaka et al. 1998; Nien et al. 2007; Shutoh et al. 2009; Yu et al. 2009; Valdez et al. 2010; Daskalos et al. 2011; Rusiecki et al. 2011; Szaumkessel et al. 2011; Fornari et al. 2012). This analysis was performed in a large number of matched tumor/non-tumor adjacent mucosa of early gastric cancer as well as non-tumor cases at different stages of the multistep cascade of gastric cancer (Carrasco et al. 2010). Among 8 genes tested, only the overexpression of p73 was higher in matched tumor/non-tumor adjacent mucosa than in chronic gastritis/intestinal metaplasia (50.5% vs. 10.8%; P < 0.0001). We also assessed a detail histopathological analysis of the precursor lessions of gastric cancer through the Sydney and OLGA systems (Dixon et al. 1996; Corvalan et al. 2011; Rugge et al. 2011). As has been described (Rugge et al. 2010) only severe atrophy and OLGA stage IV were the most relevant features to identified high-risk gastritis (Fig. 4). However, the most interesting finding come after our attempt to integrated protein expression and histopathological assessments. This integration was performed by Significance Analysis of Microarrays (SAM), a multiple testing approach method that has been extensively applied in genomic research (Tusher et al. 2001) and confirmed by logistic regression (Nick et al. 2007). This integrative approach led us to identified that overexpression of p73 was even more significant than severe atrophy and OLGA stage IV in identifying high-risk premalignant gastritis (Carrasco et al. 2010). Therefore, we believe that the identification of the overexpression of p73 might contribute greatly to risk assessment of chronic gastritis to the development of gastric cancer.

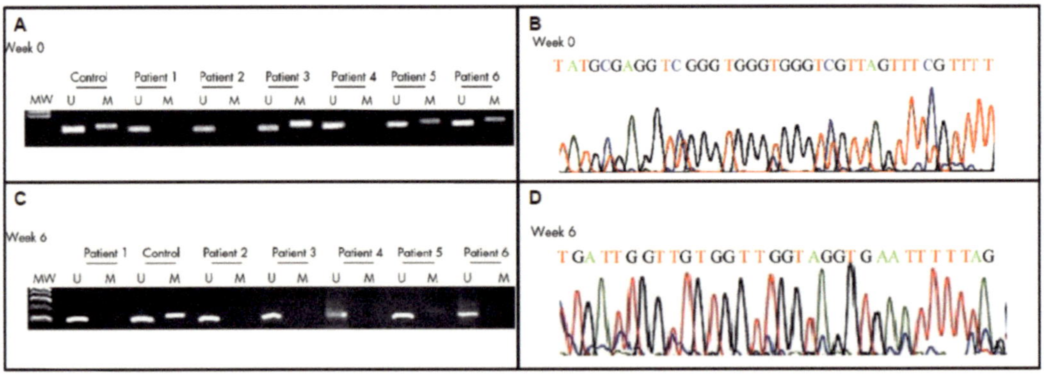

Figure 3. The effect of the eradication of H. pylori in the pattern of DNA methylation as an example of environmental factors and the susceptibility of gastric cancer. (A) Before eradication of H. pylori (week 0), methylation was present in patients 3, 5 and 6. (B) Bisulfite sequencing confirm the methylated product. (C) After eradication of H. pylori (week 6), methylation was not present in any patient. (D) Bisulfite sequencing confirm the absence of methylated cytosine. MW: molecular weight marker, U: unmethylated band, M: methylated band, red color: unmethylated cytosines converted to thymidine, blue color: methylated cytosines. Taken from Chan et al., Gut 2006;55:463-8 with permission from BMJ Publishing Group Ltd.

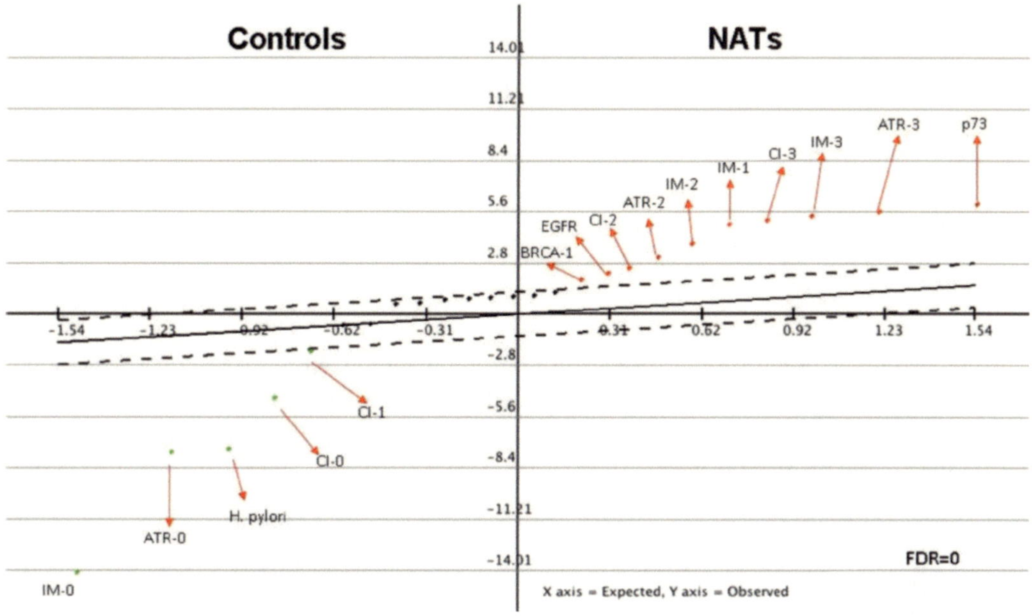

Figure 4. Serial Analysis for Microarray from Non-tumor adjacent mucosa (NTAM) and chronic gastritis controls. NTAM group is significantly characterized by the overexpression of p73, OLGA stages III to IV, and severe atrophy (ATR-3), intestinal metaplasia (IM-3), and chronic inflammation (CI-3) according to the Sydney System. Control group cases were significantly characterized by lack of intestinal metaplasia (IM-0), atrophy (ATR-0), and chronic inflammation (CI-0). False discovery rate = 0. Taken from Carrasco et al., Clin.Cancer Res 2010;16:3253-9.

4. Conclusion

Data presented here suggests that genetic, epigenetic by means of DNA methylation might play a role in the dinamics of the progression of chronic gastritis and premalignant cascade to gastric cancer. DNA methylation works in both ways, inactivating or activating tumor-related genes through the hypermethylation or hypomethylation of the promoter regions of specific genes. The integration of these molecular bases of chronic gastritis with histopathological assessment by Sydney and OLGA systems will contribute to the better risk assessment for the development of gastric cancer.

Acknowledgements

Grant Support: Grants-in-Aid for Fondo Nacional de Ciencia y Tecnologia (FONDECYT) #1111014 and Fondo de Fomento al Desarrollo Científico y Tecnológico (FONDEF) #D09i1137 to A.H. Corvalan from the Government of Chile.

Author details

Alejandro H. Corvalan, Gonzalo Carrasco and Kathleen Saavedra

Ponfiticia Universidad Catolica de Chile, Chile

References

[1] Akiyama Y, Maesawa C, Ogasawara S, et al. (2003). Cell-type-specific repression of the maspin gene is disrupted frequently by demethylation at the promoter region in gastric intestinal metaplasia and cancer cells. Am J Pathol, Vol.163; No.5: pp. 1911-1919. ISSN: 0002-9440.

[2] Bariol C, Suter C, Cheong K, et al. (2003). The relationship between hypomethylation and CpG island methylation in colorectal neoplasia. Am J Pathol, Vol.162; No.4: pp. 1361-1371. ISSN: 0002-9440.

[3] Bernal C, Aguayo FR, Villarroel C, et al. (2008). Reprimo as a potential biomarker for early detection in gastric cancer. Clin Cancer Res, Vol.14; No.19: pp.6264-6269. ISSN: 1078-0432..

[4] Boccia S, De Lauretis A, Gianfagna F, et al. (2007). CYP2E1PstI/RsaI polymorphism and interaction with tobacco, alcohol and GSTs in gastric cancer susceptibility: A meta-analysis of the literature. Carcinogenesis, Vol.28; No.1: pp.101-106. ISSN: 0143-3334.

[5] Borges Bdo N, Santos Eda S, Bastos CE, et al. (2010). Promoter polymorphisms and methylation of E-cadherin (CDH1) and KIT in gastric cancer patients from northern Brazil. Anticancer Res, Vol.30; No.6: pp.2225-2233. ISSN: 1791-7530.

[6] Callinan PA and Feinberg AP. (2006). The emerging science of epigenomics. Hum Mol Genet, Vol.15 Spec No 1: pp.R95-101. ISSN: 0964-6906.

[7] Capelle LG, de Vries AC, Haringsma J, et al. (2010). The staging of gastritis with the OLGA system by using intestinal metaplasia as an accurate alternative for atrophic gastritis. Gastrointest Endosc, Vol.71; No.7: pp.1150-1158. ISSN: 1097-6779.

[8] Carrasco G, Diaz J, Valbuena JR, et al. (2010). Overexpression of p73 as a tissue marker for high-risk gastritis. Clin Cancer Res, Vol.16; No.12: pp.3253-3259. ISSN: 1078-0432.

[9] Chalitchagorn K, Shuangshoti S, Hourpai N, et al. (2004). Distinctive pattern of LINE-1 methylation level in normal tissues and the association with carcinogenesis. Oncogene, Vol.23; No.54: pp.8841-8846. ISSN: 0950-9232.

[10] Chan AO, Lam SK, Wong BC, et al. (2003). Promoter methylation of E-cadherin gene in gastric mucosa associated with Helicobacter pylori infection and in gastric cancer. Gut, Vol.52; No.4: pp.502-506. ISSN: 0017-5749.

[11] Chan AO, Peng JZ, Lam SK, et al. (2006). Eradication of Helicobacter pylori infection reverses E-cadherin promoter hypermethylation. Gut, Vol.55; No.4: pp.463-468. ISSN: 0017-5749.

[12] Cho B, Lee H, Jeong S, et al. (2003). Promoter hypomethylation of a novel cancer/testis antigen gene CAGE is correlated with its aberrant expression and is seen in premalignant stage of gastric carcinoma. Biochem Biophys Res Commun, Vol.307; No.1: pp.52-63. ISSN: 0006-291X.

[13] Christman JK, Price P, Pedrinan L, et al. (1977). Correlation between hypomethylation of DNA and expression of globin genes in Friend erythroleukemia cells. Eur J Biochem, Vol.81; No.1: pp.53-61. ISSN: 0014-2956.

[14] Coma del Corral MJ, Pardo-Mindan FJ, Razquin S, et al. (1990). Risk of cancer in patients with gastric dysplasia. Follow-up study of 67 patients. Cancer, Vol.65; No.9: pp.2078-2085. ISSN: 0008-543X.

[15] Conchillo JM, Houben G, de Bruine A, et al. (2001). Is type III intestinal metaplasia an obligatory precancerous lesion in intestinal-type gastric carcinoma? Eur J Cancer Prev, Vol.10; No.4: pp.307-312. ISSN: 0959-8278.

[16] Correa P, Cuello C, Duque E, et al. (1976). Gastric cancer in Colombia. III. Natural history of precursor lesions. J Natl Cancer Inst, Vol.57; No.5: pp.1027-1035. ISSN: 0027-8874.

[17] Correa P, Haenszel W, Cuello C, et al. (1990). Gastric precancerous process in a high risk population: cross-sectional studies. Cancer Res, Vol.50; No.15: pp.4731-4736. ISSN:0008-5472.

[18] Correa P and Houghton J. (2007). Carcinogenesis of Helicobacter pylori. Gastroenterology, Vol.133; No.2: pp.659-672. ISSN: 0016-5085.

[19] Corvalán AH, Carrasco C and Olivares W (2011). Molecular Pathology of Gastritis. In: Gastritis and Gastric Cancer - New insights in gasroprotection, diagnosis and treatments.

[20] Rijeka, Croatia, Intech. ISBN:978-953-307-375-0.

[21] Corvalán AH and Maturana MJ. (2010). Recent Patents of DNA Methylation Biomarkers in Gastrointestinal Oncology. Recent Pat DNA Gene Seq, Vol.4; No.3: pp. 202-209. ISSN: 1872-2156.

[22] Corvalan A, Villarroel C, Ibanez P, et al. (2008). Demethylation of promoter region of p73 gene as a mechanism of overexpression of p73 protein in gastric carcinoma: Analysis by demethylation, microdissection of gastric epithelial cells and tissue mi-

croarray. Proceedings of the 98th Annual Meeting of the American Association for Cancer Research; Washington, DC, USA. Abstract #4461

[23] Cravo M, Pinto R, Fidalgo P, et al. (1996). Global DNA hypomethylation occurs in the early stages of intestinal type gastric carcinoma. Gut, Vol.39; No.3: pp.434-438. ISSN: 0017-5749.

[24] Cuello C, Correa P, Haenszel W, et al. (1976). Gastric cancer in Colombia. I. Cancer risk and suspect environmental agents. J Natl Cancer Inst, Vol.57; No.5: pp. 1015-1020. ISSN: 0027-8874.

[25] Daskalos A, Logotheti S, Markopoulou S, et al. (2011). Global DNA hypomethylation-induced DeltaNp73 transcriptional activation in non-small cell lung cancer. Cancer Lett, Vol.300; No.1: pp.79-86. ISSN: 1872-7980.

[26] de Oliveira JG and Silva AE. (2012). Polymorphisms of the TLR2 and TLR4 genes are associated with risk of gastric cancer in a Brazilian population. World J Gastroenterol, Vol.18; No.11: pp.1235-1242. ISSN: 1007-9327.

[27] Dixon MF, Genta RM, Yardley JH, et al. (1996). Classification and grading of gastritis. The updated Sydney System. International Workshop on the Histopathology of Gastritis, Houston 1994. Am J Surg Pathol, Vol.20; No.10: pp.1161-1181. ISSN:0147-5185 .

[28] El-Omar EM, Carrington M, Chow WH, et al. (2000). Interleukin-1 polymorphisms associated with increased risk of gastric cancer. Nature, Vol.404; No.6776: pp.398-402. ISSN: 0028-0836.

[29] El-Omar EM, Ng MT and Hold GL. (2008). Polymorphisms in Toll-like receptor genes and risk of cancer. Oncogene, Vol.27; No.2: pp.244-252. ISSN: 1476-5594.

[30] Esteller M and Herman JG. (2002). Cancer as an epigenetic disease: DNA methylation and chromatin alterations in human tumours. J Pathol, Vol.196; No.1: pp.1-7. ISSN: 0022-3417.

[31] Fang JY, Zhu SS, Xiao SD, et al. (1996). Studies on the hypomethylation of c-myc, c-Ha-ras oncogenes and histopathological changes in human gastric carcinoma. J Gastroenterol Hepatol, Vol.11; No.11: pp.1079-1082. ISSN: 0815-9319.

[32] Figueiredo C, Machado JC, Pharoah P, et al. (2002). Helicobacter pylori and interleukin 1 genotyping: an opportunity to identify high-risk individuals for gastric carcinoma. J Natl Cancer Inst, Vol.94; No.22: pp.1680-1687. ISSN: 0027-8874.

[33] Fornari F, Milazzo M, Chieco P, et al. (2012). In hepatocellular carcinoma miR-519d is up-regulated by p53 and DNA hypomethylation and targets CDKN1A/p21, PTEN, AKT3 and TIMP2. J Pathol, Vol.227; No.3: pp.275-285. ISSN: 1096-9896.

[34] Gherardi E, Birchmeier W, Birchmeier C, et al. (2012). Targeting MET in cancer: rationale and progress. Nat Rev Cancer, Vol.12; No.2: pp.89-103. ISSN: 1474-1768.

[35] Goelz SE, Vogelstein B, Hamilton SR, et al. (1985). Hypomethylation of DNA from benign and malignant human colon neoplasms. Science, Vol.228; No.4696: pp. 187-190. ISSN: 0036-8075.

[36] Gonzalez CA, Sala N and Capella G. (2002). Genetic susceptibility and gastric cancer risk. Int J Cancer, Vol.100; No.3: pp.249-260. ISSN: 0020-7136.

[37] Haenszel W, Correa P, Cuello C, et al. (1976). Gastric cancer in Colombia. II. Case-control epidemiologic study of precursor lesions. J Natl Cancer Inst, Vol.57; No.5: pp. 1021-1026. ISSN: 0027-8874.

[38] Hamilton JP, Sato F, Jin Z, et al. (2006). Reprimo methylation is a potential biomarker of Barrett's-Associated esophageal neoplastic progression. Clin Cancer Res, Vol.12; No.22: pp.6637-6642. ISSN: 1078-0432.

[39] Herman JG and Baylin SB. (2003). Gene silencing in cancer in association with promoter hypermethylation. N Engl J Med, Vol.349; No.21: pp.2042-2054. ISSN: 1533-4406.

[40] Hiyama T, Tanaka S, Kitadai Y, et al. (2002). p53 Codon 72 polymorphism in gastric cancer susceptibility in patients with Helicobacter pylori-associated chronic gastritis. Int J Cancer, Vol.100; No.3: pp.304-308. ISSN: 0020-7136.

[41] Honda T, Tamura G, Waki T, et al. (2004). Demethylation of MAGE promoters during gastric cancer progression. Br J Cancer, Vol.90; No.4: pp.838-843. ISSN: 0007-0920.

[42] Hull J, Thomson A and Kwiatkowski D. (2000). Association of respiratory syncytial virus bronchiolitis with the interleukin 8 gene region in UK families. Thorax, Vol.55; No.12: pp.1023-1027. ISSN: 0040-6376.

[43] Hwang IR, Kodama T, Kikuchi S, et al. (2002). Effect of interleukin 1 polymorphisms on gastric mucosal interleukin 1beta production in Helicobacter pylori infection. Gastroenterology, Vol.123; No.6: pp.1793-1803. ISSN: 0016-5085.

[44] Ichinose M, Miki K, Tatematsu M, et al. (1988). Cell-specific hypomethylation of the pepsinogen gene in pepsinogen-producing cells. Biochem Biophys Res Commun, Vol.155; No.2: pp.670-677. ISSN: 0006-291X.

[45] Jones PA and Baylin SB. (2002). The fundamental role of epigenetic events in cancer. Nat Rev Genet, Vol.3; No.6: pp.415-428. ISSN: 1471-0056.

[46] Jung EJ, Kim MA, Lee HS, et al. (2005). Expression of family A melanoma antigen in human gastric carcinoma. Anticancer Res, Vol.25; No.3B: pp.2105-2111. ISSN: 0250-7005.

[47] Kaneda A, Tsukamoto T, Takamura-Enya T, et al. (2004). Frequent hypomethylation in multiple promoter CpG islands is associated with global hypomethylation, but not with frequent promoter hypermethylation. Cancer Sci, Vol.95; No.1: pp.58-64. ISSN: 1347-9032.

[48] Kang GH, Lee HJ, Hwang KS, et al. (2003). Aberrant CpG island hypermethylation of chronic gastritis, in relation to aging, gender, intestinal metaplasia, and chronic inflammation. Am J Pathol, Vol.163; No.4: pp.1551-1556. ISSN: 0002-9440.

[49] Kang GH, Shim YH, Jung HY, et al. (2001). CpG island methylation in premalignant stages of gastric carcinoma. Cancer Res, Vol.61; No.7: pp.2847-2851. ISSN: 0008-5472.

[50] Katoh T, Boissy R, Nagata N, et al. (2000). Inherited polymorphism in the N-acetyltransferase 1 (NAT1) and 2 (NAT2) genes and susceptibility to gastric and colorectal adenocarcinoma. Int J Cancer, Vol.85; No.1: pp.46-49. ISSN: 0020-7136.

[51] Koch HK, Oehlert M and Oehlert W. (1990). An evaluation of gastric dysplasia in the years 1986 and 1987. Pathol Res Pract, Vol.186; No.1: pp.80-84. ISSN: 0344-0338.

[52] Kopelovich L, Crowell JA and Fay JR. (2003). The epigenome as a target for cancer chemoprevention. J Natl Cancer Inst, Vol.95; No.23: pp.1747-1757. ISSN: 1460-2105.

[53] Leung WK, Man EP, Yu J, et al. (2006). Effects of Helicobacter pylori eradication on methylation status of E-cadherin gene in noncancerous stomach. Clin Cancer Res, Vol.12; No.10: pp.3216-3221. ISSN: 1078-0432.

[54] Lin CH, Hsieh SY, Sheen IS, et al. (2001). Genome-wide hypomethylation in hepatocellular carcinogenesis. Cancer Res, Vol.61; No.10: pp.4238-4243. ISSN: 0008-5472.

[55] Maekita T, Nakazawa K, Mihara M, et al. (2006). High levels of aberrant DNA methylation in Helicobacter pylori-infected gastric mucosae and its possible association with gastric cancer risk. Clin Cancer Res, Vol.12; No.3 Pt 1: pp.989-995. ISSN: 1078-0432.

[56] Mesquita P, Peixoto AJ, Seruca R, et al. (2003). Role of site-specific promoter hypomethylation in aberrant MUC2 mucin expression in mucinous gastric carcinomas. Cancer Lett, Vol.189; No.2: pp.129-136. ISSN: 0304-3835.

[57] Narayan A, Ji W, Zhang XY, et al. (1998). Hypomethylation of pericentromeric DNA in breast adenocarcinomas. Int J Cancer, Vol.77; No.6: pp.833-838. ISSN: 0020-7136.

[58] Nick TG and Campbell KM. (2007). Logistic regression. Methods Mol Biol, Vol.404: pp.273-301. ISSN: 1064-3745.

[59] Nien WL, Dauphinee SM, Moffat LD, et al. (2007). Overexpression of the mTOR alpha4 phosphoprotein activates protein phosphatase 2A and increases Stat1alpha binding to PIAS1. Mol Cell Endocrinol, Vol.263; No.1-2: pp.10-17. ISSN: 0303-7207.

[60] Nishigaki M, Aoyagi K, Danjoh I, et al. (2005). Discovery of aberrant expression of R-RAS by cancer-linked DNA hypomethylation in gastric cancer using microarrays. Cancer Res, Vol.65; No.6: pp.2115-2124. ISSN:0008-5472.

[61] Ohata H, Kitauchi S, Yoshimura N, et al. (2004). Progression of chronic atrophic gastritis associated with Helicobacter pylori infection increases risk of gastric cancer. Int J Cancer, Vol.109; No.1: pp.138-143. ISSN: 0020-7136.

[62] Oshimo Y, Nakayama H, Ito R, et al. (2003). Promoter methylation of cyclin D2 gene in gastric carcinoma. Int J Oncol, Vol.23; No.6: pp.1663-1670. ISSN: 1019-6439.

[63] Ramesar KC, Sanders DS and Hopwood D. (1987). Limited value of type III intestinal metaplasia in predicting risk of gastric carcinoma. J Clin Pathol, Vol.40; No.11: pp. 1287-1290. ISSN: 0021-9746.

[64] Rokkas T, Filipe MI and Sladen GE. (1991). Detection of an increased incidence of early gastric cancer in patients with intestinal metaplasia type III who are closely followed up. Gut, Vol.32; No.10: pp.1110-1113. ISSN: 0017-5749.

[65] Rugge M, Cassaro M, Di Mario F, et al. (2003). The long term outcome of gastric non-invasive neoplasia. Gut, Vol.52; No.8: pp.1111-1116. ISSN: 0017-5749.

[66] Rugge M, de Boni M, Pennelli G, et al. (2010). Gastritis OLGA-staging and gastric cancer risk: a twelve-year clinico-pathological follow-up study. Aliment Pharmacol Ther, Vol.31; No.10: pp.1104-1111. ISSN: 1365-2036.

[67] Rugge M, Kim JG, Mahachai V, et al. (2008). OLGA gastritis staging in young adults and country-specific gastric cancer risk. Int J Surg Pathol, Vol.16; No.2: pp.150-154. ISSN: 1066-8969.

[68] Rugge M, Meggio A, Pennelli G, et al. (2007). Gastritis staging in clinical practice: the OLGA staging system. Gut, Vol.56; No.5: pp.631-636. ISSN: 0017-5749.

[69] Rugge M, Pennelli G, Pilozzi E, et al. (2011). Gastritis: the histology report. Dig Liver Dis, Vol.43 Suppl 4: pp.S373-384. ISSN: 1878-3562.

[70] Ruggiero P. (2012). Helicobacter pylori infection: what's new. Curr Opin Infect Dis, Vol.25; No.3: pp.337-344. ISSN: 1473-6527.

[71] Rusiecki JA, Al-Nabhani M, Tarantini L, et al. (2011). Global DNA methylation and tumor suppressor gene promoter methylation and gastric cancer risk in an Omani Arab population. Epigenomics, Vol.3; No.4: pp.417-429. ISSN: 1750-192X.

[72] Sapari NS, Loh M, Vaithilingam A, et al. (2012). Clinical potential of DNA methylation in gastric cancer: a meta-analysis. PLoS One, Vol.7; No.4: pp.e36275. ISSN: 1932-6203.

[73] Saraga EP, Gardiol D and Costa J. (1987). Gastric dysplasia. A histological follow-up study. Am J Surg Pathol, Vol.11; No.10: pp.788-796. ISSN: 0147-5185.

[74] Schneider BG, Peng DF, Camargo MC, et al. (2010). Promoter DNA hypermethylation in gastric biopsies from subjects at high and low risk for gastric cancer. Int J Cancer, Vol.127; No.11: pp.2588-2597. ISSN: 1097-0215.

[75] Shutoh Y, Takeda M, Ohtsuka R, et al. (2009). Low dose effects of dichlorodiphenyltrichloroethane (DDT) on gene transcription and DNA methylation in the hypothalamus of young male rats: implication of hormesis-like effects. J Toxicol Sci, Vol.34; No. 5: pp.469-482. ISSN: 1880-3989.

[76] Silva S, Filipe MI and Pinho A. (1990). Variants of intestinal metaplasia in the evolution of chronic atrophic gastritis and gastric ulcer. A follow up study. Gut, Vol.31; No.10: pp.1097-1104. ISSN: 0017-5749.

[77] Szaumkessel M, Richter J, Giefing M, et al. (2011). Pyrosequencing-based DNA methylation profiling of Fanconi anemia/BRCA pathway genes in laryngeal squamous cell carcinoma. Int J Oncol, Vol.39; No.2: pp.505-514. ISSN: 1791-2423.

[78] Tahara T, Arisawa T, Shibata T, et al. (2009). Effect of polymorphisms in the 3'-untranslated region (3'-UTR) of VEGF gene on gastric pre-malignant condition. Anticancer Res, Vol.29; No.2: pp.485-489. ISSN: 0250-7005.

[79] Tanaka H, Shimada Y, Harada H, et al. (1998). Methylation of the 5' CpG island of the FHIT gene is closely associated with transcriptional inactivation in esophageal squamous cell carcinomas. Cancer Res, Vol.58; No.15: pp.3429-3434. ISSN: 0008-5472.

[80] Trzyna E, Duleba M, Faryna M, et al. (2012). Regulation of transcription in cancer. Front Biosci, Vol.17: pp.316-330. ISSN: 1093-4715.

[81] Tusher VG, Tibshirani R and Chu G. (2001). Significance analysis of microarrays applied to the ionizing radiation response. Proc Natl Acad Sci U S A, Vol.98; No.9: pp. 5116-5121. ISSN: 0027-8424.

[82] Valdez BC, Li Y, Murray D, et al. (2010). 5-Aza-2'-deoxycytidine sensitizes busulfan-resistant myeloid leukemia cells by regulating expression of genes involved in cell cycle checkpoint and apoptosis. Leuk Res, Vol.34; No.3: pp.364-372. ISSN: 1873-5835.

[83] Vannella L, Lahner E and Annibale B. (2012). Risk for gastric neoplasias in patients with chronic atrophic gastritis: a critical reappraisal. World J Gastroenterol, Vol.18; No.12: pp.1279-1285. ISSN: 1007-9327.

[84] Whiting JL, Sigurdsson A, Rowlands DC, et al. (2002). The long term results of endoscopic surveillance of premalignant gastric lesions. Gut, Vol.50; No.3: pp.378-381. ISSN: 0017-5749.

[85] Wu DL, Sui FY, Jiang XM, et al. (2006). Methylation in esophageal carcinogenesis. World J Gastroenterol, Vol.12; No.43: pp.6933-6940. ISSN: 1007-9327.

[86] Xue H, Liu J, Lin B, et al. (2012). A meta-analysis of interleukin-8 -251 promoter polymorphism associated with gastric cancer risk. PLoS One, Vol.7; No.1: pp.e28083. ISSN: 1932-6203.

[87] Yanagawa N, Tamura G, Honda T, et al. (2004). Demethylation of the synuclein gamma gene CpG island in primary gastric cancers and gastric cancer cell lines. Clin Cancer Res, Vol.10; No.7: pp.2447-2451. ISSN: 1078-0432.

[88] Yu Y, Kanwar SS, Patel BB, et al. (2009). Elimination of Colon Cancer Stem-Like Cells by the Combination of Curcumin and FOLFOX. Transl Oncol, Vol.2; No.4: pp. 321-328. ISSN: 1936-5233.

[89] Yuzhalin A. (2011). The role of interleukin DNA polymorphisms in gastric cancer. Hum Immunol, Vol.72; No.11: pp.1128-1136. ISSN: 1879-1166.

[90] Zaika E, Wei J, Yin D, et al. (2011). p73 protein regulates DNA damage repair. FASEB J, Vol.25; No.12: pp.4406-4414. ISSN: 1530-6860.

[91] Zendehdel K, Bahmanyar S, McCarthy S, et al. (2009). Genetic polymorphisms of glutathione S-transferase genes GSTP1, GSTM1, and GSTT1 and risk of esophageal and gastric cardia cancers. Cancer Causes Control, Vol.20; No.10: pp.2031-2038. ISSN: 1573-7225.

[92] Zhou Y, Li N, Zhuang W, et al. (2007). P53 codon 72 polymorphism and gastric cancer: a meta-analysis of the literature. Int J Cancer, Vol.121; No.7: pp.1481-1486. ISSN: 0020-7136.

Chapter 6

Intestinal Metaplasia Related to Gastric Cancer: An Outcome Analysis of Biomarkers for Early Detection

Jiro Watari, Kentaro Moriichi, Hiroki Tanabe,
Mikihiro Fujiya, Hiroto Miwa, Yutaka Kohgo and
Kiron M. Das

Additional information is available at the end of the chapter

http://dx.doi.org/10.5772/52958

1. Introduction

Although the overall incidence of gastric cancer is decreasing worldwide, it is the main cause of cancer death both worldwide and in East Asia including Japan. Gastric cancer is histologically divided into two types, intestinal and diffuse types (Lauren, 1965). Helicobacter pylori (*H. pylori*) infection is considered to be a major risk factor for the development of intestinal-type gastric cancer (Correa, 1990; Sipponen & Hyvärinen, 1993; International Agency for Research on Cancer [IARC], 1994; Graham, 2000; Uemura et al., 2001). It has been postulated that *H. pylori* infection causes chronic gastritis, gastric atrophy, usually with gastric intestinal metaplasia (IM) and dysplasia, and finally gastric cancer. The stepwise course of this inflammatory process, which usually continues over decades, has been defined as a sequence of histological events that confer an increasing risk of malignant transformation, as described in Correa's hypothesis (Correa, 1995). Long-term interactions between *H. pylori* infection and human increase the risk for precancerous lesions such as atrophic gastritis and IM (Peek & Blaser, 2002; Mera et al., 2005). Based on several long-term prospective studies involving large groups of patients, it is believed that eradication of *H. pylori* infection may prevent the development of gastric cancer (Uemura et al., 2001; Mera et al., 2005; You et al., 2000; Take et al., 2005). According to a prospective, randomized, placebo-controlled, population-based study from China, *H. pylori* eradication significantly decreased the development of gastric cancer in participants without precancerous lesions, i.e., gastric atrophy, IM, or gastric dysplasia (Wong et al., 2004). Furthermore, it has been reported from Japan that *H. pylori* treatment reduces the risk of developing new gastric carcinoma in patients who have a history of gastric cancer and are thus at high risk for such development (Fukase et al., 2008). On the other hand, it is evident that gastric cancer still occurs to some degree after endoscopic resection and successful eradication of *H. pylori* (Wong et al., 2004; Fukase et al., 2008). Therefore, establishment of predictable markers for the identification of patients at high risk for recurrent gastric cancer development despite eradication of *H. pylori* infection is clinically needed.

Gastric cancer develops through the accumulation of molecular alterations (Tamura, 2006). Current knowledge of the molecular mechanisms underlying gastric carcinogenesis indicates that two major genetic instability pathways are involved in the pathogenesis of gastric cancer: microsatellite instability (MSI), and chromosome instability, including loss of heterozygosity (Lengauer et al., 1998). We have recently reported that genetic instability in IM may be associated with gastric carcinogenesis (Tanaka A et al., 2006; Zaky et al., 2008; Watari et al., 2012). Previous reports have shown that MSI may play an important role in the development of synchronous or metachronous gastric cancer (MGC) and that it may be used clinically as a molecular marker for the prediction of multiple gastric cancers (Miyoshi et al., 2001; Hasuo et al., 2007). DNA methylation changes in cancer cells are characterized by regional CpG island hypermathylation and generalized genomic hypomethylation. Epigenetic inactivation of tumor-related genes by promoter hypermethylation is increasingly recognized to play an important role on tumorigenesis (Laird, 2005; Robertson, 2005). Previous reports on promoter hypermethylation showed that epigenetic alterations are frequently observed in precancerous lesions as well as in gastric cancer (Kang et al., 2001; To et al., 2002; Chan et al., 2006; Leung et al., 2006; Perri et al., 2007; Dong et al., 2009; Park et al., 2009).

Das et al. have developed a novel monoclonal antibody (mAb), Das-1 (formerly known as $7E_{12}H_{12}$, IgM isotype), which specifically reacts with the colonic epithelium (Das et al., 1987). We have reported that IM of a colonic phenotype detected by mAb Das-1, is strongly associated with gastric cancer, thus suggesting that mAb Das-1 positivity in IM could be a sensitive and specific marker related to gastric carcinogenesis (Mirza et al., 2003; Watari et al., 2008). Furthermore, we have recently shown that *H. pylori* eradication does not reduce the histological IM score, but changes the cellular phenotype of IM, as identified by this mAb in a prospective, 4-year follow-up study (Watari et al., 2008).

Epidemiological data on pre-malignant lesions such as *H. pylori*-related IM are relevant for predicting intestinal-type gastric cancer and for evaluating screening and surveillance practices (Mirza et al., 2003; Watari et al., 2008). We followed patients who received and did not receive *H. pylori* treatment after endoscopic resection for early gastric cancer for 1 year, and then examined the changes in MSI and mAb Das-1 in IM in response to *H. pylori* therapy. Here we show our study as to whether these biomarkers are predictive markers of MGC development after *H. pylori* treatment.

2. Patients and methods

We performed a hospital-based, case-control study of 75 patients, including 50 mucosal cancer patients who had undergone endoscopic resection (Group DYS), and 25 age- and sex-

http://dx.doi.org/10.5772/52958

matched chronic gastritis patients for whom *H. pylori* had been successfully eradicated (control). In this study, the patients with duodenal ulcer only were excluded because most of duodenal ulcers were categorized as 'antral predominat gastritis' (Uemura et al., 2001) or 'non-atrophic gastritis' (Mera et al., 2005), which is considered to be a low risk group of gastric cancer. Additionally, Group DYS patients were divided into 2 groups: 25 successfully *H. pylori*-eradicated (eradicated group) and 25 un-eradicated patients (persistent group). Mucosal gastric cancer was defined as any cancer in which invasion was limited to the mucosa based on Japanese criteria (Japanese Gastric Cancer Association. Japanese Classification of Gastric Carcinom, 2010). In all patients, biopsy specimens were taken to assess *H. pylori* infection, two each from the greater curvature of the antrum and the greater curvature of the corpus. The presence of *H. pylori* status was determined by a positive result for either or both Wartin-Starry staining or *H. pylori* culture. For eradication, patients were treated with lansoprazole (30 mg), amoxicillin (750 mg), and clarithromycin (400 mg), each taken twice daily for 1 week. All patients in the eradicated group underwent endoscopic resection for their mucosal cancer and then received treatment for *H. pylori*. All patients were followed for 1 year. In patients from the eradicated group and control (chronic gastritis), clearance of *H. pylori* was confirmed by negative results by both Wartin-Starry staining and *H. pylori* culture at a follow-up endoscopy.

3. Intestinal metaplasia

All IM cases investigated here were goblet cell metaplasia, namely incomplete-type IM obtained from the antrum (Filipe et al., 1994). Serial sections (4 μm) were made, and consecutive sections were used for histologic examination by H&E staining and for immunohistochemistry.

3.1. DNA extraction

From paraffin-embedded blocks, two 7-μm tissue sections were cut. DNA was extracted from the IM samples. In this DNA extraction procedure, the sample was precisely microdissected under microscopic visualization using a PALM MG III Laser Capture Microdissection System (MEIWAFOSIS, Tokyo, Japan) to avoid DNA contamination of inflammatory or stromal cell nuclei based on the previously described methodology (Tanaka et al., 2006; Zaky et al., 2008; Watari et al., 2012).

3.2. Analysis of MSI

The MSI was analyzed as reported previously (Tanaka et al., 2006; Zaky et al., 2008; Watari et al., 2012). We examined five microsatellite markers (two mono- and three dinucleotide repeats) for MSI based on the revised Bethesda panel (Umar et al., 2004) as follows: 2p (BAT26), 4q (BAT25), 2p (D2S123), 5q (D5S346), and 17p (D17S250). Briefly, polymerase chain reaction (PCR) amplification was carried out in a reaction volume of 10 μL, which contained 100 ng of genomic DNA, 1X PCR buffer (Perkin Elmer Applied Biosystems, Foster

City, CA), 200 μmol/L of dNTP, 600 μmol/L of each primer, and 1.5 units of AmpliTaq Gold polymerase (Perkin Elmer). The MgCl2 concentration was 1.5 mmol/L. The following PCR cycle conditions were used for amplification: 95°C for 10 min, 30 cycles of 95°C for 45 sec, 55°C for 1 min, and 72°C for 30 sec. The PCR products were evaluated for MSI by capillary electrophoresis using an ABI prism 310 Genetic Analyzer (Perkin Elmer) and automatic sizing of the alleles using a Gene Scan (Applied Biosystems). The MSI status was judged according to previous reports (Tanaka et al., 2006; Zaky et al., 2008; Watari et al., 2012). MSI was defined as positive when unequivocal extra peak bands in tumor DNA were observed that differed by multiples of 2 base pairs in dinucleotide markers or 1 base pair in mononucleotide markers from DNA in normal mucosa, and was also characterized by the appearance of additional alleles in the tumor DNA. The former type MSI was judged as the minor pattern (Figure 1A) and the latter type as the major pattern (Figure 1B), as reported previously (Tanaka et al., 2006; Zaky et al., 2008; Watari et al., 2012). IM was defined as having high MSI (MSI-H) when unstable loci were observed in two or more of five microsatellite markers and as having low MSI (MSI-L) when an unstable locus was observed in only one of the five markers studied based on the criteria established in 2002 (Umar et al., 2004). The lesion was considered microsatellite stable (MSS) if no unstable loci were found. The MSI phenotype was categorized into two groups, MSI-H and MSI-L/MSS. In our study, a sample was defined as MSI only when it qualified as MSI-H.

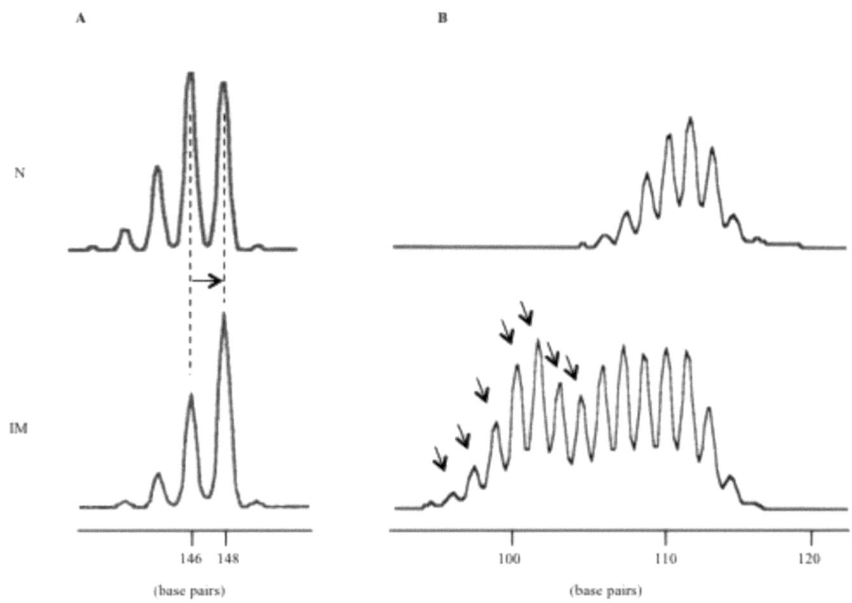

Figure 1. Examples of microsatellite instability (MSI) were detected in intestinal metaplasia (IM) by high-resolution fluorescent microsatellite analysis. DNA was isolated from IM and matching normal mucosa without IM (N). (A) Representative case of a minor pattern of MSI on D17S250. MSI is seen as an unequivocal extra peak shift (arrow) compared with normal mucosa. (B) Representative case of a major pattern of MSI on BAT26. MSI is characterized by the appearance of multiple additional alleles (arrows).

4. Immunoperoxidase assays with mAb Das-1

Serial sections were stained with mAb Das-1 using sensitive immunoperoxidase assays as described previously (Watari et al., 2012; Das et al. 1987; Mirza et al., 2003; Watari et al., 2008). Reactivity to mAb Das-1 was considered positive if cells were stained a crisp golden brown. A substantial number of cells and more than one gland had to be reactive to this mAb before a specimen was considered positive. If only an occasional goblet cell was stained, the sample was defined as negative (Watari et al., 2012; Das et al. 1987; Mirza et al., 2003; Watari et al., 2008; Das et al., 1994).

4.1. Statistical analysis

The data were assessed by the Mann-Whitney *U*-test, the chi-square test, and Fisher's exact test. Statistical significance was defined by a p value of <0.05. Odds ratios (ORs) and corresponding 95% confidence intervals (CIs) for each biomarker (MSI and mAb Das-1 reactivity) by a case-control study were calculated using StatView Ver. 5.0 for Macintosh (SAS Institute Inc., North Carolina, USA). Risk factors with a p value of < 0.10 in univariate analyses were included in a multiple logistic regression model and analyzed using the backward approach. The 95% CI of the OR was used to assess the statistical significance at the conventional level of 0.05.

4.2. Results

4.2.1. Patient characteristics

The mean ages of patients in the eradicated, persistent, and control groups were 70.8 (range 54-79), 70.9 (range 59-80), and 69.5 (range 62-77), respectively. Male patients made up 76% of the eradicated group, 92% of the persistent group, and 80% of the control group. There were no significant differences in age and gender among the three groups.

5. MSI and mAb Das-1 reactivity in IM

The observed incidences of MSI were 28.0% (14 of 50) in Group DYS and 8.0% (2 of 25) in the control; these results were significantly different (p<0.05). Similarly, mAb Das-1 reactivity of IM was also more frequently observed in Group DYS (66.0%, 33 of 50) than in the control (32.0%, 8 of 25) (p=0.07) (Table 1). We analyzed the strength of the association between gastric cancer and advanced age (70 years or older), male gender, MSI and mAb Das-1 reactivity by calculating univariate and multivariate logistic regression (Table 2). MSI and mAb Das-1 reactivity were associated with gastric cancer in the univariate analysis. In the multivariate logistic regression analysis, MSI and Das-1 reactivity were strong and independent factors (OR=7.09, 95% CI 1.27-39.6, p=0.03 in MSI; OR=4.96, 95% CI 1.64-15.0, p=0.005 in Das-1 reactivity). The sensitivity, specificity, and positive predictive value of MSI and mAb Das-1 reactivity of IM for gastric cancer were 28.0% (14 of 50), 92.0% (23 of 25), 87.5% (14 of

16), and 66.0% (33 of 50), 68.0% (17 of 25), 80.5% (33 of 41), respectively. If at least one of these 2 biomarkers was expressed in IM, those statistical calculations for gastric cancer became 78.0% (39 of 50), 60.0% (15 of 25) and 79.6% (39 of 49), respectively.

	Microsatellite instability		Das-1 reactivity	
	At initial	After 1-year	At initial	After 1-year
Group DYS (n=50)	14 (28.0) *	-	33 (66.0) **	-
Eradicated group (n=25)	7 (28.0) †	2 (8.0) †	16 (64.0)	12 (48.0) §
Persistent group (n=25)	7 (28.0)	6 (24.0)	17 (68.0)	18 (72.0) §
Control (n=25)	2 (8.0) *	1 (4.0)	8 (32.0) **	4 (16.0)

* p<0.05, ** p<0.01, † p=0.07, § p=0.08, Numbers in parentheses are percentages.

Table 1. Changes in microsatellite instability and Das-1 reactivity in Group DYS and control before and after *H. pylori* eradication

Variable	Univariate	Multivariate analysis		
	p	Odds ratio	95% CI	*p*
Microsatellite instability	0.06	7.09	1.27-39.6	0.03
Das-1 reactivity	0.007	4.96	1.64-15.0	0.005

Table 2. Predictors for development of gastric cancer

6. Changes in MSI and mAb Das-1 reactivity after *H. pylori* treatment

The incidence of MSI in IM 1 year after *H. pylori* treatment tended to decrease from 28.0% (7 of 25) to 8.0% (2 of 25) in the eradicated group (p=0.07), while there was no significant change in the persistent group during the follow-up period. The incidence of MSI also declined in the control, but the difference between pre- and post-eradication rates was not significant (Table 1). Similarly, the immunoreactivity of IM against mAb Das-1 decreased from 64.0% (16 of 25) to 48.0% (12 of 25) in the eradicated group, and from 32.0% (8 of 25) to 16.0% (4 of 25) in the control in response to *H. pylori* treatment; the difference in each group between pre- and post-treatment rates was not significant. In contrast, the incidence of the reactivity in the persistent group showed no changes at the 1-year follow-up. One year after treatment, the incidence of mAb Das-1 reactivity tended to be lower in the eradicated group than in the persistent group (p=0.08) (Table 1).

7. Newly developed gastric cancer after treatment

MGC was defined as a new carcinoma occurring at a previously uninvolved site in the stomach found more than 1 year after endoscopic resection. We encountered 13 MGCs that developed after endoscopic resection from January 1996 to July 2008, which included 3 (3.8%) of 79 patients for whom *H. pylori* had been eradicated and 10 (9.4%) of 106 patients who were un-eradicated. However, no newly developed gastric cancer was identified in 290 chronic gastritis patients in the same period. Three of 13 cases did not reveal IM in the biopsy at the time of MGC detection. The characteristics of the remaining 10 patients that developed gastric cancer after endoscopic treatment are shown in Table 3. Intriguingly, all patients showed positive for either MSI or mAb Das-1 reactivity in IM.

						At the time of MGC detection	
No.	Group	Age	Gender	Yrs after eradication	Yrs after endoscopic resection	Microsatellite instability	Das-1 reactivity
1	Eradicated group	77	M	2.5	5.2	+	+
2	Eradicated group	78	M	2.7	3.4	-	+
3	Eradicated group	68	M	1.1	1.8	-	+
4	Persistent group	65	M	NA	1.8	+	-
5	Persistent group	71	F	NA	1.8	+	-
6	Persistent group	76	M	NA	1.1	+	+
7	Persistent group	74	M	NA	1.2	+	+
8	Persistent group	79	M	NA	1.3	-	+
9	Persistent group	71	M	NA	1.0	-	+
10	Persistent group	81	M	NA	7.3	+	-

Table 3. Clinical characteristics of metachronous gastric cancer (MGC) after endoscopic resection

One of the patients (Case 1) in Group DYS presented a flat, elevated lesion at the antrum (Figure 2A). Endoscopic resection was performed on this lesion, and the histological diagnosis was mucosal cancer. Then, the patient received treatment for *H. pylori*. Thirty months after eradication, at the follow-up endoscopy, a new cancer was found at the lesser curvature of the corpus (Figure 2B and 2C). Interestingly, this patient lacked MSI prior to eradication but exhibited MSI after *H. pylori* therapy, while mAb Das-1 reactivity was positive both before and after eradication (Figure 2D and 2E).

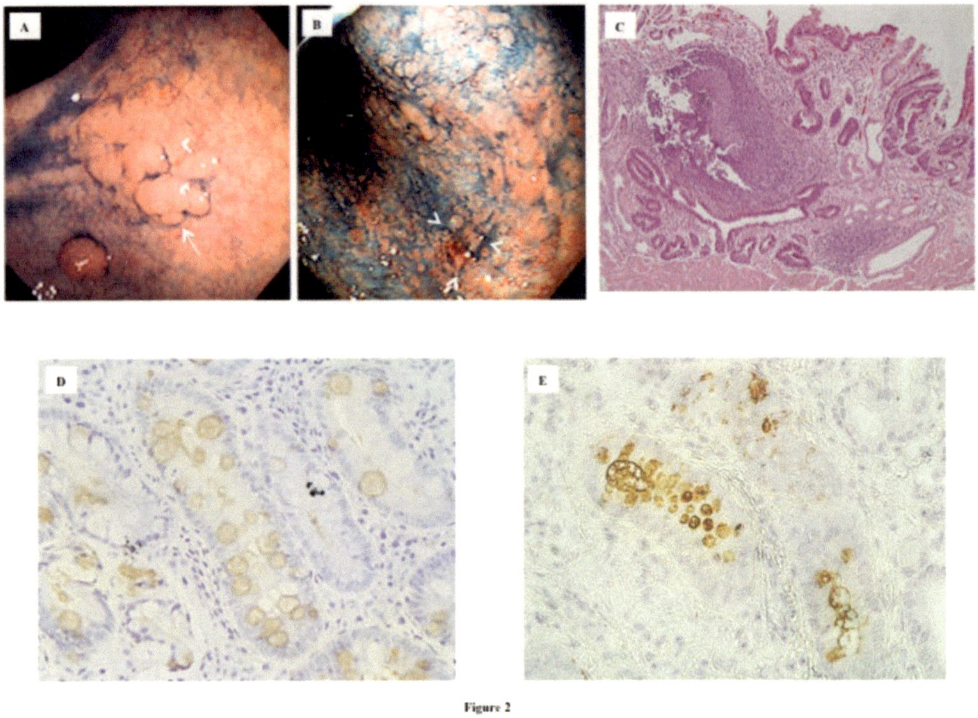

Figure 2. A) Endoscopic findings showed a flat elevated gastric cancer (arrow) at the posterior wall of the antrum. *H. pylori* was eradicated after endoscopic resection to the lesion. (B) At 30 months after eradication, a new lesion was found at the lesser curvature of the lower body of the stomach (arrowhead). (C) The resected sample was diagnosed histologically as mucosal cancer (×100). (D) IM in biopsy obtained from the antrum reacted with Das-1 (×200) prior to *H. pylori* treatment, and (E) the reactivity of Das-1 in IM was also demonstrated at the time a new gastric cancer was found following eradication (×200).

8. Discussion

Recent prospective randomized trial from Japan proved that *H. pylori* eradication significantly prevents the development of MGC after endoscopic mucosal resection to early gastric cancer (Fukase et al., 2008). In contrast, another Japanese retrospective study showed that the incidence of MGC did not differ between the eradicated group and the persistent groups during a follow-up period of as long as 11.1 years (Maehata et al. 2012). Nonetheless, new gastric cancer does sometimes develop after successful treatment of *H. pylori* infection in both reports (Wong et al., 2004; Maehata et al. 2012). These results indicate that once gastric cancer has developed in the stomach a first time, the background mucosa has increased potential of developing MGC (Wong et al., 2004; Zaky et al., 2008; Maehata et al. 2012). Therefore, efficient strategies to identify individuals who are at a "high risk" for MGC after *H. pylori* treatment are very much needed. We found in this study that MSI or mAb Das-1 reactivity in IM may serve independently as biomarkers to predict the development of gastric cancer regardless of *H. pylori* eradication.

It has previously been reported that MSI possibly plays a role in early events leading to gastric carcinogenesis (Chung et al., 1996; Buonsanti et al., 1997). Until now, we have also reported that genetic instability is frequently observed in the progression of IM in chronic gastritis patients and of IM in patients with gastric cancer and a cancerous area (Tanaka et al., 2006; Zaky et al., 2008). In this case-control study, the frequency of MSI in IM was significantly higher in Group DYS than in the control. These findings indicate that MSI may be a useful marker in identifying "high risk" IM that may develop into gastric cancer. It has since been reported that MSI may be associated with the inflammation from the standpoint of view of the investigation from patients with ulcerative colitis (Brentnall et al., 1996) or chronic hepatitis (Kondo et al., 2000). In the present study, MSI changed, becoming stable in response to the improvement of inflammation following eradication; these findings may indicate that inflammation of the stomach affects the presence of MSI. On the other hand, there is an interesting report by Kashiwagi et al. (Kashiwagi et al., 2000) in which MSI in gastritis, adenoma, and adenocarcinoma were examined retrospectively. According to their results, in all patients (n=6) with gastric adenoma or adenocarcinoma showing MSI, identical MSI patterns had been observed at the stage of gastritis, 1.5 to 7 years before the final diagnosis of adenocarcinoma. Thus, they concluded that MSI in chronic gastritis mucosa may identify patients at risk of developing gastric adenoma and cancer. Taking into account their results and ours, MSI expressed in IM, regardless of successful *H. pylori* eradication may be a predictor for the risk of MGC development.

Consistent with our previous reports (Mirza et al., 2003; Watari et al., 2008), the current study demonstrated that IM reactivity to mAb Das-1 is strongly associated with gastric cancer. However, the reactivity did not show a statistically significant decrease at 1 year after *H. pylori* eradication in the current study although our previous study showed a significant decline in mAb Das-1 positivity following treatment, up to 4 years (Watari et al., 2008). One of the explanations for this discrepancy may be the difference in the length of follow-up. It may be the case that a cellular phenotypic change by *H. pylori* treatment requires substantial time in comparison with MSI. However, mAb Das-1 reactivity declined significantly more in the eradicated group more than in the persistent group as of 1 year after *H. pylori* treatment. Some individuals actually showed persistent immunoreactivity to mAb Das-1 after treatment as shown in the previous report (Watari et al., 2008). Importantly, seven (70%) of 10 newly developed gastric cancers after endoscopic resection were positive for mAb Das-1 reactivity after eradication of *H. pylori*.

Based on our results, then, lesions that are newly or persistently positive for the markers including MSI or mAb Das-1 after *H. pylori* eradication are at a certain stage of progression of IM, and may have passed the "point of no return" (Wong et al., 2004; Wright, 1998). It remains possible, therefore, that these are patients who are at high risk of developing gastric cancer that may warrant more intensive endoscopic surveillance to detect early gastric cancer. Wong et al. reported that eradication of *H. pylori* did not decrease the development of gastric cancer in participants with precancerous lesions such as IM (Wong et al., 2004). In contrast to their report, our results may provide an important clue to the pathogenesis of the observed reduction of gastric cancer following *H. pylori* eradication in some patients with IM from the perspective of MSI or the cellular phenotype related to carcinogenesis.

It is intriguing that all newly developed cancers occurred only from Group DYS, with none from the control, although the number of cases investigated was small. This result indicates that IM in the background mucosa in patients from Group DYS is in an advanced stage compared to that in the control (chronic gastritis), and has more malignant potential. Accordingly, the accumulation of genetic alterations may be continued during the progression of IM. Considering the results in a Japanese population from Take et al., gastric cancer developed in 0.8% (8 of 944) of peptic ulcer patients cured of infection for up to 8.6 yr (mean 3.4 yr) (Take et al., 2005). Moreover, a recent report from a multi-center, open-label, randomized controlled trial from the Japan GastStudy Group suggested that eradication of *H. pylori* reduced by approximately one-third the risk of new gastric cancer in patients with a history of gastric cancer, but could not completely prevent cancer development (Fukase et al., 2008). According to this report, the incidence of new gastric cancer development was 3.5% (9 of 255) during 3 yrs of follow-up after endoscopic resection, significantly different from that reported by Take et al. Taking the findings of these reports and ours into consideration, the background gastric mucosa in patients who have a history of cancer may have more malignant potency in comparison to that in chronic gastritis patients. Thus, the molecular and cellular phenotypic backgrounds of IM can explain the pathogenesis of MGCs, even after resection of tumors due to persistent uncorrected accumulated errors of DNA mismatch repair and colonic phenotype on IM.

Newly developed gastric cancers may be the result of occult gastric cancers that are not detectable at the previous endoscopy, but that have grown enough to be diagnosed at the follow-up. Regarding the definition of MGC after endoscopic resection, therefore, it may be necessary to conduct follow-up for a long time, more than 1 year. In the current study, however, the subset of IM with MSI or mAb Das-1 positivity has the possibility of developing gastric cancer after even this relatively short period of time. Indeed, all patients who developed new cancer showed positive for MSI or mAb Das-1 reactivity in IM (Table 3). The persistence of DNA damage and the colonic phenotype, as detected by mAb Das-1, may identify the "at risk" group of patients with histological IM; thus, these biomarkers in the biopsy specimens of gastric mucosa may predict MGC development following *H. pylori* therapy. In the current study, the number of patients analyzed may be small, particularly for the comparison of MSI and cellular phenotypes in the three different groups. Further investigations on a larger series will be required in the future.

First of all, *H. pylori* should be absolutely eradicated for the prevention of MGC development. The efficacy of standard 7-14 day triple therapies is decreasing, mainly due to increasing primary bacterial resistance to antibiotics. Currently, the most effective treatments are either the sequential regimen or the concomitant therapy. The sequential therapy was first introduced in Italy in 2000 (Zullo et al., 2000). This regimen is a 10-day therapy, including a simple dual therapy with a proton pump inhibitor (PPI) plus amoxicillin 1 g (both twice daily) given for the first 5 days, followed by a triple therapy including a PPI, clarithromycin 500 mg, and tinidazole 500 mg (all given twice daily) for the remaining 5 days. Different antibiotic combinations, administered together with a PPI, have been proposed in the last decades. Unfortunately, no available therapy is able to eradicate *H. pylori* in all treated patients. Therefore, new drugs and novel therapeutic approaches are needed. It has been recently reported by a randomized clinical trial that simvastatin as adjuvant to standard therapy improves significantly the *H. pylori* eradication rate (Nseir et al., 2012). The search for novel antibacterial therapies against *H. pylori* is a "work in progress" driven by the goal of preventing gastric cancer, and by worldwide increasing antibiotic resistance (Fiorini et al., 2012).

We believe that MSI and mAb Das-1 reactivity may be reliable biomarkers to identify a subgroup of patients at sufficiently high risk of MGC after endoscopic resection to justify endoscopic surveillance. According to recent reports, *H. pylori* eradication is able to significantly reduce gene methylation thus delaying or reversing *H. pylori*-induced-gastric carcinogenesis (Chan et al., 2006; Leung et al., 2006; Perri et al., 2007). It has been also reported that sonic hedgehog methylation was detected more frequently in the high-risk group for gastric cancer after *H. pylori* treatment (Shiotani et al., 2012). Further studies on genetic and epigenetic alterations, are necessary to clarify the credibility of the markers in different regional populations.

Author details

Jiro Watari[1], Kentaro Moriichi[2], Hiroki Tanabe[2], Mikihiro Fujiya[2], Hiroto Miwa[1],
Yutaka Kohgo[2] and Kiron M. Das[3]

1 Division of Upper Gastroenterology, Department of Internal Medicine, Hyogo College of Medicine, Nishinomiya, Japan

2 Division of Gastroenterology and Hematology/Oncology, Department of Medicine, Asahikawa Medical University, Asahikawa, Japan

3 Crohn's and Colitis Center of New Jersey, Division of Gastroenterology and Hepatology, Department of Medicine, UMDNJ-Robert Wood Johnson Medical School, New Brunswick, New Jersey, USA

References

[1] Brentnall, T. A., Crispin, D. A., Bronner, M. P., et al. (1996). Microsatellite instability in nonneoplastic mucosa from patients with chronic ulcerative colitis. Cancer Res, , 56, 1237-1240.

[2] Buonsanti, G., Calistri, D., Padovan, L., et al. (1997). Microsatellite instability in intestinal- and diffuse-type gastric carcinoma. *J Pathol,* , 182, 167-173.

[3] Chan, A. O., Peng, J. Z., Lam, S. K., et al. (2006). Eradication of *Helicobacter pylori* infection reverses E-cadherin promoter hypermethylation. *Gut,* , 55, 463-468.

[4] Chung, Y. J., Song, J. M., Lee, J. Y., et al. (1996). Microsatellite instability-associated mutations associate preferentially with the intestinal type of primary gastric carcinomas in a high-risk population. *Cancer Res,* , 56, 4662-4665.

[5] Correa, P., Fox, J., Fontham, E., et al. (1990). *Helicobacter pylori* and gastric carcinoma. Serum antibody prevalence in populations with contrasting cancer risks. *Cancer,* , 66, 2569-2574.

[6] Correa, P. (1995). *Helicobacter pylori* and gastric carcinogenesis. *Am J Surg Pathol,* , 19, S37-S43.

[7] Das, K. M., Prasad, I., Garla, S., et al. (1994). Detection of a shared colon epithelial epitope on Barrett epithelium by a novel monoclonal antibody. *Ann Intern Med,* , 120, 753-756.

[8] Das, K. M., Sakamaki, S., Vecchi, M., et al., & (19987, . The production and characterization of monoclonal antibodies to a human colonic antigen associated with ulcerative colitis: cellular localization of the antigen by using the monoclonal antibody. *J Immunol,* , 139, 77-84.

[9] de Vries, A. C., Meijer, G. A., Looman, C. W., et al. (2007). Epidemiological trends of pre-malignant gastric lesions: a long-term nationwide study in the Netherlands. Gut, , 56, 1665-1670.

[10] Dong, C. X., Deng, D. J., Pan, K. F., et al. (2009). Promoter methylation of p16 associated with Helicobacter pylori infection in precancerous gastric lesions: a population-based study. *Int J Cancer,* , 124, 434-439.

[11] Filipe, M. I., Munoz, N., Matko, I., et al. (1994). Intestinal metaplasia types and the risk of gastric cancer: a cohort study in Slovenia. *Int J Cancer,* , 57, 324-329.

[12] Fiorini, G., Zullo, A., Gatta, L., et al. (2012). Newer agents for Helicobacter pylori eradication. *Clin Exp Gastroenterol,* , 5, 109-112.

[13] Fukase, K., Kato, M., Kikuchi, S., et al., Japan, Gast., & Study, Group. (2008). Effect of eradication of *Helicobacter pylori* on incidence of metachronous gastric carcinoma after endoscopic resection of early gastric cancer: an open-label, randamised controlled trial. *Lancet,* , 372, 392-397.

[14] Graham, D. Y. (2000). *Helicobacter pylori* infection is the primary cause of gastric cancer. *J Gastroenterol*, suppl 12), , 35, 90-97.

[15] Hasuo, T., Semba, S., Li, D., et al. (2007). Assessment of microsatellite instability status for the prediction of metachronous recurrence after initial endoscopic submucosal dissection for early gastric cancer. *Br J Cancer*, , 96, 89-94.

[16] International Agency for Research on Cancer.(1994). IARC monographs on the evaluation of carcinogenic risks to humans. Schistosomes, liver flukes and *Helicobacter pylori*. Lyon: IARC, , 61, 177-240.

[17] Japanese Gastric Cancer Association.(2010). Japanese Classification of Gastric Carcinoma, the 12th ed. Tokyo: Kinbara Publication

[18] Kang, G. H., Shim, Y. H., Jung, H. Y., et al. (2001). CpG island methylation in premalignant stages of gastric carcinoma. Cancer Res, , 61, 2847-2851.

[19] Kashiwagi, K., Watanabe, M., Ezaki, T., et al. (2000). Clinical usefulness of microsatellite instability for the prediction of gastric adenoma or adenocarcinoma in patients with chronic gastritis. *Br J Cancer*, , 82, 1814-1418.

[20] Kondo, Y., Kanai, Y., Sakamoto, M., et al. (2000). Genetic instability and aberrant DNA methylation in chronic hepatitis and cirrhosis-A comprehensive study of loss of heterozygosity and microsatellite instability at 39 loci and DNA hypermethylation on 8 CpG islands in microdissected specimens from patients with hepatocellular carcinoma. *Hepatology*, , 32, 970-979.

[21] Laird, P. W. (2005). Cancer epigenetics. *Hum Mol Genet*, , 14, R65-R76.

[22] Lauren, P. (1965). The two histological main type of gastric carcinoma: Diffuse and so-called intestinal type carcinoma: An attempt at a histo-clinical classification. *Acta Pathol Microbiol Scand*, , 64, 31-49.

[23] Lengauer, C., Kinzler, K. W., & Vogelstein, B. (1998). Genetic instabilities in human cancers. Nature, , 396, 643-649.

[24] Leung, W. K., Man, E. P., Yu, J., et al. (2006). Effects of Helicobacter pylori eradication on methylation status of E-cadherin gene in noncancerous stomach. Clin Cancer Res, , 12, 3216-3621.

[25] Maehata, Y., Nakamura, S., Fujisawa, K., et al. Long-term effect of Helicobacter pylori eradication on the development of metachronous gastric cancer after endoscopic resection of early gastric cancer. Gastrointest Endosc, , 75, 39-46.

[26] Mera, R., Fontham, E. T., Bravo, L. E., et al. (2005). Long term follow up of patients treated for Helicobacter pylori infection. *Gut*, , 54, 1536-1540.

[27] Mirza, Z. K., Das, K. K., Slate, J., et al. (2003). Gastric intestinal metaplasia as detected by a novel biomarker is highly associated with gastric adenocarcinoma. *Gut*, , 52, 807-812.

[28] Miyoshi, E., Haruma, K., Hiyama, T., et al. (2001). Microsatellite instability is a genetic marker for the development of multiple gastric cancers. *Int J Cancer*, , 95, 350-353.

[29] Nseir, W., Diab, H., Mahamid, M., et al. (2012). Randomised clinical trial: simvastatin as adjuvant therapy improves significantly the Helicobacter pylori eradication rate- a placebo-controlled study. *Aliment Pharmacol Ther*, , 36, 231-238.

[30] Park, S. Y., Yoo, E. J., Cho, N. Y., et al. (2009). Comparison of CpG island hypermethylation and repetitive DNA hypomethylation in premalignant stages of gastric cancer, stratified for Helicobacter pylori infection. *J Pathol*, , 219, 410-416.

[31] Peek, R. M., Jr , , & Blaser, . (2002). *Helicobacter pylori* and gastrointestinal tract adenocarcinomas. *Nat Rev Cancer*, , 2, 28-37.

[32] Perri, F., Cotugno, R., Piepoli, A., et al. (2007). Aberrant DNA methylation in non-neoplastic gastric mucosa of *H. pylori* infected patients and effect of eradication. *Am J Gastroenterol*, , 102, 1361-1371.

[33] Robertson, K. D. (2005). DNA methylation and human disease. *Nat Rev Genet*, , 6, 597-610.

[34] Shiotani, A., Murao, T., Uedo, N., et al. (2011). Eradication of *H. pylori* did not improve abnormal sonic hedgehog expression in the high risk group for gastric cancer. *Dig Dis Sci*, , 57, 643-649.

[35] Sipponen, P., & Hyvärinen, H. (1993). Role of *Helicobacter pylori* in the pathogenesis of gastritis, peptic ulcer and gastric cancer. *Scand J Gastroenterol*, suppl), , 196, 3-6.

[36] Take, S., Mizuno, M., Ishiki, K., et al. (2005). The effect of eradicating Helicobacter pylori on the development of gastric cancer in patients with peptic ulcer disease. *Am J Gastroenterol*, , 100, 1037-1042.

[37] Tamura, G. (2006). Alterations of tumor suppressor and tumor-related genes in the development and progression of gastric cancer. *World J Gastroenterol*, , 12, 192-198.

[38] Tanaka, A., Watari, J., Tanabe, H., et al. (2006). Effect of eradication of *Helicobacter pylori* on genetic instabilities in gastric intestinal metaplasia. *Aliment Pharmacol Ther*, Supple 4), , 24, 194-202.

[39] To, K. F., Leung, W. K., Lee, T. L., et al. (2002). Promoter hypermethylation of tumor-related genes in gastric intestinal metaplasia of patients with and without gastric cancer. *Int J Cancer*, , 102, 623-628.

[40] Uemura, N., Okamoto, S., Yamamoto, S., et al. (2001). *Helicobacter pylori* infection and the development of gastric cancer. *N Engl J Med*, , 345, 784-789.

[41] Umar, A., Boland, C. R., Terdiman, J. P., et al. (2004). Revised Bethesda Guidelines for hereditary nonpolyposis colorectal cancer (Lynch syndrome) and microsatellite instability. *J Natl Cancer Inst*, , 96, 261-268.

[42] Watari, J., Das, K. K., Amenta, P. S., et al. (2008). Effect of eradication of *Helicobacter pylori* on the histology and cellular phenotype of gastric intestinal metaplasia. *Clin Gastroenterol Hepatol*, , 6, 409-417.

[43] Watari, J., Moriichi, K., Tanabe, H., et al. (2012). Biomarkers predicting development of metachronous gastric cancer after endoscopic resection: an analysis of molecular pathology of *Helicobacter pylori* eradication. *Int J Cancer*, , 130, 2349-2358.

[44] Wong, B. C., Lam, S. K., Wong, W. M., et al. (2004). Helicobacter pylori eradication to prevent gastric cancer in a high-risk region of China: a randomized controlled trial. JAMA, , 291, 187-194.

[45] Wright, N. A. (1998). Gastric carcinogenesis: when is the point of no return? In: Hunt RH, Tytgat GNJ, eds. Helicobacter pylori: Basic Mechanisms to Clinical Cure. Boston, Mass: Kluwer Academic Publishers, , 325-335.

[46] Yanaoka, K., Oka, M., Ohata, H., et al. (2009). Eradication of *Helicobacter pylori* prevents cancer development in subjects with mild gastric atrophy identified by serum pepsinogen levels. *Int J Cancer*, , 125, 2697-2703.

[47] You, W. C., Zhang, L., Gail, M. H., et al. (2000). Gastric dysplasia and gastric cancer: *Helicobacter pylori*, serum vitamin C, and other risk factors. *J Natl Cancer Inst*, 92, , 1607-1612.

[48] Zaky, A., Watari, J. ., Tanabe, H., et al. (2008). Clinicopathological implications of genetic instability in intestinal type gastric cancer and intestinal metaplasia as a precancerous lesion: Proof of field cancerization in the stomach. *Am J Clin Pathol*, , 129, 613-621.

[49] Zullo, A., Rinaldi, V., Winn, S., et al. (2000). A new highly effective short-term therapy schedule for *Helicobacter pylori* eradication. *Aliment Pharmacol Ther*, , 14, 715-718.

Chapter 7

Unveiling the Intricacies of *Helicobacter pylori*-Induced Gastric Inflammation: T Helper Cells and Matrix Metalloproteinases at a Crossroad

Avisek Banerjee**, Asish K. Mukhopadhyay**,
Sumit Paul, Arindam Bhattacharyya and
Snehasikta Swarnakar

Additional information is available at the end of the chapter

http://dx.doi.org/10.5772/54193

1. Introduction

For most of the 20th century, the human stomach has been considered an environment that is inhospitable for the growth of any bacteria. But the first isolation of a curved, microaerophilic, gram-negative bacterium, *H. pylori* by Marshall and Warren in 1982 is responsible for provoking a rupture in contemporary popular medical doctrines, thereby enforcing changes in global conceptions of gastroduodenal disorders. *H. pylori* is of growing concern today because of its crucial role in the pathogenesis of chronic gastritis, peptic ulcer diseases and in the multi-step carcinogenic processess of gastric cancer, a fourth most common cancer worldwide while the second cause of cancer related deaths. Epidemiologically, more than 50% of the world population is infected by this bacterium and develops persistent inflammation in their stomachs, which lasts for decades unless treated with antibiotics. About 60-95% of peptic ulcer diseases are thought to be idiopathic and *H. pylori* is one of the causative agents of nearly all of these cases in adults. About 15% of infected individuals become symptomatic for peptic ulcer (duodenal or gastric) as a long-term consequence of infection. The apparent paradox suggests that the mere presence of *H. pylori* in the stomach is insufficient to cause gastric disease, rather requiring additional conditions. Beside bacterial genetics, host genetic factors, hygiene, microbiome, medication, food habits along with life-style might be additional reasons for *H. pylori*-induced pathogenecity.

Progression of gastric inflammation by long term association of *H. pylori* in stomach can broadly be viewed in two ways. The first being the antigenic stimulation of *H. pylori* and the second one is the host immune response to microbe that is necessary for bacterial clearance yet causing injury to the host. Besides, *H. pylori* must bear an arsenal of specific virulence factor such as the cytotoxin-associated gene-pathogenicity island (*cag*-PAI), vacuolating associated cytotoxin gene A (*vacA*), outer membrane protein A (*oip*A), blood group antigen binding adhesin (*bab*A), lipases and lipopolysaccharides (LPS) be potentially toxigenic to initiate the process of inflammation in the host gastric tissues. These antigens can interact with specific host proteins, initiating a cascade of signaling processes which ultimately affect many abnormalities like loss-of-function of tumour suppressor genes, gain-of-function of oncogenes, dysregulation of miRNAs and several defects in cytoskeleton and cell-cell junctions.

On the other hand, the host immune response is characterized by the cardinal signs of inflammation. Both innate and adaptive immune systems are activated by inhabiting *H. pylori*. The principal mechanism of innate immunity includes complement activation, phagocytosis and the inflammatory response. The adaptive immune response is guided mainly by T cells including T regulatory cells (Tregs), T helper (T_H1) cells and more recently reported T_H17 cells and their corresponding cytokines. *H. pylori* has evolved with unique features to evade immune response. It also exhibits multiple strategies to reside within the host yet escaping host immune response (refer Box 1). Thus, it remains a mystery as to why some infected patients are susceptible to disease manifestation compared to others who remain asymptomatic throughout their lives in spite of infection.

- *Acidic milieu:* Gastric niche is acidic, while *H. pylori* grow normally at neutral pH but fails to grow at pH below 4. To overcome this problem, the bacteria secrete urease, which breaks urea into water and ammonia. This property has been successfully exploited for disease diagnosis known as urea breath test.
- *Non-Adherence:* For successful colonization, the bacterium has to successfully adhere to the gastric wall, but the peristaltic movements of the stomach provide a hostile barrier. However, *H. pylori* possess spiral shaped polar flagella, which permit proficient hydrodynamic movement within gastric mucous. About 20% bacterial population adheres to gastric epithelial cells but majority remains within mucous layer. *H. pylori* express several outer membrane proteins (OMPs) which bind to their receptors on gastric epithelial cells. For example, BabA is an adhesion molecule that binds to the fucosylated Lewis ^{b} receptor, SabA binds to sialyl Lewis^{X} receptor and OipA not only adhere onto gastric epithelial cells but also triggers β-catenin activation and secretion of proinflammatory cytokines.
- *Host Immune Response:* Activation of host immune system results in inflammation. Interestingly, this gram-negative bacterium has evolved with anergic lipopolysaccharide (LPS) and flagelin due to its modification of lipid a component that has about 10^3 times less endotoxin activity in comparison to LPS of other gram-negative bacteria. Moreover, *H. pylori* can acquire molecular mimicry by taking cholesterol from its host into its own membrane. Furthermore, Tregs upregulation following infection may suppress antibacterial immune response.

Box 1. Barriers overcome by *H. pylori* for colonization and infection in host.

It is known from several studies that MMP, a family of zinc-dependent endopeptidases that selectively degrade or remodel most of ECM components and other structural molecules are intimately associated to different diseases including gastric ulcer and cancer. At present, both *in vivo* and *in vitro* studies have established the activation of several MMPs during *H. pylori* association. However, very few studies have been made till date dissecting the significant role of T_H cell subsets and MMPs during the progression of *H. pylori* related gastric inflammation. In this review, we aim at to highlight the influence of T_H cells on modulation of MMPs activity during *H. pylori* induced gastric inflammation that further open up new avenues both in research and clinical perspectives in future. Since the present scenario failed to generate much hope on *H. pylori* vaccination we will emphasise on how *H. pylori* behave within gastric niche and how do they trigger inflammation?

2. Gastric inflammation: An overview

Persistent association of microaerophilic, gram-negative enteric bacteria results in chronic gastric inflammation which in turn leads to gastric cancer. Accumulating evidences suggest that *H. pylori*-induced inflammation is initiated both by host and bacterial factors. In addition, environmental factors also play potent role in disease progression. However, the actual pathogenesis behind chronic inflammation is not well understood. *H. pylori* enter inside stomach via fecal-oral route mainly by contaminated food and water (Klein et al., 1991, Hopkins et al., 1993). The most probable mode of transmission is via direct contact with the infected patient within the family or a common source of contaminated water or food of a locality (Hopkins et al., 1993) (Nurgalieva et al., 2002).

Gastric inflammation is accompanied by induction of oxidative stress by reactive oxygen species (ROS), inducible nitric oxide synthase (iNOS) and subsequent secretion of proinflammatory cytokines like interleukin (IL)-1β, IL-6 and tumor necrosis factor (TNF)-α (Yamaoka et al., 1996). Gastric epithelial cells also secrete IL-8 (Jung et al., 1997) which attracts the polymorphonuclear (PMN) cells. Local inflammation is also associated to reduced prostaglandin synthesis and increased infiltration of mast cells, neutrophils, macrophages and *H. pylori* specific IgA and IgG antibodies (Warren, 2000). The dendritic cells (DCs), which are present in the epithelial layer, present the antigens with their Toll-like receptors (TLRs) to naïve T cells and thereby initiate humoral immune response. Moreover, *H. pylori* infection stimulates iNOS and other enzymes including myeloperoxidases, NADPH oxidases, eosinophil peroxidases. These enzymes trigger ROS and reactive nitrogen species (RNS) production, which induce DNA damage (Wang et al., 2005).Therefore, *H. pylori*-mediated inflammation is complex and no single factor can be targeted for successful clinical therapy. For example the study on mast cell-deficient $Kitl^{Sl}/Kitl^{Sl-d}$ mice reported that mast cells also contribute to neutrophil recruitment and inflammatory response due to *H. pylori* infection thereby contributing a part though are not essential for vaccine-induced immunity (Ding et al., 2009).

Over-secretion of pro-inflammatory cytokines and growth factors promote neovascularisation, which cause invasion and metastasis. Vascular endothelial growth factor (VEGF), the main mediator of angiogenesis is reported to be over-expressed in 54% of severe gastric cancer patients with lymph node and liver metastasis (Saukkonen et al., 2003). Along with

VEGF, other pro-angiogenic factors like IL-6, IL-8 and iNOS are also upregulated in tumor cells. IL-8 promotes angiogenesis in gastric tumor by interacting with its receptors CXCR1 and CXCR2, present on surface of endothelial cells. Over expression of iNOS has been observed in both primary tumors as well as lymph node metastases compared to normal mucosa (Wang et al., 2005). Excess nitric oxide increases the activity of VEGF thereby promoting blood flow, vascular permeability and endothelial cell proliferation and migration (Wang et al., 2005). Other than stimulating angiogenesis, iNOS promotes gastric carcinoma through various ways including inhibiting DNA repair enzymes, inducing oxidative DNA damage, oncogene expression and apoptosis deregulation (Ohshima et al., 2003). The niche of *H. pylori* colonization is also a determinant factor for the severity of the disease. For example; chronic corpus-predominant gastritis leads to mainly gastric adenocarcinoma, in contrast antrum-predominant gastritis may promote duodenal ulceration. Also patients with *H. pylori* infection in the distal part (antrum) of the stomach may develop duodenal ulcer but are somewhat protective from gastric cancer. Thus, duodenal ulcer may have a protective role from development of gastric adenocarcinoma (Saukkonen et al., 2003).

In cancer tissues, there is very less information available regarding the association between a specific factor and methylation of a gene. Aberrant DNA methylation is frequently associated with different human cancers. DNA methylation is involved with change in gene expression pattern, which can be confirmed by measuring the mRNA levels of the corresponding genes. Nakajima *et al,* in human gastric cancer cell lines showed that DNA methylation pattern due to *H. pylori* infection was conserved in the promoter region of 48 genes. Interestingly, this methylation pattern remained in gastric cancer patients; who were previously infected with *H. pylori* but later eradicated (Nakajima et al., 2009). Similarly from *Mongolian gerbils* (Niwa et al., 2010) 10 CpG islands showed specific methylation pattern after *H. pylori* infection, which sustained the inflammatory response of the host towards *H. pylori* infection rather than *H. pylori* itself. Therefore with reduction of inflammation, there was reduction in DNA methylations, even as *H. pylori* load remained unchanged. So, long term *H. pylori* infection induces chronic inflammation, the later maintain epigenetic changes inside host's genome.

From evolutionary view point, the successful adaptability of *H. pylori* within the host can be attributed to their versatile genetic diversity, which has specifically evolved for a habitat, population or geographical locations. The virulence of *H. pylori* depends on what specific antigens they possess. Interestingly, nature selected both Cag A^+ (high virulence) as well as $CagA^-$ (less virulent) bacteria during the course of evolution. Possibly, high-virulence implies successful host attack; while less-virulence implies their innovative masking strategy from host's immune response. So, diversity seems to help bacteria to keep the host alive even with infection, in turn preserving them. Therefore, one of the most intriguing aspects of *H. pylori* is its genetic diversity, the biological significance of which is enigmatic (Covacci and Rappuoli, 1998, Logan and Berg, 1996). The bacteria colonize the gastric mucus layer and persist livelong in close vicinity with epithelial cells. Though bacterial colonization depends on their secreting system, which they use as molecular syringes to inject their virulent component into the host (Kamada et al., 2012), yet competition also play crucial role for *H. pylori* colonization inside the gut and hence, the gut microbiota is often referred to as the forgotten organ (Sperandio, 2012). The human gastrointestinal tract hosts bacterial cells as many as 10 times more than total number of cells of human body (Hooper and Gordon, 2001). These bacteria compete with pathogens like *H. pylori* for food source. Therefore, changes in microenvironments like high salt-intake, change in life-style or food-habits give stress on normal gut microbiota and helping *H. pylori* to proliferate and induce infection.

3. Genetics of *H. pylori* and gastropathy

H. pylori are a highly heterogeneous bacterial species, both genotypically and phenotypically, and are highly adapted for survival in the gastric niche. The genomic diversity of *H. pylori* parallels that of its host species, consistent with colonization of the earliest humans and co-migration out of east Africa at least 60,000 years ago (Censini et al., 1996). *H. pylori* colonize the stomach for almost the entire lifetime of the host. *H. pylori* colonization of the gastric mucosa typically occurs in early childhood and may persist for decades or for life, unless eradicated by antimicrobial treatment.

The clinical outcome of *H. pylori* infection is determined by multiple factors, including host genetic predisposition (especially certain cytokine polymorphisms (Amieva and El–Omar, 2008), *H. pylori* strain heterogeneity and environmental factors such as dietary salt intake (Fox et al., 1999, Beevers et al., 2004, Hwang et al., 1994). *H. pylori* heterogeneity and the association with *H. pylori* virulence factors have been intensively investigated over the past two decades (Covacci et al., 1993, Atherton et al., 1995, Argent et al., 2004). One possible problem that has complicated the identification of definite disease-specific *H. pylori* virulence factors is the considerable geographic diversity in the prevalence of *H. pylori* virulence factors. The major *H. pylori* candidate virulence factors include cagA, vacA, babA and dupA.

cagA was the first reported gene that varies in *H. pylori* strains and considered as a marker for the presence of cag-PAI, which include a number of other genes associated with increased virulence (Broutet et al., 2001). The gene that encodes CagA is part of a ~40 kb horizontally acquired DNA segment in the *H. pylori* genome known as cag-PAI (Censini et al., 1996). The cag-PAI also contain genes encoding a type IV secretion system, to ensure efficient translocation of the CagA protein into the host epithelium.The CagA also disrupts the tight junctions and causes loss of apical-basolateral polarity in epithelial cells (Amieva et al., 2003).

The extent of biological activity of CagA is directly associated with the number of phosphorylation sites or the number of EPIYA motifs present at the C-terminal region of CagA (Higashi et al., 2002b, Azuma, 2004, Azuma et al., 2004). Thus, molecular weight of the CagA protein varies from 128 kDa -148 kDa and the *cagA* gene shows extensive length polymorphism at the 3′ end. Several attempts were made to type the distinct CagA proteins and the *cagA* genes on the basis of its length polymorphism at the C-terminal and 3' ends, respectively (Argent et al., 2005, Dong et al., 2002, Owen et al., 2003). Mutational analyses revealed that the first two EPIYA motifs (Y1 and Y2 positions) have little, if any, biological function while the other motifs are responsible for the CagA phosphorylation and CagA-SHP-2 complex formation (Higashi et al., 2002a). Moreover, the amino acid sequences, which are repeated among the third, fourth and fifth EPIYA motifs differ among strains isolated from west and east Asia. Accordingly, CagA was typed as Western-CagA-specific sequences (WSS) and East Asian-CagA-specific sequences (ESS) and this difference may account for differences in disease outcome between the two geographical regions. Recent study suggested that EPIYA motifs as well as the spacer sequence units were present as distinct insertions and deletions, which possibly have arisen from extensive recombination events (Chattopadhyay et al., 2012). Moreover, several new CagA types have been identified, a new typing system has been proposed. It is hypothesized that a *cagA* gene encoding higher number EPIYA motifs may perhaps have arisen from *cagA* genes that encode lesser EPIYA motifs by acquisition of DNA segments through recombination events (*refer figure 1a)*. Chattopadhyay *et al* also described that carrying a particular type of CagA is not the only determinant for the disease outcome especially in the developing countries like India, where multiple infections with different CagA primary structures are possible. Recent study regarding the multiple infections and microdiversity among the colonies from individual patient in Indian population suggested that most of the patients have acquired *H. pylori* due to repeated exposure to this pathogen with different genetic make-up, which may increase the possibility of super infections(Patra et al., 2012). Genetic exchanges between these unrelated *H. pylori* strains may support certain *H. pylori* variant to grow better in a given host than the parental strain and thereby increasing the possibility for the severity of the infection (Patra et al., 2012) (*refer figure 1)*. Additional isolates of the sequenced *H. pylori* strain J99 from its human source patient after a 6-year interval was analyzed in another study (Israel et al., 2001). Patterns of genetic diversity were distinct among the additional J99 isolates, both when compared with each other and to the original prototype isolate. Their results indicated that within an apparently homogeneous population remarkable genetic differences existed among single-colony isolates of *H. pylori*. Direct evidence that *H. pylori* has the capacity to lose and possibly acquire exogenous DNA is consistent with a model of continuous microevolution within its cognate host (Israel et al., 2001).

Soon after *H. pylori*'s discovery, it was reported that a protein in *H. pylori* broth culture filtrates could cause the formation of large intracellular vacuoles in cultured mammalian cells (Leunk et al., 1988). The *H. pylori* protein responsible for this effect (designated VacA) is encoded by a chromosomal gene known as *vacA*. The *vacA* gene encodes a precursor protein of 140 kDa (Cover et al., 1994, Telford et al., 1994, Lupetti et al., 1996). Proteolytic processing of the protoxin during secretion yields the mature toxin (~90 kDa). Secreted VacA can be further processed into an N-terminal fragment of 33 kDa (p33) and a C-terminal fragment of 55 kDa (p55), but cleavage does not seem to be necessary for VacA activity. Although the p33 domain exhibits pore-forming activity necessary for vacuole formation (McClain and Cover, 2003), and the p55 domain is responsible for target cell binding (Reyrat et al., 1999), Several families of *vacA* alleles can be distinguished on the basis of diversity near the 5′ terminus of *vacA* (which is known as the s-region s1a-c and s2), the intermediate region (i1, i2) and in the mid-region of the gene (known as the m-region m1, m2) (Atherton et al., 1995, Rhead et al., 2007). Most strains with s1/m1 genotype and some of the s1/m2 express the cytotoxin while strains with s2/m2 genotype do not express a toxic VacA (Cover and Blanke, 2005). Studies have shown that VacA contributes to *H. pylori* colonization, persistence and disease outcome *in vivo*. *H. pylori* strains that contain *vacA* alleles of the s1 type are associated with an increased risk for development of peptic ulcer disease and gastric cancer compared with strains containing *vacA* alleles of the s2 type (Atherton et al., 1995, Van Doorn et al., 1999, van Doorn et al., 1998, Figueiredo et al., 2002). However, east Asian strains are almost universally s1/m1 and are not associated with any specific clinical outcome (Ito et al., 1997, Ito et al., 1998).

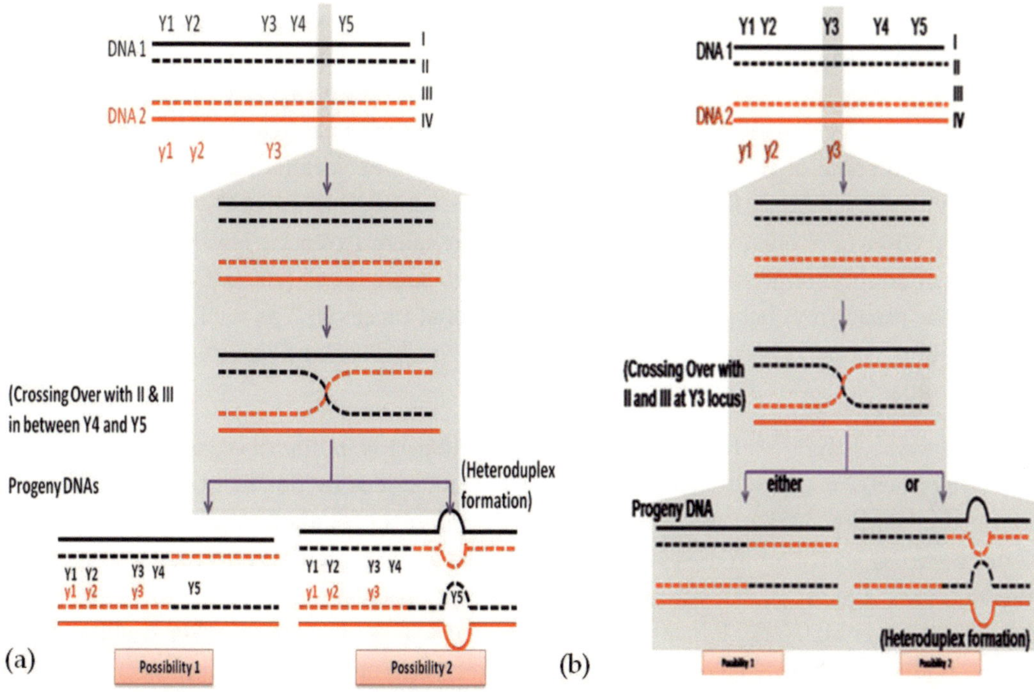

Figure 1. Schematic representation of generation of genetic diversity in cagA gene involving EPIYA motifs (Ys): **(a)** genetic diversity arise within a cagA gene from another cagA gene that encode lesser EPIYA motifs by acquisition of DNA segments through homologous recombination events or **(b)** genetic variation within a cagA gene may also result from crossing over within any particular EPIYA motif (for example Y3 as shown in the figure). In all the events, crossing over can also happen involving DNA strands I and IV, as mentioned above and therefore can generate more genetic variation within cagA gene. It is to be noted that DNA 1 and 2 are genetically different. The rationale behind making the two strands of a DNA dissimilar due to acquision of new mutations is highlighted.

Approximately 4% of the *H. pylori* genome encodes a diverse repertoire of outer membrane proteins (OMPs), the largest of which is the 21-gene Hop family. Several of the Hop proteins have been identified as adhesins, the best studied of which is BabA (Ilver et al., 1998, Guruge et al., 1998). It is an adherence factor expressed in a subgroup of *H. pylori* strains and binds to difucosylated Lewis b (Leb) blood group antigens found on gastric epithelial cells. The *babA* gene was cloned initially from strain CCUG17875, which contains a silent *babA1* gene and an expressed *babA2* gene. The sequence of these two genes differs only by presence of a 10bp deletion in the signal peptide sequence of *babA1* that eliminates its translational initiation codon (Prinz et al., 2001). Initial studies indicated that *H. pylori babA2*$^{+}$ strains are associated with an increased risk of peptic ulcers and distal gastric adenocarcinoma, whereas *babA2*$^{-}$ strains are more often associated with uncomplicated forms of gastritis (Gerhard et al., 1999, Prinz et al., 2001). *babA2*-genopositive *H. pylori* usually coexists with other disease-related *H. pylori* virulence-factor genes, such as *vacA s1* and *cagA*. Tripositive strains, which have *cagA*$^+$, *vacA s1*, *babA2*$^+$in a single *H. pylori* species, further increase the risk of developing gastroduodenal ulcers and distal gastric cancer(Prinz et al., 2001, Gerhard et al., 1999).

Recent studies have proposed the possibility of using genetic markers in the plasticity zone as indicators of pathogenicity for *H. pylori* infection, in spite of a lack of credible knowledge regarding the functions of the putatively encoded proteins in this cluster. It seems that these determinants may play a key role in determining the virulence capacity of *H. pylori* strains either directly or by encoding factors that may lead to varying clinical outcomes. The association between some of the ORFs in the plasticity zone and various disease categories has been previously reported. For instance, Occhialini *et al.* (Occhialini et al., 2000) found that two single ORFs (*jhp0940* and *jhp0947*) were more prevalent in strains isolated from patients with gastric adenocarcinoma in Costa Rica. However, Santos *et al.* (2003) (Santos et al., 2003) showed the association between *jhp0947* and duodenal ulcer (DU) as well as gastric cancer in Brazilian patients. This was once more confirmed for *jhp0947* and *jhp0949* genes in DU patients from the Netherlands (de Jonge et al., 2004).

Recently, a novel duodenal ulcer promoting gene (*dupA*) was described, which consists of two ORFs *jhp0917* and *jhp0918* and form one continuous gene by the insertion of a base T or C after the position 1385 of the *jhp0917* in the 3' region (Lu et al., 2005). This gene (homologues to *virB*4) is located in the plasticity region and is associated with increased risk of DU and protective against gastric atrophy, intestinal metaplasia and gastric carcinoma in Japan and Korea (Lu et al., 2005). However, the role of *dupA* as a virulence marker is still controversial. Some researchers have supported the interpretations of Lu *et al.* (2005) (Lu et al., 2005) but others did not find any association. Hussein *et al.* (2008) (Hussein et al., 2008) have reported that *dupA* gene is associated with peptic ulcer but they did not find any negative association with gastric cancer in Iraqi population. In Chinese and north Indian populations significant association of *dupA* with DU was established (Arachchi et al., 2007). In contrast, Argent *et al.* (2007)(Argent et al., 2007) showed no association of *dupA* gene with DU in population from Belgium, South Africa, China and the United States. Meta-analysis based study by Shiota *et al.* (2010) (Shiota et al., 2010) has shown that the presence of *dupA* gene was significantly associated with DU. Another systematic review confirmed that *dupA* was associated with gastro duodenal diseases (Hussein, 2010). Study in southeast Indian population demonstrated that *dupA* gene was 6.5 times more prevalent in duodenal ulcer patients than non-ulcer patients (Alam et al., 2012). Infection with the *dupA*-positive *H. pylori* increased the risk for DU overall and this evidence was significant in Indian study (Alam et al., 2012). The discrepancy of *dupA* association with diseases outcome could be related to the limitation of PCR techniques for detecting the intact *dupA* gene or may be a consequence of the genetic diversity of *H. pylori*, which is at a level as yet unseen among other bacterial pathogens (Covacci and Rappuoli, 1998, Logan and Berg, 1996, Blaser 1998).

http://dx.doi.org/10.5772/54193

4. Immunobiology of host and *H. pylori* interaction in both *in vivo* and *in vitro*

Through evolution, *H. pylori* have gradually developed highly sophisticated adaptation for successful colonization and better adaptation inside the host's microenvironment. Interestingly, humans too show some tricky adaptation to check *H. pylori* colonization inside the stomach. The *in vitro* studies documented (Linden et al., 2009) that human gastric cell-surface mucin MUC1, a large glycoprotein, prevents the adhesion of the bacterium with the epithelial layer. *H. pylori* usually bind to MUC1 through their cell surface receptor BabA and SabA adhesion proteins, but the human gastric cells shed these MUC1 glycoproteins by MUC1 sheddases ADAM17 and MMP-14. Similarly, in murine model too, MUC1 prevents *H. pylori* colonization (McGuckin et al., 2007).

After entering the gastric milieu, most of the bacteria remain in the gastric mucosa and only about 10% *H. pylori* bind with the gastric epithelial cells (Oh et al., 2005, Semino-Mora et al., 2003). So it becomes difficult to eradicate the bacteria with antibiotics. *H. pylori* adhere via BabA (Ilver et al., 1998) with histo-blood group antigen Le^b expressed over gastric epithelial cell surface. The other protein that significantly contribute stable adherence of *H. pylori* is sialic acid-binding adhesion protein (SabA) which bind to $Lewis^X$ (Mahdavi et al., 2002), a glycosphingolipid that is significantly expressed during gastric dysplasia (Hansson et al., 1993).

The genetic study in relation to the virulence factor has been extensively studied in relation to *cagA* and *vacA* (Peek and Crabtree, 2006). CagA positive *H. pylori* strains impart higher risk for gastric cancer (GC) than infection of strains that devoid of *cag*PAI (Parsonnet et al., 1997, Enroth et al., 2000). After stable adherence, *H. pylori* with its type IV secreting system translocate CagA into the gastric epithelial cells (Segal et al., 1999). Once inside, Cag A is differentiately phosphorylated at its specific tyrosine residues in their EPIYA (Glu-Pro-Ile-Tyr-Ala) motifs located at the C-terminal region of the protein (Higashi et al., 2002a). This phosphorylation is carried out by host's Src and Abl family kinases (Selbach et al., 2002, Poppe et al., 2007). A variety of tyrosine phosphorylation motifs results in difference in virulence and consequently host infection(Higashi et al., 2002a).This overall difference in phosphorylation of the tyrosine motifs may be the reason for diversity of GC incidence in the global scenario (*refer figure 1)*. Phosphorylated CagA can interact with several other host proteins and ultimately targets specific proteins including oncoprotein, tumor suppressing protein, junction proteins, cell cycle regulators and several other transcription factors. These collectively affect the cell's normal physiology and propel the cells toward carcinoma. The phosphorylated CagA protein binds to SH2 domain of tyrosine phosphatase and increases its phosphatase activity (Higashi et al., 2002b, Hatakeyama, 2004). SHP-2 is an important component involved in intracellular signaling during development and haematopoiesis whose gain-of-function lead to lymphoid and myeloid malignancy (Tartaglia and Gelb, 2005). Due to the intrinsic membrane tethering property of CagA the CagA-SHP-2 complex localizes to the plasma membrane of the host epithelium (Higashi et al., 2002b), leading to deregulation of the SHP-2. This event is necessary and sufficient to change the gastric epithelium to a transformed epithelium, which is characterized by altered cellular proliferation, migration and elongated cell morphology known as hummingbird phenotype (Higashi et al., 2002b, Yamazaki et al., 2003). So, transgenic expression of CagA also manifest gastrointestinal as well as hematopoietic abnormalities (Ohnishi et al., 2008). *H. pylori* having a functional *cag* PAI also stimulate cultured gastric epithelial cells to secrete the pro-inflammatory cytokine or chemokine IL-8 (Crabtree et al., 1995). CagA binds to SHP-2 and induces 'humming bird phenotype' in AGS cell line involving extracellular signal-regulated kinase (Erk), mitogen-activated protein (MAP) kinase pathway and dephosphorylating focal adhesion kinase (FAK) (Tartaglia and Gelb, 2005) (Higashi et al., 2004). Cag A also interacts with Crk and thereby promotes loss of adhesion in gastric epithelial cells (Suzuki et al., 2005). In addition, Cag A also interacts with other factors including c-Met and Grb2 (Churin et al., 2003, Mimuro et al., 2002). In addition to the above components, *H. pylori* also secrete nucleotide-binding oligomerization domain-1 (NOD1), a specific peptidoglycan of gram-negative bacteria (Viala et al., 2004), a potent molecule involved in stimulating the host innate immune response (Fox and Wang, 2007).

The other virulence factor in *H. pylori* is VacA. The intra-luminal environment of VacA-induced vacuoles is acidic, and the vacuoles are endocytically active (Cover et al., 1991, Papini et al., 1994). A current model to explain the mechanism by which VacA induces vacuole formation proposes that VacA binds to the plasma membrane of cells, is internalized by cells, forms anion-selective channels in endosomal membranes and alters the permeability of these compartments. Within 10 minutes of addition of VacA to a human gastric adenocarcinoma cell line (AZ-521), two classes of mitogen-activated protein kinases (p38 and ERK1/2) and the activating transcription factor 2 (ATF2) signalling pathway are activated (Nakayama et al., 2004). Within 30–60 minutes of the binding of VacA to BHK-21 cells expressing receptor protein tyrosine phosphatase β (RPTPβ, also known as Ptprz), tyrosine phosphorylation of G-protein-coupled receptor kinase interactor (Git1) can be detected (Fujikawa et al., 2003). In another model system, binding of of VacA to a mast cell line (RBL-2H3) cells results in a rapid change in cytosolic calcium concentrations (de Bernard et al., 2005). VacA is also reported to induce pro-inflammatory effects. It stimulates the production of TNF-α and IL-6 by mast cells and induces chemotaxis and degranulation of these cells (de Bernard et al., 2005). Moreover, VacA treatment stimulates expression of cyclooxygenase-2, a proinflammatory enzyme, in neutrophils and macrophages (Boncristiano et al., 2003). Thus, the effects of VacA on immune cells are complex and are characterized by both immnostimulatory and immnosuppressive actions.

5. Role of T cells in *H. pylori* infection

Very limited information is available on how the host immune system; particularly the adaptive immune system is modulated by *H. pylori* infection to promote gastric diseases. Chronic inflammation associated to *H. pylori* infection is known to promote gastric cancer in some individuals (Suerbaum and Michetti, 2002, El-Serag and Rudolph, 2007). In contrast to earlier notion that T cells generate antitumor responses, as supported by the fact that $Rag^{-/-}$ mice and mice with mutated interferon signaling promote more tumor development, recent advances establish new insights into T cells particularly TH17 response in aggravating gastric cancer due to *H. pylori* colonization (Erdman et al., 2003, Dunn et al., 2006).

Bacterial chemotaxis is their inherent property by which it can migrate from a harsh environment towards more favorable environment. Genetically modified *H. pylori* (Che^{-}) cannot respond to environmental stimulus although they retain power of locomotion. In animal models, they manifest marginal colonization abnormalities and relatively less inflammation severity. Interestingly, Che^{-} *H. pylori* fail to colonize epithelial cells and gastric glands vigorously. This support the fact that chemotaxis helps the bacteria to successfully cross the thick mucus layer with their unipolar flagella and adhere to gastric epithelial cells which are resident of antigen presenting cells (APCs); thus promoting antigen presentation to naïve T cells (Rolig et al., 2011). In the process, epithelial cells also secrete chemokines for recruiting APCs like DCs. DCs with their Toll-like receptors recognize specific antigens of the bacteria; and in turn presents those antigenic peptide fragments to T cells to promote class switching and differentiation in TH1 subsets, T regs or more recently classified TH17 cells (*refer figure 2*). Specific cytokines secreted by these cells regulate host immune response leading towards chronic inflammation.

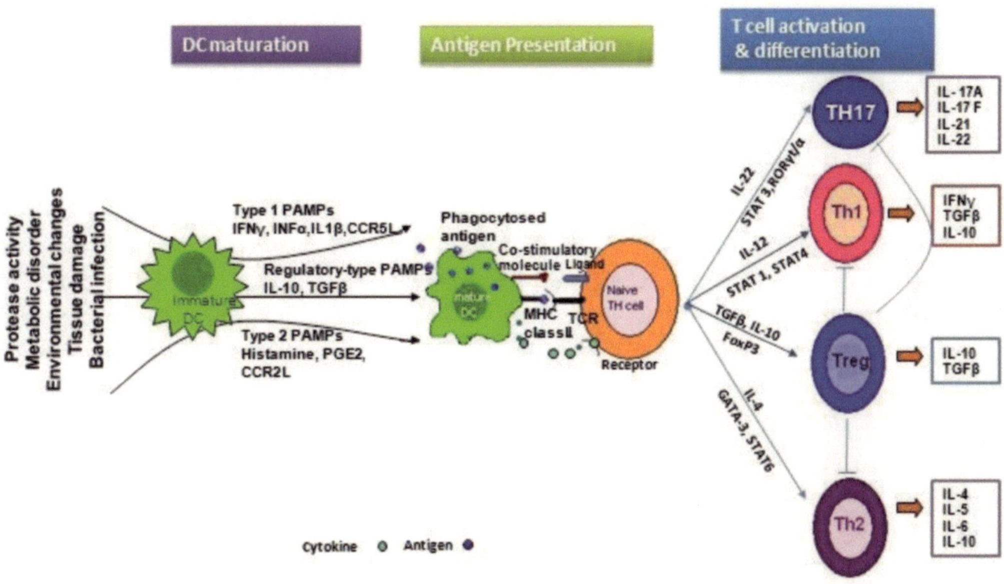

Figure 2. Maturation of DC and formation of T cell subsets following exogeneous stimuli: Maturation of dendritic cell (DC) occurs under the influence of different pathogen-associated molecular patterns and specific host cytokines.Various physiological and environmental factors also trigger DC for successful antigen presentation. Upon maturation, DC expresses MHC II and co-stimulatory molecules including cytokines and growth factors which enhance antigen presentation, naïve T cells activation followed by differentiation into TH1, TH2, TH17 and regulatory T cell (Treg). Each T cell subtypes has its own signature cytokines which perform effector functions as well as maintain balance among various other T cell subtypes.

The mechanism underlying differentiation of T cell has been intensively investigated: Stat1 and Stat4 signaling drive TH1 response; Stat6 signaling promotes TH2 whereas Stat3 signaling drives TH17 responses. IL-2 drives TH1 responses and results in (interferon) IFNγ production; that may have carcinogenic effect. However, role of TH2 and TH17 are not well known (Dunn et al., 2006) until recent reports suggest that TH17 may play a pivotal role in *H. pylori*-mediated gastric cancer (Rolig et al., 2011). In addition, nuclear transcription factors, NF-κB are normally activated during *H. pylori* infection. This is not unusual since conditional knock-out mice have shown that NF-κB not only signals epithelial cells to undergo transformation but also myeloid cells which are source of inflammation (Greten et al., 2004, Karin and Greten, 2005). NF-κB in turn promotes IL-6 expression and contribute to carcinogenesis (Naugler and Karin, 2008). Key features that appear to be IL-6 specific are triggering proliferative, pro-angiogenic and anti-apoptotic genes including Stat3 (Yu and Jove, 2004). Under Stat3 signaling, the role of TH17 in case of an enteric bacteria like *H. pylori* become significant. Recent studies have focused on the post-transcriptional modification within naive T cells that are ultimately primed by APCs for proliferation and differentiation into effecter T cell subtypes. Posttranscriptional regulation rather repressions of target genes may be responsible for development of T cell subtypes. On this account miRNA has received much attention in various diseases including cancer. miR-155 is expressed in variety of immune cell type's namely DCs, macrophages, TH1 and TH17 cells. In myeloid cells, miR-155 is induced by TLR and TNFα that in turn activate AP-1 and NF-κB transcription factors (Oertli et al., 2011). miR-155$^{-/-}$ mice show TH2 bias development, signifying miR-155 mediated TH1 response. miRNA is also reported to be involved in TH17 differentiation (O'Connell et al., 2010). It was demonstrated that miR-155$^{-/-}$ mice were incapable of spontaneously arresting *H. pylori* load, lacked vaccine-induced protective immunity and failed to induce infection-associated preneoplastic pathology (Oertli et al., 2011).

The role of Tregs in modulating host immune response during *H. pylori* infection has been speculated for quite a sometime. Tregs are a subset of T cells that suppresses the host immune response and are associated with cancer and parasite infection. These specialized T cells express markers like CD4, CD25, and FoxP3. Tregs increase the tolerance towards self-antigens and at the same time facilitates the growth of tumors through immunosupression. Once differentiated Tregs proliferate and maintain their population through autocrine signaling pathway and starts secreting immunosuppressive cytokines like IL-10 and TGFβ (Joetham et al., 2007). Reports indicate that reduction of Tregs can actually stimulate the immune response against other microbial infections (Belkaid et al., 2002). In recent years, the observation shows that the rate of Treg infiltration in human stomach is proportionate to the degree of inflammation and *H. pylori* density. Interestingly, this study also concluded that Treg infiltration parallels the increased expression of programmed cell death 1(PD-1), a negative regulatory molecule belonging to CD28/B7 family (Wu et al., 2001).

It has been hypothesized that better hygiene in Europe and America has inversely proportional with the rise of asthma, due to lack of early exposure to microbial antigens. Arnold *et al* reported that prior infection with *H. pylori* in neonatal mice increases the number of long lived Treg cells in the airways and thereby checks the development of asthma. In support, the experiments were performed to sensitized mice with ovalbumin to generate primary T cell response, following feeding virulent *H. pylori* to both neonatal and adult mice prior to application of aerosolized allergic antigens. This showed *H. pylori* infected neonatal mice have reduced airway hypersensitivity and less number of immune cells in bronchoalveolar lavage in compared to the control; even to adult mice infected with *H. pylori* (Papatriantafyllou, 2011).

H. pylori induced gastric inflammation relates to both TH1 and TH2 mediated phenomena. *H. pylori* infection was looked out as predominantly TH1 mediated inflammatory pathway. But recent reports show deviation from the earlier notion. Kido et al (2010) demonstrated that in humans, an epithelial derived cytokine, thymic stromal lymphopoitein (TSLP), induces DC-mediated TH2 inflammatory response and thereby triggering B cell activation in *H. pylori*-induced gastritis. *H. pylori* infection results in mixed T cell response. Several studies established the upregulation of TH1 (Bimczok et al., 2011), TH2 (Kido et al., 2010), Treg (Mitchell et al., 2012), TH17 (Shi et al., 2010) subtypes suggesting seems a host immunomodulatory balance for inflammation. TH17 followed by TH1 (Shi et al., 2010) upregulation may promote acute inflammation via IL-17 and gelatinase activity (*refer figure 3)*. The above inflammatory condition is counter balanced by Treg's IL-10 to promote chronic infection by partial immunosuppression. Thus, TH17 plays a significant role to develop inflammation due to *H. pylori* infection, though better understanding of how TH17 is activated during post infection along with its exact role during infection remains open for further investigation. However, post infection when inflammation begin the order of T cell subset activation may be first through TH17, TH1 lymphocytes (Shi et al., 2010) and finely counterbalanced by immunosuppressive Treg activation. Thus, the frequency of tumor-infiltrated Th17 cells decreases in advanced disease human patients. In contrast, tumor-infiltrated Treg increases compared with early disease human patients. Therefore, maintenance of fine tune balance between Treg and TH17 seems crucial (Kao et al., 2010, Maruyama et al., 2010).

6. Tracking the matrix metalloproteinases during infection

Proteinase are a class of enzymes capable of hydrolysing peptide bonds. These biocatalysts are largely classified into two major groups: exopeptidases and endopeptidases, depending on the site of cleaving a peptide bond either proximal or distal to the amino or carboxy termini of the substrate respectively. They are further subdivided into serine proteases, threonine proteases, cysteine proteases, aspartate proteases, metalloproteases, glutamic acid proteases based on their catalytic properties (Hartley, 1960). Source of proteases are mainly restricted to stomach, pancreas and small intestine; where they are utilized for digestion of protein. Matrix metalloproteinases (MMPs) are Zn-requiring endopeptidases, the essential player for ECM remodeling of tissues. The function of MMPs are tightly regulated at several levels by via different mechanisms including synthesis in zymogen, localization in cellular compartments like granules or lysosomes, inhibition by protease inhibitors and inactivation in response to change in pH and/or temperature. However, virulent bacteria colonizing the gut sometime secrete proteases that can directly activate host MMPs, thereby increasing their biochemical efficiency to degrade host's ECM (Löwer et al., 2008). Therefore, disbalance of proteases and/or protease inhibitors play decisive role in chronic inflammation and cancer (Wex et al., 2004). In this chapter we will limit our discussion to MMPs as their role in gastric inflammation as well as in gastric cancer is just relevant (Knapinska and Fields). MMPs comprise more than 29 different proteases that differ in the expression profile, substrate specificity, subcellular localisation and functional implications (Birkedal-Hansen et al., 1993). Among them, gelatinases, (MMP-2 and MMP-9) and stromelysin-1 (MMP-3) collectively cleave gelatins (types I and V), collagens (type IV, V, VII, IX and X), elastin, fibronectin, laminin and proteoglycan core proteins. The activities of MMPs are regulated by the endogenous tissue inhibitors of metalloproteinases (TIMPs), while cytokines, growth factors, tumour promoters and transcription factors including nuclear factor NF-κB and activator protein AP-1 modulate their gene expressions. The balance between MMPs and TIMPs is a critical factor for diverse cellular functions including cellular proliferation, migration, adhesion and apoptosis (Somerville et al., 2003). Based on the important role of certain members of MMPs in cancer, including gastric cancer, they have been studied to a large extent in chronic gastritis and premalignant lesions in the stomach (Pender and MacDonald, 2004, Schuppan and Hahn, 2000).

To explore the role of host proteinases during *H. pylori* infection, *in vivo* models are essential. Although, a majority of *H. pylori* strains do not colonize mouse, the few that do have substantially contributed in understanding the pathogenic mechanism of this bacterium and helped largely in the development of therapeutic strategies against it (Kundu et al., 2011). Because of the ease with which gelatinases MMP-2 and -9 can be assayed in a zymography, host MMP-9 and MMP-2 activities were reported to be first up regulated in *H. pylori* infected gastric mucosa (Kundu et al., 2006, Mori et al., 2003, Kubben et al., 2007). However, reports regarding the expression of TIMP-1 and TIMP-2 in course of *H. pylori* infection are not straightforward. Several studies have reported unchanged or even increased expression of both TIMP-1 and TIMP-2 (Cheng et al. 2012) while a few others claimed decreased expression of TIMP-1 in course of *H. pylori* infection and augmentation of TIMP-1 expression following a course of *H. pylori* eradication therapy (Kundu et al., 2006, Kundu et al., 2011). Reports of other studies soon followed and workers identified several other MMPs including MMP-3, MMP-7, MMP-1, MMP-13 and MT1- MMP as target genes in *H. pylori* infection (Schuppan and Hahn, 2000). While ascribing functionality to these enzymes, localization of MMP-9 expression was observed in the macrophages infiltrating the gastric mucosa that elicited the inflammatory response in the host through activation of cytokine networks (Kundu et al., 2011). A correlation was observed between the expression of MMP-7 and bacterial virulence factor CagA and functionally the MMP-7 upregulation was shown to be involved in the degradation of insulin-like growth factor binding protein-5, leading to higher insulin-like growth factor-II levels that explained epithelial hyper proliferation and stromal expansion in *H. pylori*-infected subjects (Steele et al., 2007). An increasing pool of evidence suggested the increased expressions of several pro-inflammatory cytokines and in *H. pylori*-associated gastro duodenal disorders. Among them, TNF-α and IL-1β are essentially involved in the activation of NF-κB in gastric epithelial cells (Münzenmaier et al., 1997), which in turn induces several inflammatory genes including IL-8, iNOS and several MMPs (Wroblewski et al., 2003). Reports suggested that IL-1β was a key mediator for the induction of

MMP- 1 and -3 in gastric adenocarcinoma (AGS) cells (Wallasch et al., 2002), whereas MMP-9 induction was regulated via the NF-κB pathway(Kundu et al., 2011). Using the ADAM-17 deficient mice, it was shown that this protease is essential for the *H.pylori*-dependent activation of epithelial growth factor receptor (EGFR) and downstream pathways including ERK 1/2 and MMP-7 production(Lee et al., 2003). In addition to the epigenetic dysregulation of MMPs in *H. pylori* infection, several gene polymorphisms in MMP-1, 3, 7 and 9 have been identified to be associated with ulcer disease or gastric cancer (Matsumura et al., 2005, Zhang et al., 2004, Alakus et al., 2010, Dey et al., 2012).

Another way of exploring host-pathogen interaction is to co-culture the parasite and the host cell that it infects. In this regard AGS cell lines co-cultured with *H. pylori* provide a good model to intensely investigate the function of bacterial as well as host secreted MMPs. The functions of bacterial MMPs are currently the focus of investigation. A typical *H. pylori* bacterium has around 1500-1600 genes in its genome, out of which at least 20 are proteases. Notably, a 200 KD zinc-dependent endopeptidase was isolated from *H. pylori* and found to be localized on the bacterial outer membrane and like other MMPs it was also secreted into the conditioned medium. *H. pylori* also co-cultured with AGS cells also expressed MMP-3 like enzyme and TIMP-3 like protein. Moreover, expression of bacterial MMPs and TIMPs suggested the involvement of bacterial type IV secretory system which might transfer Cag A protein into gastric epithelial cells allowing *H. pylori* to modulate host MMP and TIMP mobilization which could trigger the onset of *H. pylori* mediated insult in the host (Windle and Kelleher, 1997, Göõz et al., 2001, Sokolova et al., 2012, Oliveira et al., 2006).

7. Th-17 governs matrix metalloproteases: A pertinent query in clinical therapy

Upon *H. pylori* infection different T cell subtypes in the host having specific surface marker, cytokine profile and transcription factor, arise from CD4+ T cells (Reiner, 2007).The pathways involved in tissue damage during gastritis or gastric adenocarcinoma are complex. However, disruption of tissue architecture is deeply associated with a class of proteases namely MMPs. MMPs are capable of cleaving almost all ECM proteins and connective tissues (Nagase and Woessner, 1999). It has been observed earlier that *H. pylori*-induced gastric ulcer and gastrointestinal diseases are associated with regulation in MMP expression profile and activity profile involved in gastric tissue (Saarialho-Kere et al., 1996, Pender and MacDonald, 2004, Hellmig et al., 2006). The major source of MMP in stomach is gastric epithelial cells (Pillinger et al., 2005, Mori et al., 2003). Several studies were mainly focused on reporting the basic changes occurring on MMPs during infection and the cell signaling cascade associated with it. At the same time, significant reports were published from the immunological perspective upon *H. pylori* infection on the host. However, the story may not complete if we don't connect the two ends of the stick. On a broader view, there are accumulating evidences that T cell secreted cytokines primarily regulate MMP secretion from the gastric epithelial cells (MacDonald et al., 1999),though *in vitro* studies support *H. pylori* can alone stimulate gastric epithelial cell lines to secrete MMPs (Crawford et al., 2003, Bebb et al.), which are collectively responsible for disrupting tissue architecture. The general view is that once *H. pylori* antigen is taken up and presented by antigen presenting cells (APCs) to naïve T cell, the later start to differentiate into specific effecter T cell subsets. These specialized subtypes of T cells start secreting specific cytokines, which ultimately activate gastric epithelial cells to produce specific MMPs.

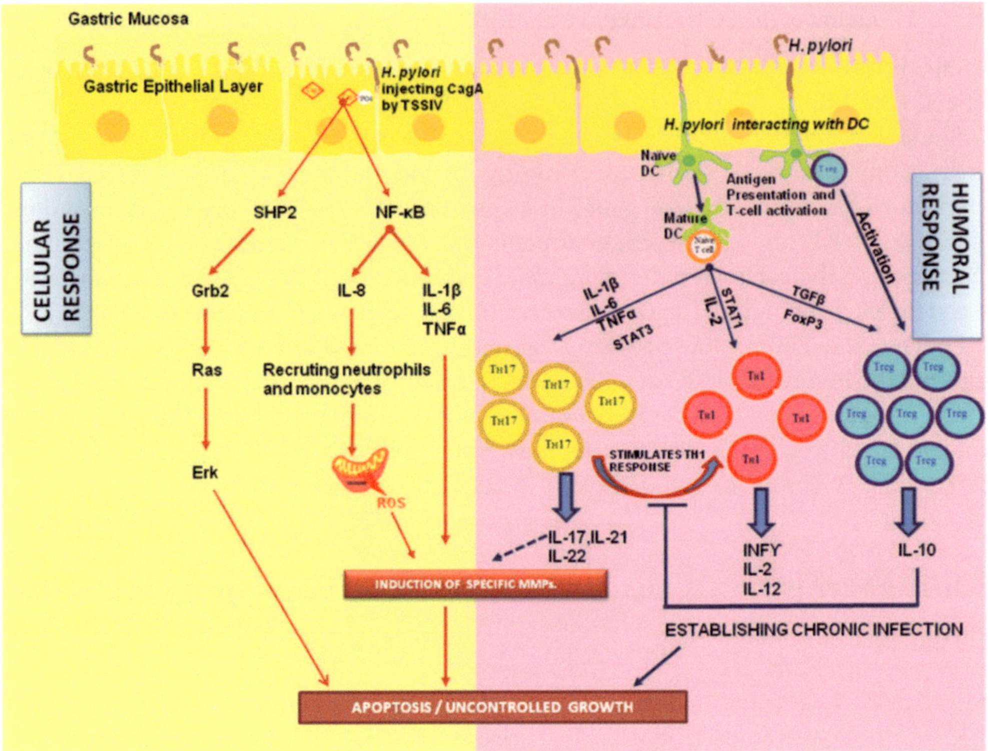

Figure 3. Schematic view of Helicobacter pylori infection and MMPs induction involving both cellular and humoral components. Cellular response: During infection H. pylori injects CagA with their type IV Secretion System (TSSIV) into the gastric epithelial cells. CagA phosphorylation occurs by host's Src/Abl kinases and phosphorylated CagA activates a series of signaling molecules including inflammatory cytokines, ROS, MMPs leading to aberrant cellular function. **Humoral response**: H. pylori prime the host immune system by various lymphocyte subsets through dendritic cells (DC)-mediated antigen presentation to naïve T cell. Under the influence of specific cytokines and foreign antigens the naïve T cells start class switching and differentiate into effector T subtypes via signature transcription factors. TH17 and TH1 promote while Treg arrests inflammatory response by secreting immunosuppressive cytokines; thereby maintaining H. pylori load inside gastric mucosa. TH17 stimulates MMPs through IL-17 and IL-21.

Studies using *in vitro* system document that *H. pylori* infection can induce apoptosis and stimulate release of chemokines from the infected gastric epithelial cells (Cover et al., 2003, Yamaoka et al., 1998, Bhattacharyya et al., 2002). Interestingly, *H. pylori* infection in lymphocyte deficient mice fails to develop gastric inflammation. However, administration of T cells into these animals induces severe gastric ulcer, suggesting T cell mediated inflammatory response play the dominant role in *H. pylori*-mediated mucosal damage (Eaton et al., 1999, Ea-

http://dx.doi.org/10.5772/54193

ton et al., 2001, Smythies et al., 2000). *H. pylori* infection has a strong Th1 response which is mediated by Th1 cytokines including IFN-γ, IL-12, and TNF-α (Ernst and Gold, 2000, D'Elios et al., 1997, Crabtree, 1998, Monteleone et al., 1999, Pender et al., 1997).

Activated CD4+ T cells secrete IL-21, which regulates the growth and functional properties of T cells, B cells, NK cells and DC (Leonard and Spolski, 2005). Of late, it is reported that IL-21 secretes from TH17 in Stat-3 dependent manner and in turn IL-21 can induce IL-17 production the maintaining TH17 cell population in an autocrine manner(Wei et al., 2007). In contrast, IL-21 is also reported as a TH2 secreted cytokine which prevents the differentiation of naive CD4+ T cells into TH1 cells (Wurster et al., 2002). Therefore the role of IL-21 though appears complex, yet it's a crucial cytokine which promotes gelatinase activities during *H. pylori* infection (Caruso et al., 2007). The other studies by Shi et al demonstrated that IL-17 stimulates MMP activity (Shi et al., 2010). Thus, TH17 acting as an initiator of inflammation and MMPs which inturn carry out the effecter function of inflammation. Though, it is yet to be understood on the backdrop of *H. pylori* infection but from the above documents a strong correlation of IL-17 and MMPs is plausible and the TH17-MMP pathway may evolve as one of the crucial one during *H. pylori*-mediated gastric inflammation (*refer figure 3).*

8. Management of *H. pylori* infection and future avenues

As, much greater percentage of the world's population are infected with *H. pylori* compared to the actual number of people developing symptoms so, it may be plausible that host's inflammation due to food habits, hygiene and lifestyle contribute to bacterial susceptibility. In view of this, host's prior inflammatory history may be a dominant issue over virulence of *H. pylori* in the development of gastric diseases. *H. pylori* are known to induce atrophic gastritis and achlorhydria. The later is associated with loss of parietal cells which leads to reduced gastric acid secretion (Fox and Wang, 2007). The rise of intragastric pH above 4.0 accelerates the growth of a range of bacterial species in gastric juice including *H. felis* (Williams and McColl, 2006). In addition to the finding of Cai X *et al.*, that *H. felis*-infected wild type mice developed antral gastric cancer, after prolonged achlorhydria along with undetectable *H. pylori*; Ekstroma *et al* reported the difficulty in detecting *H. pylori* from patients with severe achlorhydria (Ekstrom et al., 2001) (Cai et al., 2005), even though achlorhydric mice develop pathophysical manifestation like gastrin-deficient ones. (Zavros et al., 2005, Zavros et al., 2002).Therefore, *H. pylori*-induced atrophic gastritis and achlorhydria, though progression to severe gastric diseases may be partly contributed by other bacteria including *H. felis*, remain open for further investigation.

The study on tribal populations in India reported that biopsy samples contain strains having *cag* PAI and putatively toxigenic s1 alleles of *vacA*, which contribute to virulence when active, and this is in accord with the high abundance (about 90%) of this strain type in mainstream Indian populations (Mukhopadhyay et al., 2000, Chattopadhyay et al., 2002, Datta et al., 2003). This abundance is also remarkable, in light of the apparent absence of *H. pylori*-associated gastrointestinal disease in these populations suggesting that *H. pylori* infections on an average are less virulent in these ethnic minorities than in mainstream Indians. Such virulence might be due to subtle features of bacterial strains or intricacies of the human host environment. For example, lesser virulence of the *H. pylori* strains themselves might be ascribed to subtle (e.g., point) mutations that affect levels of expression of virulence genes or the potencies of their products, which do not, however, affect outcomes of diagnostic PCR tests (Kersulyte et al., 1999, Philpott et al., 2002).

Antibiotics along with proton pump inhibitors (PPIs) known as 'Triple therapy' have been used for *H. pylori*-infected patients by most physicians for high effectiveness and negligible side effects However, long term 'Triple therapy' in *H. pylori*-infected patients may increase atrophic gastritis (Kuipers et al., 1996). Omeprazole, the potent PPI used to treat reflux esophagitis in *H. pylori*-infected patients, increase the proportion of atrophic gastritis compared to those patients receiving alternative treatments (Berstad et al., 1997, Eissele et al., 1997, Klinkenberg-Knol et al., 2000). In addition, omeprazole initiates dysplasia in *H. felis*-infected mice with over expressed gastrin (Takaishi et al., 2005). Therefore, the effect of long-term PPI treatment over gastric microbiome needs further investigation. Antibiotic treatments not only remove *H. pylori* but also other bacteria from gut microbiota some of which may exacerbate disease condition. In theory, screening and treating patients for *H. pylori* eradication by antibiotics would be economical; only if the probability of reducing gastric disorder is 30% or more (Parsonnet et al., 1996). Studies involving *H. pylori* eradication by antibiotic treatment have shown reduced risk for tumor recurrence (Uemura et al., 1997), or development of gastric cancer (Uemura et al., 2001, Wong et al., 2004) though little or no significant improvement of gastric atrophy with *H. pylori* eradication has been reported (Ruiz et al., 2001). In contrast, even increasing gastro-esophageal reflux is reported after *H. pylori* eradication (Labenz et al., 1997), though other studies do not agree (Moayyedi et al., 2001, Schwizer et al., 2001, Kuipers et al., 2004, Vaira et al., 2003). Therefore, antibiotic treatment to eradicate *H. pylori* in early infected patients may prevent the development of disease; though it still remains unclear whether patients with advanced stages of the disease can benefit from antibiotic intervention. In addition, long-term use of antibiotics kills the beneficial bacteria thereby changing gut microbiota. The later would in turn affect host's metabolic and immunological functions, which may disrupt gut, liver and brain functions (Nicholson et al., 2012). Moreover, the consequence in disease progression yet remains to be explored in the context of modalities of *H. pylori* treatment. Therefore, gut microbiota influence significantly on the host immune system and vice versa (Hooper et al., 2012).

Although, 'Triple therapy' is successful in individual cases, yet the recurrence of bacterial infection especially in highly endemic countries makes vaccination as an alternative approach to standard therapy. However, till date vaccination against *H. pylori* has not shown much promise. Vaccination in various clinical trials of either preventive or therapeutic has failed to generate successful immune response. Vaccination has been tested in many ways. Firstly, intra-gastric immunization has been used in some studies to could efficiently stimulate gastrointestinal immune response. However, this method requires large amount of antigen and adjuvant injection in gastric milieu which potentially raises other side-effects (Wu et al., 2008). Secondly, intranasal immunization against *H. pylori* prove ineffective as it fails to stimulate immune system in stomach and intestine. Moreover, it increases the chance of infection of olfactory bulb of brain (van Ginkel et al.). Finally, sublingual immunization emerges as another approach, in which the vaccine or antigen do not enter the brain (Song et al., 2008). Indeed, sublingual immunization against *H. pylori* strongly induces IFNγ, IL-17 along with increased expression of various integrins and chemokines facilitating the migration of lymphocytes into stomach mucosa (Raghavan et al.).

Though large-scale research is going around the world in relation to *H. pylori* infection, yet day by day the result is becoming exhaustive without a conclusive direction. The bacteria colonize the gastric mucus layer and are continuously faced with harsh physiological conditions and a vigorous immune response. The need for adaptation to the extremely changing micro-environment and to individual hosts (Van Vliet et al., 2002) is probably the cause of a high degree of inter strain genetic variation observed in the *H. pylori* population worldwide. (Blaser, 1994). So, identification of subpopulations at high risk of developing deleterious *H-pylori*-related diseases remains a mainstream challenge for clinicians and basic researchers. In relation to treatment, nothing absolute promising therapeutic has yet arrived in the market. So, the fundamental question that arises is should we treat infection or inflammation with more priority? Since neither antibiotic treatment nor vaccine development have shown much promise in recovery of infected patients. The approach of reducing inflammation may arrest the development of gastric diseases. Epigenetic studies reveal that changes in the DNA methylation pattern during infection are due to inflammation. One possibility entails concurrent infection with particular parasites that may down regulate inflammatory responses to infection, as has been documented in a mouse infection model (Martin et al., 2000). Features of human host genotype might also determine resistance to pathogenic effects of putatively virulent *H. pylori* strains (Ferrero and Fox, 2001, Ferrero and Jenks, 2001). Also, inflammatory cytokines generates ROS within the cells and activate several MMPs that further aggravate the inflammatory response leading towards disease progression. Finally, while many studies have investigated the host genetic factors involved in gastric carcinogenesis (Hishida et al.), but there is an urgent need for extensive studies that will investigate the genetic traits associated with the risk of gastric precancerous conditions. Particularly, studies on polymorphism in the genes involved in host immunity against *H. pylori* infection or the genes essential for the development/ differentiation of the gastric epithelial cells, are the need of the time.

Abbreviations

H. pylori: *Helicobacter pylori*

MMP: matrix metalloproteinase

ECM: extracellular matrix

ROS: reactive oxygen species

TSSIV: type IV Secretion System

IL: interleukin

IFNγ: interferon gamma

DC: dendritic cell

NK cell: natural killer cell

APC: antigen presenting cell

TIMP: tissue inhibitor of metalloproteinase

EGFR: epidermal growth factor receptor

Erk: extracellular signal-regulated kinase

iNOS: inducible nitric oxide species.

NF-κB: nuclear factor kappa B

AP-1: activator protein 1

Treg: regulatory T cell

TH: T helper cell

TGF-β: transforming growth factor beta

miRNA: micro-RNA

SabA: sialic acid-binding protein

VacA: vacuolating associated cytotoxin gene

CagA: cytotoxin-associated gene A

Cag-PAI: cytotoxin-associated gene-pathogenicity island

NOD1: nucleotide-binding oligomerization domain-1

FAK: focal adhesion kinase

dupA: duodenal ulcer promoting gene

BabA: Lewis blood group antigen binding adhesin

ORF: open reading frame

VEGF: vascular endothelial growth factor

TNFα: tumor necrosis factor alpha

GC: gastric cancer

DU: duodenal ulcer

MAPK: mitogen-activated protein kinase

http://dx.doi.org/10.5772/54193

Acknowledgements

The authors are indeed grateful to Prof. Siddhartha Roy, Director, CSIR-IICB, Kolkata, for encouraging and supporting. The authors are thankful to Mr. Sayantan Jana and Mr. Somnath Chatterjee for assisting in referencing and drawing figure respectively.

Author details

Avisek Banerjee**[1], Asish K. Mukhopadhyay**[2], Sumit Paul[1], Arindam Bhattacharyya[3] and Snehasikta Swarnakar[1*]

*Address all correspondence to: snehasiktas@hotmail.com

1 Drug Development Diagnostics and Biotechnology Division, CSIR-Indian Institute of Chemical Biology, Jadavpur, Kolkata, India

2 National Institute of Cholera and Enteric Diseases, Kolkata, India

3 Immunology Lab, Department of Zoology, University of Calcutta, Kolkata, India

**These authors contributed equally to this work.

References

[1] Alakus, H., Afriani, N., Warnecke-Eberz, U., Bollschweiler, E., Fetzner, U., Drebber, U., Metzger, R., Hölscher, A. & Mönig, S. 2010. Clinical Impact of MMP and TIMP Gene Polymorphisms in Gastric Cancer. *World Journal of Surgery*, 34, 2853-2859.

[2] Alam, J., Maiti, S., Ghosh, P., De, R., Chowdhury, A., Das, S., Macaden, R., Devarbhavi, H., Ramamurthy, T. & Mukhopadhyay, A. K. 2012. Significant association of the dupA gene of *Helicobacter pylori* with duodenal ulcer development in a South-east Indian population. *J Med Microbiol*, 61, 1295-302.

[3] Amieva, M. R. & El–Omar, E. M. 2008. Host-Bacterial Interactions in *Helicobacter pylori* Infection. *Gastroenterology*, 134, 306-323.

[4] Amieva, M. R., Vogelmann, R., Covacci, A., Tompkins, L. S., Nelson, W. J. & Falkow, S. 2003. Disruption of the epithelial apical-junctional complex by *Helicobacter pylori* CagA. *Science*, 300, 1430-4.

[5] Arachchi, H. S., Kalra, V., Lal, B., Bhatia, V., Baba, C. S., Chakravarthy, S., Rohatgi, S., Sarma, P. M., Mishra, V., Das, B. & Ahuja, V. 2007. Prevalence of duodenal ulcer-promoting gene (dupA) of *Helicobacter pylori* in patients with duodenal ulcer in North Indian population. *Helicobacter*, 12, 591-7.

[6] Argent, R. H., Burette, A., Miendje Deyi, V. Y. & Atherton, J. C. 2007. The presence of dupA in *Helicobacter pylori* is not significantly associated with duodenal ulceration in Belgium, South Africa, China, or North America. *Clin Infect Dis,* 45, 1204-6.

[7] Argent, R. H., Kidd, M., Owen, R. J., Thomas, R. J., Limb, M. C. & Atherton, J. C. 2004. Determinants and consequences of different levels of CagA phosphorylation for clinical isolates of *Helicobacter pylori*. *Gastroenterology,* 127, 514-23.

[8] Argent, R. H., Zhang, Y. & Atherton, J. C. 2005. Simple method for determination of the number of *Helicobacter pylori* CagA variable-region EPIYA tyrosine phosphorylation motifs by PCR. *J Clin Microbiol,* 43, 791-5.

[9] Atherton, J. C., Cao, P., Peek, R. M., Jr., Tummuru, M. K., Blaser, M. J. & Cover, T. L. 1995. Mosaicism in vacuolating cytotoxin alleles of *Helicobacter pylori*. Association of specific vacA types with cytotoxin production and peptic ulceration. *J Biol Chem,* 270, 17771-7.

[10] Azuma, T. 2004. *Helicobacter pylori* CagA protein variation associated with gastric cancer in Asia. *J Gastroenterol,* 39, 97-103.

[11] Azuma, T., Yamazaki, S., Yamakawa, A., Ohtani, M., Muramatsu, A., Suto, H., Ito, Y., Dojo, M., Yamazaki, Y., Kuriyama, M., Keida, Y., Higashi, H. & Hatakeyama, M. 2004. Association between diversity in the Src homology 2 domain--containing tyrosine phosphatase binding site of *Helicobacter pylori* CagA protein and gastric atrophy and cancer. *J Infect Dis,* 189, 820-7.

[12] Backert, S., Ziska, E., Brinkmann, V., Zimny-Arndt, U., Fauconnier, A., Jungblut, P. R., Naumann, M. & Meyer, T. F. 2000. Translocation of the *Helicobacter pylori* CagA protein in gastric epithelial cells by a type IV secretion apparatus. *Cell Microbiol,* 2, 155-64.

[13] Bebb, J. R., Letley, D. P., Thomas, R. J., Aviles, F., Collins, H. M., Watson, S. A., Hand, N. M., Zaitoun, A. & Atherton, J. C. *Helicobacter pylori* upregulates matrilysin (MMP-7) in epithelial cells in vivo and in vitro in a Cag dependent manner. *Gut. 2003 Oct;52(10):1408-13.*

[14] Beevers, D. G., Lip, G. Y. & Blann, A. D. 2004. Salt intake and *Helicobacter pylori* infection. *Journal of Hypertension,* 22, 1475-1477.

[15] Belkaid, Y., Piccirillo, C. A., Mendez, S., Shevach, E. M. & Sacks, D. L. 2002. CD4+CD25+ regulatory T cells control Leishmania major persistence and immunity. *Nature,* 420, 502-7.

[16] Berstad, A. E., Hatlebakk, J. G., Maartmann-Moe, H., Berstad, A. & Brandtzaeg, P. 1997. *Helicobacter pylori* gastritis and epithelial cell proliferation in patients with reflux oesophagitis after treatment with lansoprazole. *Gut,* 41, 740-7.

[17] Bhattacharyya, A., Pathak, S., Datta, S., Chattopadhyay, S., Basu, J. & Kundu, M. 2002. Mitogen-activated protein kinases and nuclear factor-kappaB regulate *Helicobacter pylori*-mediated interleukin-8 release from macrophages. *Biochem J,* 368, 121-9.

[18] Bimczok, D., Grams, J. M., Stahl, R. D., Waites, K. B., Smythies, L. E. & Smith, P. D. 2011. Stromal Regulation of Human Gastric Dendritic Cells Restricts the Th1 Response to *Helicobacter pylori*. *Gastroenterology,* 141, 929-938.

[19] Birkedal-Hansen, H., Moore, W. G. I., Bodden, M. K., Windsor, L. J., Birkedal-Hansen, B., Decarlo, A. & Engler, J. A. 1993. Matrix Metalloproteinases: A Review. *Critical Reviews in Oral Biology & Medicine,* 4, 197-250.

[20] Blaser, M. J. 1994. *Helicobacter pylori* phenotypes associated with peptic ulceration. *Scand J Gastroenterol Suppl,* 205, 1-5.

[21] Blaser , M. J. 1998. Helicobacters are indigenous to the human stomach: duodenal ulceration is due to changes in gastric microecology in the modern era. *Gut,* 43, 721-727.

[22] Boncristiano, M., Paccani, S. R., Barone, S., Ulivieri, C., Patrussi, L., Ilver, D., Amedei, A., D'elios, M. M., Telford, J. L. & Baldari, C. T. 2003. The *Helicobacter pylori* vacuolating toxin inhibits T cell activation by two independent mechanisms. *J Exp Med,* 198, 1887-97.

[23] Broutet, N., Marais, A., Lamouliatte, H., De Mascarel, A., Samoyeau, R., Salamon, R. & Megraud, F. 2001. cagA Status and eradication treatment outcome of anti-*Helicobacter pylori* triple therapies in patients with nonulcer dyspepsia. *J Clin Microbiol,* 39, 1319-22.

[24] Cai, X., Carlson, J., Stoicov, C., Li, H., Wang, T. C. & Houghton, J. 2005. *Helicobacter felis* eradication restores normal architecture and inhibits gastric cancer progression in C57BL/6 mice. *Gastroenterology,* 128, 1937-52.

[25] Caruso, R., Fina, D., Peluso, I., Fantini, M. C., Tosti, C., Del Vecchio Blanco, G., Paoluzi, O. A., Caprioli, F., Andrei, F., Stolfi, C., Romano, M., Ricci, V., Macdonald, T. T., Pallone, F. & Monteleone, G. 2007. IL-21 is highly produced in *Helicobacter pylori*-infected gastric mucosa and promotes gelatinases synthesis. *J Immunol,* 178, 5957-65.

[26] Censini, S., Lange, C., Xiang, Z., Crabtree, J. E., Ghiara, P., Borodovsky, M., Rappuoli, R. & Covacci, A. 1996. cag, a pathogenicity island of *Helicobacter pylori,* encodes type I-specific and disease-associated virulence factors. *Proc Natl Acad Sci U S A,* 93, 14648-53.

[27] Chattopadhyay, S., Datta, S., Chowdhury, A., Chowdhury, S., Mukhopadhyay, A. K., Rajendran, K., Bhattacharya, S. K., Berg, D. E. & Nair, G. B. 2002. Virulence Genes in Helicobacter pylori Strains from West Bengal Residents with Overt *H. pylori*-Associated Disease and Healthy Volunteers. *Journal of Clinical Microbiology,* 40, 2622-2625.

[28] Chattopadhyay, S., Patra, R., Chatterjee, R., De, R., Alam, J., Ramamurthy, T., Chowdhury, A., Nair, G. B., Berg, D. E. & Mukhopadhyay, A. K. 2012. Distinct repeat motifs at the C-terminal region of CagA of *Helicobacter pylori* strains isolated from diseased patients and asymptomatic individuals in West Bengal, India. *Gut Pathog,* 4, 4.

[29] Cheng, H. C., Yang, H. B., Chang, W. L., Chen, W. Y., Yeh, Y. C. & Sheu, B. S. Expressions of MMPs and TIMP-1 in gastric ulcers may differentiate *H. pylori*-infected from NSAID-related ulcers. *ScientificWorldJournal,* 2012, 539316.

[30] Churin, Y., Al-Ghoul, L., Kepp, O., Meyer, T. F., Birchmeier, W. & Naumann, M. 2003. *Helicobacter pylori* CagA protein targets the c-Met receptor and enhances the motogenic response. *J Cell Biol,* 161, 249-55.

[31] Covacci, A., Censini, S., Bugnoli, M., Petracca, R., Burroni, D., Macchia, G., Massone, A., Papini, E., Xiang, Z., Figura, N. & et al. 1993. Molecular characterization of the 128-kDa immunodominant antigen of *Helicobacter pylori* associated with cytotoxicity and duodenal ulcer. *Proc Natl Acad Sci U S A,* 90, 5791-5.

[32] Covacci, A. & Rappuoli, R. 1998. *Helicobacter pylori*: molecular evolution of a bacterial quasi-species. *Curr Opin Microbiol,* 1, 96-102.

[33] Cover, T. L. & Blanke, S. R. 2005. *Helicobacter pylori* VacA, a paradigm for toxin multifunctionality. *Nat Rev Microbiol,* 3, 320-32.

[34] Cover, T. L., Krishna, U. S., Israel, D. A. & Peek, R. M., JR. 2003. Induction of gastric epithelial cell apoptosis by *Helicobacter pylori* vacuolating cytotoxin. *Cancer Res,* 63, 951-7.

[35] Cover, T. L., Puryear, W., Perez-Perez, G. I. & Blaser, M. J. 1991. Effect of urease on HeLa cell vacuolation induced by *Helicobacter pylori* cytotoxin. *Infect Immun,* 59, 1264-70.

[36] Cover, T. L., Tummuru, M. K., Cao, P., Thompson, S. A. & Blaser, M. J. 1994. Divergence of genetic sequences for the vacuolating cytotoxin among *Helicobacter pylori* strains. *J Biol Chem,* 269, 10566-73.

[37] Crabtree, J. E. 1998. Role of cytokines in pathogenesis of *Helicobacter pylori*-induced mucosal damage. *Dig Dis Sci,* 43, 46S-55S.

[38] Crabtree, J. E., Xiang, Z., Lindley, I. J., Tompkins, D. S., Rappuoli, R. & Covacci, A. 1995. Induction of interleukin-8 secretion from gastric epithelial cells by a cagA negative isogenic mutant of *Helicobacter pylori. J Clin Pathol,* 48, 967-9.

[39] Crawford, H. C., Krishna, U. S., Israel, D. A., Matrisian, L. M., Washington, M. K. & Peek, R. M., JR. 2003. *Helicobacter pylori* strain-selective induction of matrix metalloproteinase-7 in vitro and within gastric mucosa. *Gastroenterology,* 125, 1125-36.

[40] Dey S, Stalin S, Gupta A, Saha D, Kesh K, Swarnakar S. Matrix metalloproteinase3 gene promoter polymorphisms and their haplotypes are associated with gastric cancer risk in eastern Indian population. Mol Carcinog. 2012 Oct;51 Suppl 1:E42-53. doi: 10.1002/mc.21837. Epub 2011 Nov 28.

[41] D'elios, M. M., Manghetti, M., De Carli, M., Costa, F., Baldari, C. T., Burroni, D., Telford, J. L., Romagnani, S. & Del Prete, G. 1997. T helper 1 effector cells specific for

Helicobacter pylori in the gastric antrum of patients with peptic ulcer disease. *J Immunol,* 158, 962-7.

[42] Datta, S., Chattopadhyay, S., Balakrish Nair, G., Mukhopadhyay, A. K., Hembram, J., Berg, D. E., Rani Saha, D., Khan, A., Santra, A., Bhattacharya, S. K. & Chowdhury, A. 2003. Virulence Genes and Neutral DNA Markers of *Helicobacter pylori* Isolates from Different Ethnic Communities of West Bengal, India. *Journal of Clinical Microbiology,* 41, 3737-3743.

[43] De Bernard, M., Cappon, A., Pancotto, L., Ruggiero, P., Rivera, J., Del Giudice, G. & Montecucco, C. 2005. The *Helicobacter pylori* VacA cytotoxin activates RBL-2H3 cells by inducing cytosolic calcium oscillations. *Cell Microbiol,* 7, 191-8.

[44] De Jonge, R., Kuipers, E. J., Langeveld, S. C., Loffeld, R. J., Stoof, J., Van Vliet, A. H. & Kusters, J. G. 2004. The *Helicobacter pylori* plasticity region locus jhp0947-jhp0949 is associated with duodenal ulcer disease and interleukin-12 production in monocyte cells. *FEMS Immunol Med Microbiol,* 41, 161-7.

[45] Ding, H., Nedrud, J. G., Wershil, B., Redline, R. W., Blanchard, T. G. & Czinn, S. J. 2009. Partial protection against *Helicobacter pylori* in the absence of mast cells in mice. *Infect Immun,* 77, 5543-50.

[46] Dong, Q., O'sullivan, M., Hall, W., Herra, C., Kean, C., O'morain, C. & Buckley, M. 2002. Identification of a new segment involved in cagA 3' region variation of *Helicobacter pylori*. *FEMS Immunol Med Microbiol,* 33, 51-5.

[47] Dunn, G. P., Koebel, C. M. & Schreiber, R. D. 2006. Interferons, immunity and cancer immunoediting. *Nat Rev Immunol,* 6, 836-48.

[48] Eaton, K. A., Mefford, M. & Thevenot, T. 2001. The role of T cell subsets and cytokines in the pathogenesis of *Helicobacter pylori* gastritis in mice. *J Immunol,* 166, 7456-61.

[49] Eaton, K. A., Ringler, S. R. & Danon, S. J. 1999. Murine splenocytes induce severe gastritis and delayed-type hypersensitivity and suppress bacterial colonization in *Helicobacter pylori*-infected SCID mice. *Infect Immun,* 67, 4594-602.

[50] Eissele, R., Brunner, G., Simon, B., Solcia, E. & Arnold, R. 1997. Gastric mucosa during treatment with lansoprazole: *Helicobacter pylori* is a risk factor for argyrophil cell hyperplasia. *Gastroenterology,* 112, 707-17.

[51] Ekstrom, A. M., Held, M., Hansson, L. E., Engstrand, L. & Nyren, O. 2001. *Helicobacter pylori* in gastric cancer established by CagA immunoblot as a marker of past infection. *Gastroenterology,* 121, 784-91.

[52] El-Serag, H. B. & Rudolph, K. L. 2007. Hepatocellular carcinoma: epidemiology and molecular carcinogenesis. *Gastroenterology,* 132, 2557-76.

[53] Enroth, H., Kraaz, W., Engstrand, L., Nyren, O. & Rohan, T. 2000. *Helicobacter pylori* strain types and risk of gastric cancer: a case-control study. *Cancer Epidemiol Biomarkers Prev,* 9, 981-5.

[54] Erdman, S. E., Poutahidis, T., Tomczak, M., Rogers, A. B., Cormier, K., Plank, B., Horwitz, B. H. & Fox, J. G. 2003. CD4+ CD25+ regulatory T lymphocytes inhibit microbially induced colon cancer in Rag2-deficient mice. *Am J Pathol,* 162, 691-702.

[55] Ernst, P. B. & Gold, B. D. 2000. The disease spectrum of *Helicobacter pylori*: the immunopathogenesis of gastroduodenal ulcer and gastric cancer. *Annu Rev Microbiol,* 54, 615-40.

[56] Ferrero, R. L. & Fox, J. G. 2001. In Vivo Modeling of Helicobacter-associated Gastrointestinal Diseases.

[57] Ferrero, R. L. & Jenks, P. J. 2001. In Vivo Adaptation to the Host.

[58] Figueiredo, C., Machado, J. C., Pharoah, P., Seruca, R., Sousa, S., Carvalho, R., Capelinha, A. F., Quint, W., Caldas, C., Van Doorn, L. J., Carneiro, F. & Sobrinho-SimoeS, M. 2002. *Helicobacter pylori* and interleukin 1 genotyping: an opportunity to identify high-risk individuals for gastric carcinoma. *J Natl Cancer Inst,* 94, 1680-7.

[59] Fox, J. G., Dangler, C. A., Taylor, N. S., King, A., Koh, T. J. & Wang, T. C. 1999. High-Salt Diet Induces Gastric Epithelial Hyperplasia and Parietal Cell Loss, and Enhances *Helicobacter pylori* Colonization in C57BL/6 Mice. *Cancer Research,* 59, 4823-4828.

[60] Fox, J. G. & Wang, T. C. 2007. Inflammation, atrophy, and gastric cancer. *J Clin Invest,* 117, 60-9.

[61] Fujikawa, A., Shirasaka, D., Yamamoto, S., Ota, H., Yahiro, K., Fukada, M., Shintani, T., Wada, A., Aoyama, N., Hirayama, T., Fukamachi, H. & Noda, M. 2003. Mice deficient in protein tyrosine phosphatase receptor type Z are resistant to gastric ulcer induction by VacA of *Helicobacter pylori*. *Nat Genet,* 33, 375-81.

[62] Gerhard, M., Lehn, N., Neumayer, N., Boren, T., Rad, R., Schepp, W., Miehlke, S., Classen, M. & Prinz, C. 1999. Clinical relevance of the *Helicobacter pylori* gene for blood-group antigen-binding adhesin. *Proc Natl Acad Sci U S A,* 96, 12778-83.

[63] Göõz, M., Göõz, P. & Smolka, A. J. 2001. Epithelial and bacterial metalloproteinases and their inhibitors in *H. pylori* infection of human gastric cells. *American Journal of Physiology - Gastrointestinal and Liver Physiology,* 281, G823-G832.

[64] Greten, F. R., Eckmann, L., Greten, T. F., Park, J. M., Li, Z. W., Egan, L. J., Kagnoff, M. F. & Karin, M. 2004. IKKbeta links inflammation and tumorigenesis in a mouse model of colitis-associated cancer. *Cell,* 118, 285-96.

[65] Guruge, J. L., Falk, P. G., Lorenz, R. G., Dans, M., Wirth, H. P., Blaser, M. J., Berg, D. E. & Gordon, J. I. 1998. Epithelial attachment alters the outcome of *Helicobacter pylori* infection. *Proc Natl Acad Sci U S A,* 95, 3925-30.

[66] Hansson, L. E., Engstrand, L., Nyren, O., Evans, D. J., Jr., Lindgren, A., Bergstrom, R., Andersson, B., Athlin, L., Bendtsen, O. & Tracz, P. 1993. *Helicobacter pylori* infection: independent risk indicator of gastric adenocarcinoma. *Gastroenterology*, 105, 1098-103.

[67] Hartley, B. S. 1960. Proteolytic Enzymes. *Annual Review of Biochemistry*, 29, 45-72.

[68] Hatakeyama, M. 2004. Oncogenic mechanisms of the *Helicobacter pylori* CagA protein. *Nat Rev Cancer*, 4, 688-94.

[69] Hellmig, S., Ott, S., Rosenstiel, P., Robert Folsch, U., Hampe, J. & Schreiber, S. 2006. Genetic variants in matrix metalloproteinase genes are associated with development of gastric ulcer in *H. pylori* infection. *Am J Gastroenterol*, 101, 29-35.

[70] Higashi, H., Nakaya, A., Tsutsumi, R., Yokoyama, K., Fujii, Y., Ishikawa, S., Higuchi, M., Takahashi, A., Kurashima, Y., Teishikata, Y., Tanaka, S., Azuma, T. & Hatakeyama, M. 2004. *Helicobacter pylori* CagA induces Ras-independent morphogenetic response through SHP-2 recruitment and activation. *J Biol Chem*, 279, 17205-16.

[71] Higashi, H., Tsutsumi, R., Fujita, A., Yamazaki, S., Asaka, M., Azuma, T. & Hatakeyama, M. 2002a. Biological activity of the *Helicobacter pylori* virulence factor CagA is determined by variation in the tyrosine phosphorylation sites. *Proc Natl Acad Sci U S A*, 99, 14428-33.

[72] Higashi, H., Tsutsumi, R., Muto, S., Sugiyama, T., Azuma, T., Asaka, M. & Hatakeyama, M. 2002b. SHP-2 tyrosine phosphatase as an intracellular target of *Helicobacter pylori* CagA protein. *Science*, 295, 683-6.

[73] Hishida, A., Matsuo, K., Goto, Y. & Hamajima, N. Genetic predisposition to Helicobacter pylori-induced gastric precancerous conditions. *World J Gastrointest Oncol*, 2, 369-79.

[74] Hooper, L. V. & Gordon, J. I. 2001. Commensal host-bacterial relationships in the gut. *Science*, 292, 1115-8.

[75] Hooper, L. V., Littman, D. R. & Macpherson, A. J. 2012. Interactions between the microbiota and the immune system. *Science*, 336, 1268-73.

[76] Hopkins, R. J., Vial, P. A., Ferreccio, C., Ovalle, J., Prado, P., Sotomayor, V., Russell, R. G., Wasserman, S. S. & Morris, J. G., JR. 1993. Seroprevalence of *Helicobacter pylori* in Chile: vegetables may serve as one route of transmission. *J Infect Dis*, 168, 222-6.

[77] Hussein, N. R. 2010. The association of dupA and *Helicobacter pylori*-related gastroduodenal diseases. *Eur J Clin Microbiol Infect Dis*, 29, 817-21.

[78] Hussein, N. R., Mohammadi, M., Talebkhan, Y., Doraghi, M., Letley, D. P., Muhammad, M. K., Argent, R. H. & Atherton, J. C. 2008. Differences in virulence markers between Helicobacter pylori strains from Iraq and those from Iran: potential importance of regional differences in *H. pylori*-associated disease. *J Clin Microbiol*, 46, 1774-9.

[79] Hwang, H., Dwyer, J. & Russell, R. M. 1994. Diet, Helicobacter pylori Infection, Food Preservation and Gastric Cancer Risk: Are There New Roles for Preventative Factors? *Nutrition Reviews,* 52, 75-83.

[80] Ilver, D., Arnqvist, A., Ogren, J., Frick, I. M., Kersulyte, D., Incecik, E. T., Berg, D. E., Covacci, A., Engstrand, L. & Boren, T. 1998. *Helicobacter pylori* adhesin binding fucosylated histo-blood group antigens revealed by retagging. *Science,* 279, 373-7.

[81] Israel, D. A., Salama, N., Krishna, U., Rieger, U. M., Atherton, J. C., Falkow, S. & Peek, R. M. 2001. *Helicobacter pylori* genetic diversity within the gastric niche of a single human host. *Proceedings of the National Academy of Sciences,* 98, 14625-14630.

[82] Ito, Y., Azuma, T., Ito, S., Miyaji, H., Hirai, M., Yamazaki, Y., Sato, F., Kato, T., Kohli, Y. & Kuriyama, M. 1997. Analysis and typing of the vacA gene from cagA-positive strains of *Helicobacter pylori* isolated in Japan. *Journal of Clinical Microbiology,* 35, 1710-4.

[83] Ito, Y., Azuma, T., Ito, S., Suto, H., Miyaji, H., Yamazaki, Y., Kohli, Y. & Kuriyama, M. 1998. Full-Length Sequence Analysis of the vacA Gene from Cytotoxic and Noncytotoxic *Helicobacter pylori. Journal of Infectious Diseases,* 178, 1391-1398.

[84] Joetham, A., Takada, K., Taube, C., Miyahara, N., Matsubara, S., Koya, T., Rha, Y.-H., Dakhama, A. & Gelfand, E. W. 2007. Naturally Occurring Lung CD4+CD25+ T Cell Regulation of Airway Allergic Responses Depends on IL-10 Induction of TGF-β. *The Journal of Immunology,* 178, 1433-1442.

[85] Jung, H. C., Kim, J. M., Song, I. S. & Kim, C. Y. 1997. *Helicobacter pylori* induces an array of pro-inflammatory cytokines in human gastric epithelial cells: Quantification of mRNA for interleukin-8, -1α/β, granulocyte-macrophage colony-stimulating factor, monocyte chemoattractant protein-1 and tumour necrosis factor-α. *Journal of Gastroenterology and Hepatology,* 12, 473-480.

[86] Kamada, N., Kim, Y. G., Sham, H. P., Vallance, B. A., Puente, J. L., Martens, E. C. & Nunez, G. 2012. Regulated virulence controls the ability of a pathogen to compete with the gut microbiota. *Science,* 336, 1325-9.

[87] Kao, J. Y., Zhang, M., Miller, M. J., Mills, J. C., Wang, B., Liu, M., Eaton, K. A., Zou, W., Berndt, B. E., Cole, T. S., Takeuchi, T., Owyang, S. Y. & Luther, J. 2010. *Helicobacter pylori* Immune Escape Is Mediated by Dendritic Cell–Induced Treg Skewing and Th17 Suppression in Mice. *Gastroenterology,* 138, 1046-1054.

[88] Karin, M. & Greten, F. R. 2005. NF-kappaB: linking inflammation and immunity to cancer development and progression. *Nat Rev Immunol,* 5, 749-59.

[89] Kersulyte, D., Chalkauskas, H. & Berg, D. E. 1999. Emergence of recombinant strains of *Helicobacter pylori* during human infection. *Molecular Microbiology,* 31, 31-43.

[90] Kido, M., Tanaka, J., Aoki, N., Iwamoto, S., Nishiura, H., Chiba, T. & Watanabe, N. 2010. *Helicobacter pylori* Promotes the Production of Thymic Stromal Lymphopoietin

by Gastric Epithelial Cells and Induces Dendritic Cell-Mediated Inflammatory Th2 Responses. *Infection and Immunity*, 78, 108-114.

[91] Klein, P. D., Graham, D. Y., Gaillour, A., Opekun, A. R. & Smith, E. O. 1991. Water source as risk factor for *Helicobacter pylori* infection in Peruvian children. Gastrointestinal Physiology Working Group. *Lancet*, 337, 1503-6.

[92] Klinkenberg-Knol, E. C., Nelis, F., Dent, J., Snel, P., Mitchell, B., Prichard, P., Lloyd, D., Havu, N., Frame, M. H., Roman, J. & Walan, A. 2000. Long-term omeprazole treatment in resistant gastroesophageal reflux disease: efficacy, safety, and influence on gastric mucosa. *Gastroenterology*, 118, 661-9.

[93] Knapinska, A. & Fields, G. B. Chemical Biology for Understanding Matrix Metalloproteinase Function. *Chembiochem*.

[94] Kubben, F. J. G. M., Sier, C. F. M., Schram, M., Witte, T. A. M. C., Veenendaal, R. A., Van Duijn, W., Verheijen, J. H., Hanemaaijer, R., Lamers, C. B. H. W. & Verspaget, H. W. 2007. Eradication of *Helicobacter pylori* Infection Favourably Affects Altered Gastric Mucosal MMP-9 Levels. *Helicobacter*, 12, 498-504.

[95] Kuipers, E. J., Lundell, L., Klinkenberg-Knol, E. C., Havu, N., Festen, H. P., Liedman, B., Lamers, C. B., Jansen, J. B., Dalenback, J., Snel, P., Nelis, G. F. & Meuwissen, S. G. 1996. Atrophic gastritis and *Helicobacter pylori* infection in patients with reflux esophagitis treated with omeprazole or fundoplication. *N Engl J Med*, 334, 1018-22.

[96] Kuipers, E. J., Nelis, G. F., Klinkenberg-Knol, E. C., Snel, P., Goldfain, D., Kolkman, J. J., Festen, H. P., Dent, J., Zeitoun, P., Havu, N., Lamm, M. & Walan, A. 2004. Cure of *Helicobacter pylori* infection in patients with reflux oesophagitis treated with long term omeprazole reverses gastritis without exacerbation of reflux disease: results of a randomised controlled trial. *Gut*, 53, 12-20.

[97] Kundu, P., De, R., Pal, I., Mukhopadhyay, A. K., Saha, D. R. & Swarnakar, S. 2011. Curcumin Alleviates Matrix Metalloproteinase-3 and -9 Activities during Eradication of *Helicobacter pylori* Infection in Cultured Cells and Mice. *PLoS ONE*, 6, e16306.

[98] Kundu, P., Mukhopadhyay, A. K., Patra, R., Banerjee, A., Berg, D. E. & Swarnakar, S. 2006. Cag Pathogenicity Island-independent Up-regulation of Matrix Metalloproteinases-9 and -2 Secretion and Expression in Mice by *Helicobacter pylori* Infection. *Journal of Biological Chemistry*, 281, 34651-34662.

[99] Labenz, J., Blum, A. L., Bayerdorffer, E., Meining, A., Stolte, M. & Borsch, G. 1997. Curing *Helicobacter pylori* infection in patients with duodenal ulcer may provoke reflux esophagitis. *Gastroenterology*, 112, 1442-7.

[100] Lee, D. C., Sunnarborg, S. W., Hinkle, C. L., Myers, T. J., Stevenson, M., Russell, W. E., Castner, B. J., Gerhart, M. J., Paxton, R. J., Black, R. A., Chang, A. & Jackson, L. F. 2003. TACE/ADAM17 Processing of EGFR Ligands Indicates a Role as a Physiological Convertase. *Annals of the New York Academy of Sciences*, 995, 22-38.

[101] Leonard, W. J. & Spolski, R. 2005. Interleukin-21: a modulator of lymphoid proliferation, apoptosis and differentiation. *Nat Rev Immunol,* 5, 688-98.

[102] Leunk, R. D., Johnson, P. T., David, B. C., Kraft, W. G. & Morgan, D. R. 1988. Cytotoxic activity in broth-culture filtrates of Campylobacter pylori. *J Med Microbiol,* 26, 93-9.

[103] Linden, S. K., Sheng, Y. H., Every, A. L., Miles, K. M., Skoog, E. C., Florin, T. H., Sutton, P. & Mcguckin, M. A. 2009. MUC1 limits *Helicobacter pylori* infection both by steric hindrance and by acting as a releasable decoy. *PLoS Pathog,* 5, e1000617.

[104] Logan, R. P. & Berg, D. E. 1996. Genetic diversity of *Helicobacter pylori. Lancet,* 348, 1462-3.

[105] Löwer, M., Weydig, C., Metzler, D., Reuter, A., Starzinski-Powitz, A., Wessler, S. & Schneider, G. 2008. Prediction of Extracellular Proteases of the Human Pathogen *Helicobacter pylori* Reveals Proteolytic Activity of the Hp1018/19 Protein HtrA. *PLoS ONE,* 3, e3510.

[106] Lu, H., Hsu, P.-I., Graham, D. Y. & Yamaoka, Y. 2005. Duodenal ulcer promoting gene of Helicobacter pylori. *Gastroenterology,* 128, 833-848.

[107] Lupetti, P., Heuser, J. E., Manetti, R., Massari, P., Lanzavecchia, S., Bellon, P. L., Dallai, R., Rappuoli, R. & Telford, J. L. 1996. Oligomeric and subunit structure of the *Helicobacter pylori* vacuolating cytotoxin. *J Cell Biol,* 133, 801-7.

[108] Macdonald, T. T., Bajaj-Elliott, M. & Pender, S. L. 1999. T cells orchestrate intestinal mucosal shape and integrity. *Immunol Today,* 20, 505-10.

[109] Mahdavi, J., Sonden, B., Hurtig, M., Olfat, F. O., Forsberg, L., Roche, N., Angstrom, J., Larsson, T., Teneberg, S., Karlsson, K. A., Altraja, S., Wadstrom, T., Kersulyte, D., Berg, D. E., Dubois, A., Petersson, C., Magnusson, K. E., Norberg, T., Lindh, F., Lundskog, B. B., Arnqvist, A., Hammarstrom, L. & Boren, T. 2002. *Helicobacter pylori* SabA adhesin in persistent infection and chronic inflammation. *Science,* 297, 573-8.

[110] Martin, S. L., Borrow, R., Van Der Ley, P., Dawson, M., Fox, A. J. & Cartwright, K. A. V. 2000. Effect of sequence variation in meningococcal PorA outer membrane protein on the effectiveness of a hexavalent PorA outer membrane vesicle vaccine. *Vaccine,* 18, 2476-2481.

[111] Maruyama, T., Kono, K., Mizukami, Y., Kawaguchi, Y., Mimura, K., Watanabe, M., Izawa, S. & Fujii, H. 2010. Distribution of Th17 cells and FoxP3(+) regulatory T cells in tumor-infiltrating lymphocytes, tumor-draining lymph nodes and peripheral blood lymphocytes in patients with gastric cancer. *Cancer Science,* 101, 1947-1954.

[112] Matsumura, S., Oue, N., Nakayama, H., Kitadai, Y., Yoshida, K., Yamaguchi, Y., Imai, K., Nakachi, K., Matsusaki, K., Chayama, K. & Yasui, W. 2005. A single nucleotide polymorphism in the <i>MMP-9</i> promoter affects tumor progression and invasive phenotype of gastric cancer. *Journal of Cancer Research and Clinical Oncology,* 131, 19-25.

[113] Mcclain, M. S. & Cover, T. L. 2003. Expression of *Helicobacter pylori* vacuolating toxin in Escherichia coli. *Infect Immun,* 71, 2266-71.

[114] Mcguckin, M. A., Every, A. L., Skene, C. D., Linden, S. K., Chionh, Y. T., Swierczak, A., Mcauley, J., Harbour, S., Kaparakis, M., Ferrero, R. & Sutton, P. 2007. Muc1 mucin limits both *Helicobacter pylori* colonization of the murine gastric mucosa and associated gastritis. *Gastroenterology,* 133, 1210-8.

[115] Mimuro, H., Suzuki, T., Tanaka, J., Asahi, M., Haas, R. & Sasakawa, C. 2002. Grb2 is a key mediator of *Helicobacter pylori* CagA protein activities. *Mol Cell,* 10, 745-55.

[116] Mitchell, P. J., Afzali, B., Fazekasova, H., Chen, D., Ali, N., Powell, N., Lord, G. M., Lechler, R. I. & Lombardi, G. 2012. *Helicobacter pylori* induces in vivo expansion of human regulatory T cells through stimulating IL-1β-production by dendritic cells. *Clinical & Experimental Immunology,* n/a-n/a.

[117] Moayyedi, P., Bardhan, C., Young, L., Dixon, M. F., Brown, L. & Axon, A. T. 2001. *Helicobacter pylori* eradication does not exacerbate reflux symptoms in gastroesophageal reflux disease. *Gastroenterology,* 121, 1120-6.

[118] Monteleone, G., Macdonald, T. T., Wathen, N. C., Pallone, F. & Pender, S. L. 1999. Enhancing Lamina propria Th1 cell responses with interleukin 12 produces severe tissue injury. *Gastroenterology,* 117, 1069-77.

[119] Mori, N., Sato, H., Hayashibara, T., Senba, M., Geleziunas, R., Wada, A., Hirayama, T. & Yamamoto, N. 2003. *Helicobacter pylori* induces matrix metalloproteinase-9 through activation of nuclear factor kappaB. *Gastroenterology,* 124, 983-92.

[120] Mukhopadhyay, A. K., Kersulyte, D., Jeong, J.-Y., Datta, S., Ito, Y., Chowdhury, A., Chowdhury, S., Santra, A., Bhattacharya, S. K., Azuma, T., Nair, G. B. & Berg, D. E. 2000. Distinctiveness of Genotypes of *Helicobacter pylori* in Calcutta, India. *Journal of Bacteriology,* 182, 3219-3227.

[121] Münzenmaier, A., Lange, C., Glocker, E., Covacci, A., Moran, A., Bereswill, S., Baeuerle, P. A., Kist, M. & Pahl, H. L. 1997. A secreted/shed product of *Helicobacter pylori* activates transcription factor nuclear factor-kappa B. *The Journal of Immunology,* 159, 6140-7.

[122] Nagase, H. & Woessner, J. F., JR. 1999. Matrix metalloproteinases. *J Biol Chem,* 274, 21491-4.

[123] Nakajima, T., Yamashita, S., Maekita, T., Niwa, T., Nakazawa, K. & Ushijima, T. 2009. The presence of a methylation fingerprint of *Helicobacter pylori* infection in human gastric mucosae. *Int J Cancer,* 124, 905-10.

[124] Nakayama, M., Kimura, M., Wada, A., Yahiro, K., Ogushi, K., Niidome, T., Fujikawa, A., Shirasaka, D., Aoyama, N., Kurazono, H., Noda, M., Moss, J. & Hirayama, T. 2004. *Helicobacter pylori* VacA activates the p38/activating transcription factor 2-mediated signal pathway in AZ-521 cells. *J Biol Chem,* 279, 7024-8.

[125] Naugler, W. E. & Karin, M. 2008. The wolf in sheep's clothing: the role of interleukin-6 in immunity, inflammation and cancer. *Trends Mol Med,* 14, 109-19.

[126] Nicholson, J. K., Holmes, E., Kinross, J., Burcelin, R., Gibson, G., Jia, W. & Pettersson, S. 2012. Host-gut microbiota metabolic interactions. *Science,* 336, 1262-7.

[127] Niwa, T., Tsukamoto, T., Toyoda, T., Mori, A., Tanaka, H., Maekita, T., Ichinose, M., Tatematsu, M. & UshijimA, T. 2010. Inflammatory processes triggered by *Helicobacter pylori* infection cause aberrant DNA methylation in gastric epithelial cells. *Cancer Res,* 70, 1430-40.

[128] Nurgalieva, Z. Z., Malaty, H. M., Graham, D. Y., Almuchambetova, R., Machmudova, A., Kapsultanova, D., Osato, M. S., Hollinger, F. B. & Zhangabylov, A. 2002. *Helicobacter pylori* infection in Kazakhstan: effect of water source and household hygiene. *Am J Trop Med Hyg,* 67, 201-6.

[129] O'connell, R. M., Kahn, D., Gibson, W. S. J., Round, J. L., Scholz, R. L., Chaudhuri, A. A., Kahn, M. E., Rao, D. S. & Baltimore, D. 2010. MicroRNA-155 Promotes Autoimmune Inflammation by Enhancing Inflammatory T Cell Development. *Immunity,* 33, 607-619.

[130] Occhialini, A., Marais, A., Alm, R., Garcia, F., Sierra, R. & Megraud, F. 2000. Distribution of open reading frames of plasticity region of strain J99 in *Helicobacter pylori* strains isolated from gastric carcinoma and gastritis patients in Costa Rica. *Infect Immun,* 68, 6240-9.

[131] Odenbreit, S., Puls, J., Sedlmaier, B., Gerland, E., Fischer, W. & Haas, R. 2000. Translocation of *Helicobacter pylori* CagA into gastric epithelial cells by type IV secretion. *Science,* 287, 1497-500.

[132] Oertli, M., Engler, D. B., Kohler, E., Koch, M., Meyer, T. F. & Muller, A. 2011. MicroRNA-155 is essential for the T cell-mediated control of *Helicobacter pylori* infection and for the induction of chronic Gastritis and Colitis. *J Immunol,* 187, 3578-86.

[133] Oh, J. D., Karam, S. M. & Gordon, J. I. 2005. Intracellular *Helicobacter pylori* in gastric epithelial progenitors. *Proc Natl Acad Sci U S A,* 102, 5186-91.

[134] Ohnishi, N., Yuasa, H., Tanaka, S., Sawa, H., Miura, M., Matsui, A., Higashi, H., Musashi, M., Iwabuchi, K., Suzuki, M., Yamada, G., Azuma, T. & Hatakeyama, M. 2008. Transgenic expression of *Helicobacter pylori* CagA induces gastrointestinal and hematopoietic neoplasms in mouse. *Proc Natl Acad Sci U S A,* 105, 1003-8.

[135] Ohshima, H., Tatemichi, M. & Sawa, T. 2003. Chemical basis of inflammation-induced carcinogenesis. *Arch Biochem Biophys,* 417, 3-11.

[136] Oliveira, M. J., Costa, A. C., Costa, A. M., Henriques, L., Suriano, G., Atherton, J. C., Machado, J. C., Carneiro, F., Seruca, R., Mareel, M., Leroy, A. & Figueiredo, C. 2006. *Helicobacter pylori* Induces Gastric Epithelial Cell Invasion in a c-Met and Type IV Secretion System-dependent Manner. *Journal of Biological Chemistry,* 281, 34888-34896.

[137] Owen, R. J., Sharp, S. I., Chisholm, S. A. & Rijpkema, S. 2003. Identification of cagA tyrosine phosphorylation DNA motifs in *Helicobacter pylori* isolates from peptic ulcer patients by novel PCR-restriction fragment length polymorphism and real-time fluorescence PCR assays. *J Clin Microbiol,* 41, 3112-8.

[138] Papatriantafyllou, M. 2011. Asthma: The secret face of *H. pylori*. *Nat Rev Immunol,* 11, 500-501.

[139] Papini, E., De Bernard, M., Milia, E., Bugnoli, M., Zerial, M., Rappuoli, R. & Montecucco, C. 1994. Cellular vacuoles induced by *Helicobacter pylori* originate from late endosomal compartments. *Proc Natl Acad Sci U S A,* 91, 9720-4.

[140] Parsonnet, J., Friedman, G. D., Orentreich, N. & Vogelman, H. 1997. Risk for gastric cancer in people with CagA positive or CagA negative *Helicobacter pylori* infection. *Gut,* 40, 297-301.

[141] Parsonnet, J., Harris, R. A., Hack, H. M. & Owens, D. K. 1996. Modelling cost-effectiveness of *Helicobacter pylori* screening to prevent gastric cancer: a mandate for clinical trials. *Lancet,* 348, 150-4.

[142] Patra, R., Chattopadhyay, S., De, R., Ghosh, P., Ganguly, M., Chowdhury, A., Ramamurthy, T., Nair, G. B. & Mukhopadhyay, A. K. 2012. Multiple Infection and Microdiversity among *Helicobacter pylori* Isolates in a Single Host in India. *PLoS ONE,* 7, e43370.

[143] Peek, R. M., Jr. & Crabtree, J. E. 2006. Helicobacter infection and gastric neoplasia. *J Pathol,* 208, 233-48.

[144] Pender, S. L. & Macdonald, T. T. 2004. Matrix metalloproteinases and the gut - new roles for old enzymes. *Curr Opin Pharmacol,* 4, 546-50.

[145] Pender, S. L., Tickle, S. P., Docherty, A. J., Howie, D., Wathen, N. C. & Macdonald, T. T. 1997. A major role for matrix metalloproteinases in T cell injury in the gut. *J Immunol,* 158, 1582-90.

[146] Philpott, D. J., Belaid, D., Troubadour, P., Thiberge, J.-M., Tankovic, J., Labigne, A. & Ferrero, R. L. 2002. Reduced activation of inflammatory responses in host cells by mouse-adapted *Helicobacter pylori* isolates. *Cellular Microbiology,* 4, 285-296.

[147] Pillinger, M. H., Marjanovic, N., Kim, S. Y., Scher, J. U., Izmirly, P., Tolani, S., Dinsell, V., Lee, Y. C., Blaser, M. J. & Abramson, S. B. 2005. Matrix metalloproteinase secretion by gastric epithelial cells is regulated by E prostaglandins and MAPKs. *J Biol Chem,* 280, 9973-9.

[148] Poppe, M., Feller, S. M., Romer, G. & Wessler, S. 2007. Phosphorylation of *Helicobacter pylori* CagA by c-Abl leads to cell motility. *Oncogene,* 26, 3462-72.

[149] Prinz, C., Schoniger, M., Rad, R., Becker, I., Keiditsch, E., Wagenpfeil, S., Classen, M., Rosch, T., Schepp, W. & GerharD, M. 2001. Key importance of the *Helicobacter pylori*

adherence factor blood group antigen binding adhesin during chronic gastric inflammation. *Cancer Res,* 61, 1903-9.

[150] Raghavan, S., Ostberg, A. K., Flach, C. F., Ekman, A., Blomquist, M., Czerkinsky, C. & Holmgren, J. Sublingual immunization protects against *Helicobacter pylori* infection and induces T and B cell responses in the stomach. *Infect Immun,* 78, 4251-60.

[151] Reiner, S. L. 2007. Development in motion: helper T cells at work. *Cell,* 129, 33-6.

[152] Ren, S., Higashi, H., Lu, H., Azuma, T. & Hatakeyama, M. 2006. Structural basis and functional consequence of *Helicobacter pylori* CagA multimerization in cells. *J Biol Chem,* 281, 32344-52.

[153] Reyrat, J. M., Lanzavecchia, S., Lupetti, P., De Bernard, M., Pagliaccia, C., Pelicic, V., Charrel, M., Ulivieri, C., Norais, N., Ji, X., Cabiaux, V., Papini, E., Rappuoli, R. & Telford, J. L. 1999. 3D imaging of the 58 kDa cell binding subunit of the *Helicobacter pylori* cytotoxin. *J Mol Biol,* 290, 459-70.

[154] Rhead, J. L., Letley, D. P., Mohammadi, M., Hussein, N., Mohagheghi, M. A., Eshagh Hosseini, M. & Atherton, J. C. 2007. A new *Helicobacter pylori* vacuolating cytotoxin determinant, the intermediate region, is associated with gastric cancer. *Gastroenterology,* 133, 926-36.

[155] Rohde, M., Puls, J., Buhrdorf, R., Fischer, W. & Haas, R. 2003. A novel sheathed surface organelle of the *Helicobacter pylori* cag type IV secretion system. *Mol Microbiol,* 49, 219-34.

[156] Rolig, A. S., Carter, J. E. & Ottemann, K. M. 2011. Bacterial chemotaxis modulates host cell apoptosis to establish a T-helper cell, type 17 (Th17)-dominant immune response in *Helicobacter pylori* infection. *Proc Natl Acad Sci U S A,* 108, 19749-54.

[157] Ruiz, B., Garay, J., Correa, P., Fontham, E. T., Bravo, J. C., Bravo, L. E., Realpe, J. L. & Mera, R. 2001. Morphometric evaluation of gastric antral atrophy: improvement after cure of *Helicobacter pylori* infection. *Am J Gastroenterol,* 96, 3281-7.

[158] Saarialho-Kere, U. K., Vaalamo, M., Puolakkainen, P., Airola, K., Parks, W. C. & Karjalainen-Lindsberg, M. L. 1996. Enhanced expression of matrilysin, collagenase, and stromelysin-1 in gastrointestinal ulcers. *Am J Pathol,* 148, 519-26.

[159] Santos, A., Queiroz, D. M. M., Ménard, A., Marais, A., Rocha, G. A., Oliveira, C. A., Nogueira, A. M. M. F., Uzeda, M. & Mégraud, F. 2003. New Pathogenicity Marker Found in the Plasticity Region of the *Helicobacter pylori* Genome. *Journal of Clinical Microbiology,* 41, 1651-1655.

[160] Saukkonen, K., Rintahaka, J., Sivula, A., Buskens, C. J., Van Rees, B. P., Rio, M. C., Haglund, C., Van Lanschot, J. J., Offerhaus, G. J. & Ristimaki, A. 2003. Cyclooxygenase-2 and gastric carcinogenesis. *APMIS,* 111, 915-25.

[161] Schuppan, D. & Hahn, E. G. 2000. MMPs in the gut: inflammation hits the matrix. *Gut,* 47, 12-14.

[162] Schwizer, W., Thumshirn, M., Dent, J., Guldenschuh, I., Menne, D., Cathomas, G. & Fried, M. 2001. *Helicobacter pylori* and symptomatic relapse of gastro-oesophageal reflux disease: a randomised controlled trial. *Lancet,* 357, 1738-42.

[163] Segal, E. D., Cha, J., Lo, J., Falkow, S. & TompkinS, L. S. 1999. Altered states: involvement of phosphorylated CagA in the induction of host cellular growth changes by *Helicobacter pylori. Proc Natl Acad Sci U S A,* 96, 14559-64.

[164] Segal, E. D., Lange, C., Covacci, A., Tompkins, L. S. & Falkow, S. 1997. Induction of host signal transduction pathways by *Helicobacter pylori. Proc Natl Acad Sci U S A,* 94, 7595-9.

[165] Selbach, M., Moese, S., Hauck, C. R., Meyer, T. F. & Backert, S. 2002. Src is the kinase of the *Helicobacter pylori* CagA protein in vitro and in vivo. *J Biol Chem,* 277, 6775-8.

[166] Semino-Mora, C., Doi, S. Q., Marty, A., Simko, V., Carlstedt, I. & Dubois, A. 2003. Intracellular and interstitial expression of *Helicobacter pylori* virulence genes in gastric precancerous intestinal metaplasia and adenocarcinoma. *J Infect Dis,* 187, 1165-77.

[167] Shi, Y., Liu, X.-F., Zhuang, Y., Zhang, J.-Y., Liu, T., Yin, Z., Wu, C., Mao, X.-H., Jia, K.-R., Wang, F.-J., Guo, H., Flavell, R. A., Zhao, Z., Liu, K.-Y., Xiao, B., Guo, Y., Zhang, W.-J., Zhou, W.-Y., Guo, G. & Zou, Q.-M. 2010. *Helicobacter pylori*-Induced Th17 Responses Modulate Th1 Cell Responses, Benefit Bacterial Growth, and Contribute to Pathology in Mice. *The Journal of Immunology,* 184, 5121-5129.

[168] Shiota, S., Matsunari, O., Watada, M., Hanada, K. & Yamaoka, Y. 2010. Systematic review and meta-analysis: the relationship between the *Helicobacter pylori* dupA gene and clinical outcomes. *Gut Pathog,* 2, 13.

[169] Smythies, L. E., Waites, K. B., Lindsey, J. R., Harris, P. R., Ghiara, P. & Smith, P. D. 2000. Helicobacter pylori-induced mucosal inflammation is Th1 mediated and exacerbated in IL-4, but not IFN-gamma, gene-deficient mice. *J Immunol,* 165, 1022-9.

[170] Sokolova, O., Vieth, M. & Naumann, M. 2012. Protein kinase C isozymes regulate matrix metalloproteinase-1 expression and cell invasion in *Helicobacter pylori* infection. *Gut.*

[171] Somerville, R., Oblander, S. & Apte, S. 2003. Matrix metalloproteinases: old dogs with new tricks. *Genome Biology,* 4, 216.

[172] Song, J. H., Nguyen, H. H., Cuburu, N., Horimoto, T., Ko, S. Y., Park, S. H., Czerkinsky, C. & Kweon, M. N. 2008. Sublingual vaccination with influenza virus protects mice against lethal viral infection. *Proc Natl Acad Sci U S A,* 105, 1644-9.

[173] Sperandio, V. 2012. Microbiology. Virulence or competition? *Science,* 336, 1238-9.

[174] Steele, I. A., Dimaline, R., Pritchard, D. M., Peek, R. M., Jr., Wang, T. C., Dockray, G. J. & Varro, A. 2007. Helicobacter and gastrin stimulate Reg1 expression in gastric epithelial cells through distinct promoter elements. *Am J Physiol Gastrointest Liver Physiol,* 293, G347-54.

[175] Stein, M., Bagnoli, F., Halenbeck, R., Rappuoli, R., Fantl, W. J. & Covacci, A. 2002. c-Src/Lyn kinases activate *Helicobacter pylori* CagA through tyrosine phosphorylation of the EPIYA motifs. *Mol Microbiol,* 43, 971-80.

[176] Stein, M., Rappuoli, R. & Covacci, A. 2000. Tyrosine phosphorylation of the *Helicobacter pylori* CagA antigen after cag-driven host cell translocation. *Proc Natl Acad Sci U S A,* 97, 1263-8.

[177] Suerbaum, S. & Michetti, P. 2002. *Helicobacter pylori* infection. *N Engl J Med,* 347, 1175-86.

[178] Suzuki, M., Mimuro, H., Suzuki, T., Park, M., Yamamoto, T. & Sasakawa, C. 2005. Interaction of CagA with Crk plays an important role in *Helicobacter pylori*-induced loss of gastric epithelial cell adhesion. *J Exp Med,* 202, 1235-47.

[179] Takaishi, S., Cui, G., Frederick, D. M., Carlson, J. E., Houghton, J., Varro, A., Dockray, G. J., Ge, Z., Whary, M. T., Rogers, A. B., Fox, J. G. & Wang, T. C. 2005. Synergistic inhibitory effects of gastrin and histamine receptor antagonists on Helicobacter-induced gastric cancer. *Gastroenterology,* 128, 1965-83.

[180] Tanaka, J., Suzuki, T., Mimuro, H. & Sasakawa, C. 2003. Structural definition on the surface of *Helicobacter pylori* type IV secretion apparatus. *Cell Microbiol,* 5, 395-404.

[181] Tartaglia, M. & Gelb, B. D. 2005. Germ-line and somatic PTPN11 mutations in human disease. *Eur J Med Genet,* 48, 81-96.

[182] Telford, J. L., Ghiara, P., Dell'orco, M., Comanducci, M., Burroni, D., Bugnoli, M., Tecce, M. F., Censini, S., Covacci, A., Xiang, Z. & et al. 1994. Gene structure of the *Helicobacter pylori* cytotoxin and evidence of its key role in gastric disease. *J Exp Med,* 179, 1653-58.

[183] Uemura, N., Mukai, T., Okamoto, S., Yamaguchi, S., Mashiba, H., Taniyama, K., Sasaki, N., Haruma, K., Sumii, K. & Kajiyama, G. 1997. Effect of *Helicobacter pylori* eradication on subsequent development of cancer after endoscopic resection of early gastric cancer. *Cancer Epidemiol Biomarkers Prev,* 6, 639-42.

[184] Uemura, N., Okamoto, S., Yamamoto, S., Matsumura, N., Yamaguchi, S., Yamakido, M., Taniyama, K., Sasaki, N. & SchlempER, R. J. 2001. *Helicobacter pylori* infection and the development of gastric cancer. *N Engl J Med,* 345, 784-9.

[185] Vaira, D., Vakil, N., Rugge, M., Gatta, L., Ricci, C., Menegatti, M., Leandro, G., Holton, J., Russo, V. M. & MigliolI, M. 2003. Effect of *Helicobacter pylori* eradication on development of dyspeptic and reflux disease in healthy asymptomatic subjects. *Gut,* 52, 1543-7.

[186] Van Doorn, L. J., Figueiredo, C., Megraud, F., Pena, S., Midolo, P., Queiroz, D. M., Carneiro, F., Vanderborght, B., Pegado, M. D., Sanna, R., De Boer, W., Schneeberger, P. M., Correa, P., Ng, E. K., Atherton, J., Blaser, M. J. & Quint, W. G. 1999. Geographic distribution of vacA allelic types of *Helicobacter pylori. Gastroenterology,* 116, 823-30.

[187] Van Doorn, L. J., Figueiredo, C., Sanna, R., Pena, S., Midolo, P., Ng, E. K., Atherton, J. C., Blaser, M. J. & Quint, W. G. 1998. Expanding allelic diversity of *Helicobacter pylori* vacA. *J Clin Microbiol,* 36, 2597-603.

[188] Van Ginkel, F. W., Jackson, R. J., Yoshino, N., Hagiwara, Y., Metzger, D. J., Connell, T. D., Vu, H. L., Martin, M., Fujihashi, K. & Mcghee, J. R. Enterotoxin-based mucosal adjuvants alter antigen trafficking and induce inflammatory responses in the nasal tract. *Infect Immun. 2005 Oct;73(10):6892-902.*

[189] Van Vliet, A. H. M., Stoof, J., Vlasblom, R., Wainwright, S. A., Hughes, N. J., Kelly, D. J., Bereswill, S., Bijlsma, J. J. E., Hoogenboezem, T., Vandenbroucke-Grauls, C. M. J. E., Kist, M., Kuipers, E. J. & Kusters, J. G. 2002. The Role of the Ferric Uptake Regulator (Fur) in Regulation of *Helicobacter pylori* Iron Uptake. *Helicobacter,* 7, 237-244.

[190] Viala, J., Chaput, C., Boneca, I. G., Cardona, A., Girardin, S. E., Moran, A. P., Athman, R., Memet, S., Huerre, M. R., Coyle, A. J., Distefano, P. S., Sansonetti, P. J., Labigne, A., Bertin, J., Philpott, D. J. & Ferrero, R. L. 2004. Nod1 responds to peptidoglycan delivered by the *Helicobacter pylori* cag pathogenicity island. *Nat Immunol,* 5, 1166-74.

[191] Wallasch, C., Crabtree, J. E., Bevec, D., Robinson, P. A., Wagner, H. & Ullrich, A. 2002. *Helicobacter pylori*-stimulated EGF receptor transactivation requires metalloprotease cleavage of HB-EGF. *Biochemical and Biophysical Research Communications,* 295, 695-701.

[192] Wang, L., Shi, G. G., Yao, J. C., Gong, W., Wei, D., Wu, T. T., Ajani, J. A., Huang, S. & Xie, K. 2005. Expression of endothelial nitric oxide synthase correlates with the angiogenic phenotype of and predicts poor prognosis in human gastric cancer. *Gastric Cancer,* 8, 18-28.

[193] Warren, J. R. 2000. Gastric pathology associated with *Helicobacter pylori*. *Gastroenterol Clin North Am,* 29, 705-51.

[194] Wei, L., Laurence, A., Elias, K. M. & O'shea, J. J. 2007. IL-21 is produced by Th17 cells and drives IL-17 production in a STAT3-dependent manner. *J Biol Chem,* 282, 34605-10.

[195] Wex, T., Treiber, G., Nilius, M., Vieth, M., Roessner, A. & Malfertheiner, P. 2004. *Helicobacter pylori*-mediated gastritis induces local downregulation of secretory leukocyte protease inhibitor in the antrum. *Infect Immun,* 72, 2383-5.

[196] Williams, C. & Mccoll, K. E. 2006. Review article: proton pump inhibitors and bacterial overgrowth. *Aliment Pharmacol Ther,* 23, 3-10.

[197] Windle, H. J. & Kelleher, D. 1997. Identification and characterization of a metalloprotease activity from *Helicobacter pylori*. *Infection and Immunity,* 65, 3132-7.

[198] Wong, B. C., Lam, S. K., Wong, W. M., Chen, J. S., Zheng, T. T., Feng, R. E., Lai, K. C., Hu, W. H., Yuen, S. T., Leung, S. Y., Fong, D. Y., Ho, J. & Ching, C. K. 2004. *Helico-*

bacter pylori eradication to prevent gastric cancer in a high-risk region of China: a randomized controlled trial. *JAMA,* 291, 187-94.

[199] Wroblewski, L. E., Noble, P.-J. M., Pagliocca, A., Pritchard, D. M., Hart, C. A., Campbell, F., Dodson, A. R., Dockray, G. J. & Varro, A. 2003. Stimulation of MMP-7 (matrilysin) by *Helicobacter pylori* in human gastric epithelial cells: role in epithelial cell migration. *Journal of Cell Science,* 116, 3017-3026.

[200] Wu, C., Shi, Y., Guo, H., Zou, W. Y., Guo, G., Xie, Q. H., Mao, X. H., Tong, W. D. & Zou, Q. M. 2008. Protection against Helicobacter pylori infection in mongolian gerbil by intragastric or intramuscular administration of *H. pylori* multicomponent vaccine. *Helicobacter,* 13, 191-9.

[201] Wu, Y. Y., Chen, J. H., Kao, J. T., Liu, K. C., Lai, C. H., Wang, Y. M., Hsieh, C. T., Tzen, J. T. & Hsu, P. N. Expression of CD25(high) regulatory T cells and PD-1 in gastric infiltrating CD4(+) T lymphocytes in patients with *Helicobacter pylori* infection. *Clin Vaccine Immunol,* 18, 1198-201.

[202] Wurster, A. L., Rodgers, V. L., Satoskar, A. R., Whitters, M. J., Young, D. A., Collins, M. & Grusby, M. J. 2002. Interleukin 21 is a T helper (Th) cell 2 cytokine that specifically inhibits the differentiation of naive Th cells into interferon gamma-producing Th1 cells. *J Exp Med,* 196, 969-77.

[203] Yamaoka, Y., Kita, M., Kodama, T., Sawai, N. & Imanishi, J. 1996. *Helicobacter pylori* cagA gene and expression of cytokine messenger RNA in gastric mucosa. *Gastroenterology,* 110, 1744-1752.

[204] Yamaoka, Y., Kita, M., Kodama, T., Sawai, N., Tanahashi, T., Kashima, K. & Imanishi, J. 1998. Chemokines in the gastric mucosa in *Helicobacter pylori* infection. *Gut,* 42, 609-17.

[205] Yamazaki, S., Yamakawa, A., Ito, Y., Ohtani, M., Higashi, H., Hatakeyama, M. & Azuma, T. 2003. The CagA protein of *Helicobacter pylori* is translocated into epithelial cells and binds to SHP-2 in human gastric mucosa. *J Infect Dis,* 187, 334-7.

[206] Yeo, H. J., Savvides, S. N., Herr, A. B., Lanka, E. & Waksman, G. 2000. Crystal structure of the hexameric traffic ATPase of the *Helicobacter pylori* type IV secretion system. *Mol Cell,* 6, 1461-72.

[207] Yu, H. & Jove, R. 2004. The STATs of cancer--new molecular targets come of age. *Nat Rev Cancer,* 4, 97-105.

[208] Zavros, Y., Eaton, K. A., Kang, W., Rathinavelu, S., Katukuri, V., Kao, J. Y., Samuelson, L. C. & Merchant, J. L. 2005. Chronic gastritis in the hypochlorhydric gastrin-deficient mouse progresses to adenocarcinoma. *Oncogene,* 24, 2354-66.

[209] Zavros, Y., Rieder, G., Ferguson, A., Samuelson, L. C. & Merchant, J. L. 2002. Genetic or chemical hypochlorhydria is associated with inflammation that modulates parietal and G-cell populations in mice. *Gastroenterology,* 122, 119-33.

[210] Zhang, J., Jin, X., Fang, S., Li, Y., Wang, R., Guo, W., Wang, N., Wang, Y., Wen, D., Wei, L., Kuang, G. & Dong, Z. 2004. The functional SNP in the matrix metalloproteinase-3 promoter modifies susceptibility and lymphatic metastasis in esophageal squamous cell carcinoma but not in gastric cardiac adenocarcinoma. *Carcinogenesis*, 25, 2519-2524.

Chapter 8

Accumulation of DNA Methylation Changes in the Progression of Gastritis to Gastric Cancer

Zheming Lu and Dajun Deng

Additional information is available at the end of the chapter

http://dx.doi.org/10.5772/53147

1. Introduction

The field of epigenetics describes information transmission through cell divisions of heritable changes of gene transcription activity without DNA sequence changes. Epigenetic information is biologically important for tissue or organ development and cell differentiation. Alteration of epigenetic information is involved in the development of cancers and other diseases. DNA methylation, histone modifications, and transmitted chromatin structure are the underlying mechanisms for epigenetic transmission. Aberrant DNA methylation is found in two distinct forms, hypermethylation and hypomethylation. Global hypomethylation and regional hypermethylation are characterized as two features of human cancer cells [1,2].

The regional hypermethylation involves CpG islands located in the promoter and 5′-exon(s). DNA methylation, the incorporation of a methyl group to the C-5 position of the cytosine ring in the context of 5′-CpG-3′ dinucleotides, which leads to the formation of 5-methylcytosine (5-mC), is the most studied epigenetic change to date in gastric carcinogenesis. Hypermethylation of CpG islands recruits methyl DNA binding proteins, and subsequently histone deacetylases. Deacetylation of the histone tails makes the DNA structure of the promoter into a closed chromatin structure that is inaccessible to transcription factors leading to transcriptional silencing of tumor suppressor genes, mimicking their genetic mutations. Thus, aberrant hypermethylation of these CpG islands acts as an alternative way to genetic changes for the inactivation of tumor suppressor genes. Global hypomethylation at repetitive sequences causes genomic instability. Both types of DNA methylation changes were implicated in the development and progression of cancers [1-3].

It is interesting to note that site-specific gene hypermethylation is an early event in *H. pylori* -related gastric carcinogenesis. Kang *et al.* [4] indicated that gastric cancer (GC) as well as its associated normal mucosa exhibited the highest number of methylated genes when compared the tissues from other organs, including the lung, breast, colon, and liver (Fig. 1). This suggests the possibility that aberrant hypermethylation of CpG islands is more involved in the carcinogenesis in the stomach than in the other human tissues or organs. Methylation changes of some CpG islands can be detected in cancer tissues and morphologically normal gastric tissues from patients with GC or precancerous lesions, including epithelium dysplasia and intestinal metaplasia, but cannot be observed in gastritis lesions or normal gastric tissues from subjects without malignant disease.

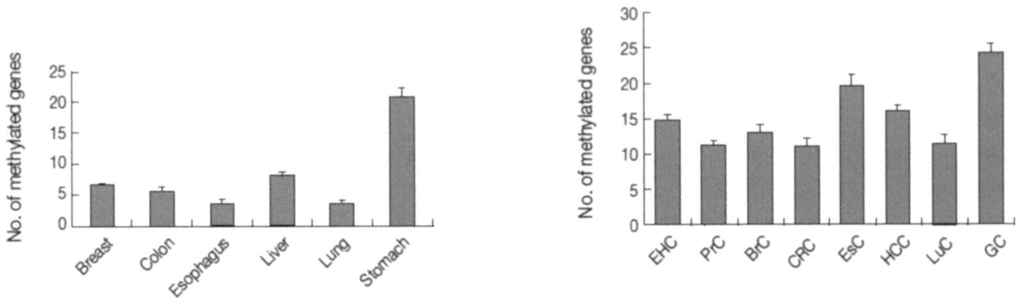

Figure 1. Bar graphs display the number of methylated genes in cancer-associated normal tissues (A) and cancer tissues (B). [4] The error bars indicate the standard error of the mean. Forty-one genes are analyzed for their methylation status in tissue samples from eight human cancer tissue types and six types of cancer-associated normal tissue using the MethyLight assay. EHC, extrahepatic bile duct cancer; PrC, prostate adenocarcinoma; BrC, breast adenocarcinoma; CRC, colorectal adenocarcinoma; EsC, esophageal adenocarcinoma; HCC, hepatocellular carcinoma; LuC, lung adenocarcinoma; GC, gastric adenocarcinoma.

2. Accumulation of DNA methylation changes in progressions of gastritis, intestinal metaplasia, and dysplasia to GC

As early as in the 19th century, a German pathologist von Waldeyer stated that 'cancer, in particular gastric cancer, may be considered an adaptive response to an adverse environment, characterized by a progressive phenotypic alteration.' Currently, it is well accepted that the phenotypic transformation preceding GC, that is, superficial gastritis, chronic atrophic gastritis (CAG), intestinal metaplasia, and dysplasia/adenoma, are the consequences of an accumulation of molecular alterations triggered by a chronic inflammatory process [5,6]. Therefore, the progressive phenotypic alteration could at times represent an altered epigenome, which is the result of host adaptive responses to environmental exposure. If hypermethylation of promoter CpG islands of some genes plays an important role in the malignant transformation of gastric epithelial cells, it's reasonable to assume that the pattern of hypermethylation could be found in premalignant lesions in the stomach. Kang *et al.* investigated the methylation profile in multistep lesions of the stomach and determined the methylation frequency of 12 genes, including APC, COX-2,DAP-kinase, E-cadherin, GSTP1, hMLH1, MGMT, p16, p14, RASSF1A, THBS1, and TIMP3, by methylation-specific PCR.They demonstrated that hypermethylation of certain promoter CpG islands occurs early in gastric carcinogenesis and accumulates during progression of the gastric lesion along the multistep carcinogenesis [7-9]. Tables 1 lists the methylation frequencies of tested CpG islands. The most tested CpG islands exhibited increase methylation tendency along the progression, such as COX-2, DAP-kinase, GSTP1, hMLH1, p14, p16, RASSF1A, THBS1, and TIMP-3. The average number of methylated genes was 2.7, 3.6, 3.4, and 5.2 per 12 tested genes in CG, IM, GA, and GC, respectively. Methylation index was defined as ratio of the number of methylated genes to the number of total tested genes. The average methylation index was 0.23, 0.3, 0.28, and 0.43 in chronic gastritis, intestinal metaplasia, adenoma, and cancer, respectively. The methylation index was significantly higher for precancerous lesions intestinal metaplasia and adenoma than for gastritis. A significant increase of methylation frequency was observed from these pre-malignant lesions to gastric cancer [8].

	CG(N=74) (%)	IM(N=57) (%)	GA(N=79) (%)	GC(N=80) (%)	p value
APC	48 (64.9)	46 (80.7)	57 (72.2)	62 (77.5)	NS[a]
COX2	1 (2.2)	5 (8.8)	3 (3.8)	37 (46.3)	< 0.001
DAP-K	26 (35.1)	28 (49.1)	27 (34.2)	45 (56.3)	0.012
E-cadherin	63 (85.1)	41 (71.9)	46 (58.2)	53 (67.5)	0.003
GSTP1	0	0	0	13 (16.3)	< 0.001
hMLH1	0	4 (7)	7 (8.9)	16 (20)	< 0.001
MGMT	11 (14.9)	5 (8.8)	8 (10.1)	17 (21.3)	NS
p14	22 (29.7)	18 (31.6)	60 (75.9)	50 (62.5)	< 0.001
p16	2 (2.7)	4 (7)	9 (11.4)	35 (43.8)	< 0.001
RASSF1A	0	0	0	6(7.5)	0.001
THBS1	13 (17.6)	28 (49.1)	27 (34.2)	45 (56.3)	< 0.001
TIMP3	17 (23)	25 (43.9)	22 (27.8)	52 (65)	< 0.001
Average number of methylated genes	2.7[b]	3.6[c,d]	3.4[b,c]	5.2[d]	
methylation index	0.23	0.3	0.28	0.43	

[a]Not significant ($p>0.05$).

[b] Chronic gastritis versus gastric adenoma; $p = 0.034$; Student's t test.

[c] Intestinal metaplasia versus gastric adenoma; $p = 0.527$; Student's t test.

[d] Intestinal metaplasia versus gastric carcinoma; $p < 0.001$; Student's t test.

Table 1. Methylation Frequency of Each Gene in CG, IM, GA, and GC [8]

During multistep gastric carcinogenesis, there is a steep rise in the number of methylated genes from chronic gastritis to intestinal metaplasia, which was a consistent finding in a series of studies. Intestinal metaplasia is a precancerous lesion with the typical characteristics of trans-differentiation of gastric progenitor cells into those committed to intestinal cell lineage, which normally present in intestinal mucosa [10]. Regardless of the status of H. pylori infection, the number of methylated genes in chronic gastritis with intestinal metaplasia was significantly higher than that in chronic gastritis without intestinal metaplasia[9]. This suggests that intestinal metaplasia is an epigenetically altered lesion. Hypermethylation of promoter CpG island in chronic gastritis without intestinal metaplasia occurs in association with *H. pylori* infection [11] and aging [12,13]. It is unknown whether trans-differentiation results in these epigenetic changes.

Although the loss of DNA methylation was the first epigenetic alteration identified in cancer[14], global hypomethylation has been overlooked in favor of gene promoter associated hypermethylation. Global DNA hypomethylation is associated with hypomethylation of normally methylated repetitive sequences, such as LINE1, Alu, and Satα, as well as centromeres and microsatellite DNA [15, 16]. In a recent study, using the immunohistochemical evaluation of 5-mC, Compare *et al.* [6] have found a gradual decrease in the global DNA methylation from *H. pylori*-negative normal gastric biopsy to *H. pylori*-positive chronic gastritis lesions, *H. pylori*-positive CAG, and GC tissues, which suggests that the global DNA hypomethylation could be implicated in *H. pylori*-related gastric carcinogenesis at an early stage. *H. pylori*-eradication can not reverse the global hypomethylation in precancerous lesions. This has been confirmed by assessing hypomethylation of repetitive sequences instead of by the global 5-methylcytosine content. Yoshida *et al.* [17] have reported increased hypomethylation of DNA repetitive elements through the multistep process of gastric carcinogenesis and suggested that *H. pylori* infection may induce hypomethylation of repetitive elements. Although the exact mechanism by which the global loss of DNA methylation contributes to the neoplastic process is unknown, it is believed that it may induce chromosomal instability and activate cellular proto-oncogenes, which leading to an increased risk of cancer. Bester *et al.* have reported that nucleotide deficiency promotes genomic instability in early stages of cancer development [18]. It is interesting to investigate if the nucleotide deficiency also leads to the global hypomethylation.

Indeed, hypomethylation and hypermethylation of CpG islands in the gene promoter region may activate proto-oncogenes or inactivate tumour suppressor genes that confer selective growth advantage leading ultimately to cell hyperproliferation and cancerous growth [19,20].

3. Dynamic DNA methylation related to progression of gastritis

The stomach is one of the organs frequently showing aberrant methylation of CpG islands in epithelial cells because it is directly contacted with chemical and biological toxic agents daily. DNA methylation changes accumulate continuously during progression of gastritis, particularly during the establishment of the methylation pattern. Dynamic changes of methylation pattern occur consistently for gastric mucosae cells adapting to the environmental causal factors such as *H. pylori* infection, high concentration of salts, and N-nitroso compounds. For example, on one hand, *p16* inactivation by methylation in cancer cells is very stable. Methylation of *p16* CpG islands can be gradually restored within about two weeks after demethylation induced by DNMT1 inhibitor treatment [21]. On the other hand, *p16* methylation in gastric tissues can be reversed after *H. pylori* eradication, which will discuss below. This fluctuation nature can be partially explained by the dynamic induction of methylation/demethylation.

3.1. Association between methylation of CpG islands and environmental/dietary factors, lifestyle, aging in gastric carcinogenesis

Despite strong evidences from observational epidemiology data and experimental animal studies suggesting that environmental/dietary factors, lifestyle, and aging are risk factors of gastric cancer, there has been limited understanding of the mechanisms through which such exposures have their effects on the molecular steps in tumorigenesis. It is now becoming apparent that altered epigenetic marks may play a fundamental role in determining not only susceptibility to cancer, but also contribute to promote neoplastic pathogenesis. Alternatively, the altered epigenome could at times represent adaptive responses to environmental exposure.

Environmental factors known to play crucial roles in the etiology of human cancer include chemical carcinogens (such as those found in cigarette smoke), microorganism infections, dietary contaminants (such as N-nitroso compounds), and lifestyles (such as alcohol consumption, excess intake of salt), deficiency of nutritional regimes. Stress may also contribute to the development of gastric cancer. Environmental and dietary factors in animals and humans inevitably affect epigenetic patterns, although a clear-cut causal relationship has yet to be established. The major obstacle in establishing such relationship is the fact that environmental and dietary factors induce changes are most likely subtle and cumulative, and culminate into a quantitative manifestation over a long period of time.

While animal and human studies have linked dietary factors to epigenetic regulation, it has been challenging to determine the exact mechanisms that nutrients may systemically affect epigenetic changes. The most studied and best-understood fact is the relationship between dietary methyl donors (including vitamins B6 and B12, methionine, and folate) and DNA methylation [22]. As an essential amino acid, methionine plays the central role in the epigenetic regulation by serving as a methyl donor for methylation reactions. In the process of cytosine methylation, DNMT enzyme converts the donor S-adenosyl-L-methionine (SAM) to S-adenosylhomocysteine (SAH), and transfers a methyl group from the donor SAM to the C-5 cytosine carbon atom. Therefore, an optimal supply of SAM or removal of SAH is essential for a normal establishment of genome-wide DNA methylation patterns. When methyl groups are in short supply, there is a competition for the limited resources. Perturbations in this system may be caused by dietary imbalances affecting the supply of methyl donors such as folate.

Because humans tend to consume foods and nutrients that are highly interrelated, study of dietary patterns may have improved the power of detecting the effect of diet on DNA methylation. In humans, studies on diet and DNA methylation have yielded inconsistent findings.Animal studies have provided direct evidence that dietary factors induce changes in DNA methylation patterns. Bai *et al.* investigated whether p16 hypermethylation is an early and frequent event in gastric carcinogenesis induced by N-methyl-N'-nitro-N-nitrosoguanidine (MNNG).The frequency and timing of *p16* hypermethylation during the multistep gastric carcinogenesis in Wistar rats were analyzed in various microdissected gastric lesions. Our group has found that *p16* methylation is a frequent and early event during MNNG-induced gastric carcinogenesis of rats [23]. The frequency of *p16* methylation is positively correlated with the severity of pathological abnormality of mucosa and negatively correlated with the expression of P16. The *p16* methylation in the distal glandular stomach epithelium was higher than that in the proximal stomach. These results suggest that hypermethylation of CpG islands may account for the silencing of *p16* in rat stomach and is an early event whose accumulation will finally lead to gastric carcinogenesis [23].(Table 2)

Pathological status	Proximal	Distal	Total
Normal	0/16(0)	1/20(5.0)	1/36(2.8)
Chronic atrophic gastritis	3/20(15.0)	1/4(25.0)	4/24(16.7)
Dysplasia	3/13(23.1)	6/11(54.5)	9/24(37.5)[a]
Adenoma II	4/6(66.7)	11/17(64.7)	15/23(65.0)[a]
Adenoma I	4/6(66.7)	10/14(71.4)	14/20(70.0)[a,b]
Adenocarcinoma	5/5(100)	18/22(81.8)	23/27(85.2)[a,b,c]
Total	19/66(28.8)	47/88(53.4)[d]	

[a]Normal vs. dysplasia, adenoma-I/II, and adenocarcinoma, $P<0.001$.

[b]Chronic atrophic gastritis vs. adenoma-I and adenocarcinoma, $P<0.001$.

[c]Dysplasia vs. adenocarcinoma, $P<0.002$.

[d]Proximal vs. distal, $P<0.001$.

Table 2. Frequency (%) of p16 methylation in tumors and various precancerous tissues of rat glandular stomach by MNNG [23]

Promoter methylation is also present in non-neoplastic cells as an age-related tissue-specific phenomenon. Aging was first revealed to be an methylation inducing factor of *ER* methylation in colonic mucosae [24]. The correlation between high incidence of gastric cancers in older people and high methylation frequency of CpG islands suggests the link of aging and cancer via increased methylation changes of CpG islands. Waki *et al.* [12] found that methylation of *E-cadherin* and *p16* was not seen in non-neoplastic cells of organs from people (n=6; ≤22 years old). In contrast, these genes were methylated in non-neoplastic gastric epithelial cells of persons (n=14; ≥45 years old) 86% and 29%, respectively. Considering that non-neoplastic gastric mucosae from GC patients harbor higher methylation levels of CpG islands than gastric mucosae from control patients without GC, these non-cancer subjects with high methylation levels of CpG islands are expected to be at increased risk of GC. The finding that the stomach is one of the organs with a high frequency of aging-related methylation is consistent with the finding that GC is one of the tumors with a high frequency of CpG island methylation. The causes for high frequency of DNA methylation in the stomach may be related to the accumulation of the gastric mucosa to exogenous agents or a set of programmed aging events.

3.2. Induction of aberrant DNA methylation in gastric mucosa by H. pylori infection

Up to 80% of GC patients have a current or past *H. pylori* infection [25]. World Health Organization has designated *H. pylori* as a human class I carcinogen for gastric malignancy. Although the exact mechanism of *H. pylori*-associated gastric carcinogenesis is still elusive, long-standing bacterial infection, perpetuated chronic inflammation, and sustained mucosal epithelial cell proliferation are thought to produce a carcinogenic environment which gradually causes epigenetic reprogramming of host cells in the stomach. Chan *et al.* [11] were the first to demonstrate *H. pylori*-associated hypermethylation in the gastric epithelia, which was consist with a recent study established the correlation between *H. pylori* infection and high levels of aberrant DNA methylation in gastric cancer. Maekita *et al.* [26] compared methylation levels in the non-cancerous gastric mucosae of GC and non-cancer patients with and without *H. pylori* infection, respectively. They found that methylation levels of several CpG islands in H. pylori-positive individuals were 5.4- to 303-fold higher than those in H. pylori-negative individuals [27]. They also found that, among *H. pylori*-negative individuals, methylation levels were 2.2- to 32-fold higher in the non-cancerous gastric mucosae of GC patients than in the normal gastric mucosa of healthy individuals. (Fig. 2)

The fraction of methylated DNA molecules was quantified for eight regions of seven genes using DNA from the antral noncancerous gastric mucosae. Methylation levels increased in individuals with *H. pylori* infection whether or not they had gastric cancer. When methylation levels were compared among individuals without *H. pylori* infection, they were clearly higher in gastric cancer patients than in healthy volunteers. *Error bars*: standard errors

Our group studied the *p16* methylation among 920 subjects with gastric lesions and its association with *H. pylori* infection. The frequency of *p16* methylation was significantly higher in *H. pylori* positive subjects than *H. pylori* negative subjects in each category of gastric lesion. Compared with *H. pylori* negative, the odd ratios (ORs) of *p16* methylation were markedly elevated in *H. pylori* positive subjects for superficial gastritis (OR, 9.45; 95% confidence interval [CI]: 2.94–30.41), chronic atrophic gastritis (OR, 15.92; 95%CI: 7.60–33.36), intestinal metaplasia (OR, 4.46; 95%CI: 2.44–8.13), indefinite dysplasia (OR, 3.67; 95%CI:,1.90–7.10), and dysplasia (OR, 2.48; 95%CI: 1.02–5.99).(table 4) Moreover, the frequencies of *p16* methylation increased steadily with the *H. pylori* density in gastric mucosa [28]. (table 3)

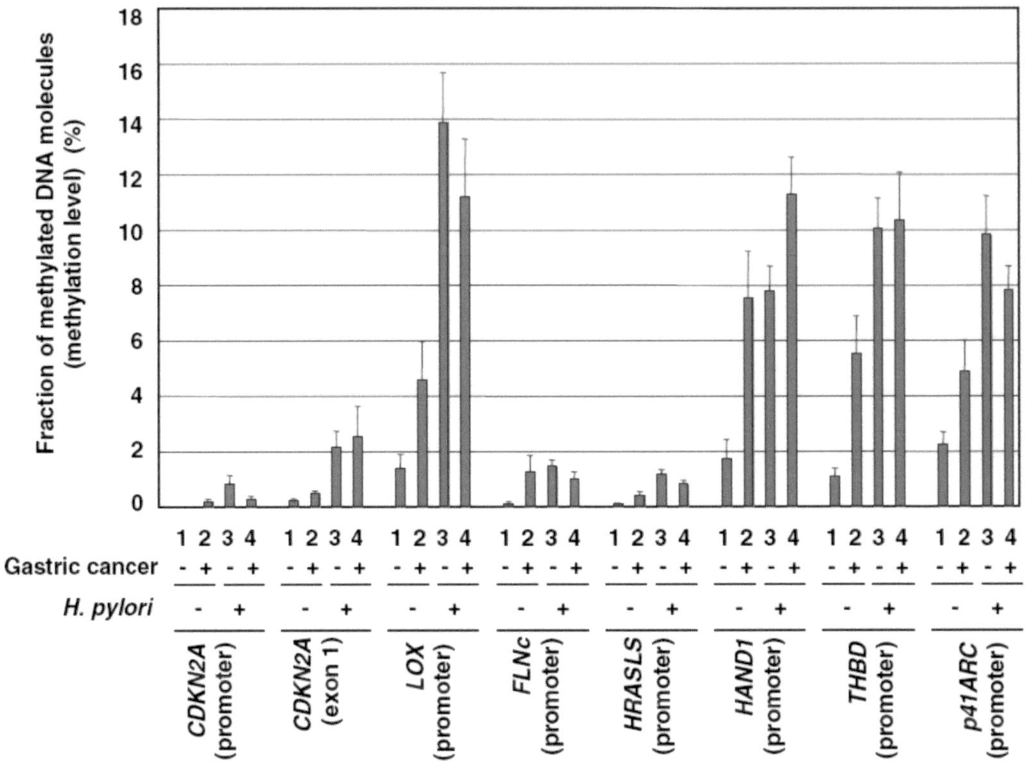

Figure 2. Methylation levels in the noncancerous gastric mucosae of individuals with and without H. pylori infection, and with and without gastric cancer[27].

Pathological category	*H.pylori* status	Methylation frequency of *p16*	*p* value[1]	OR[2](95%CI)
SG	No	18.6% (11/59)	<0.001	1.00
	Yes	68.4%(13/19)		9.45(2.94-30.41)
CAG	No	21.5%(14/65)	<0.001	1.00
	Yes	81.8%(108/132)		15.92(7.60-33.36)
IM	No	23.3%(20/86)	<0.001	1.00
	Yes	57.0%(81/142)		4.46(2.44-8.13)
Ind DYS	No	36.7%(18/49)	<0.001	1.00
	Yes	67.4%(145/215)		3.67(1.90-7.10)
DYS	No	24.3%(9/37)	<0.001	1.00
	Yes	45.5%(35/77)		2.48(1.02-5.99)

[1]Pearson's x^2 test.-[2]adjusted for gender, age, smoking and drinking.

Table 3. p16 Methylation Associated With H. Pylori Infection by Paathological Category [28]

Eradiation of *H. pylori* infection could not reverse all epigenetic changes in gastric mucosae. Leung *et al.* [29] have reported that one year after *H. pylori* eradication, there is a marked reduction in the mean methylation density of the *CDH1* gene in both the promoter region and exon-1. Perri *et al.* [30] have observed partial regression of epigenetic events one year after successfully eradicating of *H. pylori* infection therapy. *CDH1*, *p16*, and *APC* methylation significantly decrease while *COX2* methylation completely disappear. Moreover, an animal model was adopted to strengthen these findings. *H. pylori* infection is best modeled in Mongolian gerbils. The incidence of gastric cancers in gerbils depends on the duration of *H. pylori* infection, and eradication of *H. pylori* significantly reduces the incidence [31]. Thus, this model is expected to be useful in analyzing detailed molecular mechanisms for induction of aberrant DNA methylation.Mongolian gerbils experimentally infected with *H. pylori* and subsequent genome-wide screening exhibited hypermethylation at several CpG islands in the gastric mucosae. Methylation levels started to increase 5-10 weeks after the infection, reached high levels by 50 weeks. Clearance of the infection resulted in markedly decreased methylation levels 10 and 20 weeks later, but they remained elevated compared with that in non-infected animals [32,33]. Thus, it is strongly in support of the potential beneficial effects of *H. pylori* eradication on the reversal of promoter hypermethylation in the non-cancerous stomach and possibly on chemoprevention of GCs. These findings also suggest that some methylation changes induced by *H. pylori* infection are temporary and some of them are persistent which is not dependent on consistent *H. pylori* infection.

The dynamic and reversible nature of methylation profile could be explained by an old concept that stem cells may be the cellular origin of cancer. Although it is unknown which methylation changes in the genome are reversible or not, one of the possible mechanisms for the diverse fates of methylation of CpG islands is that the fates of methylation is dependent on the fates of host cells in which the methylation occurs. The aberrant methylations are likely temporary events if they occur in fully or partially differentiated epithelial cells, because most gastric epithelial cells will quickly drop off from the gastric epithelium through regular regeneration within several days. The methylation changes are likely permanent if they occur in tissue stem cells, because these cells will remain for life-time in the stomach and even benefit from these changes. It is reported that the temporary component is the one that disappears after eradicating the infection [34-36]. Further works have demonstrated the existence of gene specificity in the DNA hypermethylation induced by infection. Methylation of specific genes that occurs in a significant number of cells in the mucosa establishes an 'epigenetic field for cancerisation' or 'epigenetic field defect', characterizing a site with high risk for subsequent malignant transformation [33, 37].

Although the mechanistic understanding of the *H. pylori*-induced alteration of DNA methylation is limited, one plausible explanation is mediated by interleukin-1 beta (IL-1β). The level of IL-1β in gastric mucosa is up-regulated in specimens infected with both cagA positive and negative *H. pylori* strains [38,39]. Furthermore, Hmadcha *et al.* [40] have found that IL-1β, through the production of nitric oxide (NO) and the subsequent activation of DNA methyltransferase, may induce CpG island methylation. NO is a gaseous free radical which can be produced intracellularly by nitric oxide synthase (NOS)-mediated oxidation of arginine or formed in the acidic stomach through the alternative nitrate-dependent NO pathway. *H. pylori* infection has been shown to be associated with up-regulation of inducible nitric oxide synthase (iNOS) both *in vivo* and *in vitro*[41,42]. Increased iNOS activity has been observed in both patients with chronic gastritis and GC patients [43]. In addition, IL-1β siRNA blocked *H. pylori*-induced methylation of the *CDH1* promoter CpG island in a gastric cancer cell line [44]. In an animal experiment by the Ushijima team, it has found that *H. pylori* infection induces hypermethylation of CpG island of candidate genes, and that the eradication leads to marked decrease of methylation levels in these genes [32]. Notably, the suppression of inflammation by treatment of the immunosuppressive drug cyclosporine, which suppresses inflammation without affecting bacterial colonization, abolishes this aberrant methylation in the candidate genes. These findings suggest that the infection-associated inflammatory process, rather than *H. pylori* itself, was responsible for the induction of the hypermethylation. However, in their subsequent gerbil study, neutrophilic inflammation caused by treatment with ethanol or NaCl does not induce DNA methylation in these genes, whereas chronic inflammation caused by *H. pylori* or *H. felis* infection leads to altered methylation in candidate genes. This finding suggests that it is not the inflammation itself, but rather specific types of inflammation, that are necessary for methylation induction[32].

3.3. Spread of *de novo* methylation of *p16* CpG island from normal mucosae, gastritis, to gastric carcinoma

It has been reported that *p16* methylation is very stable in cultured cancer cell lines based on its efficient recovery after the removal of a DNA methylation inhibitor treatment [21]. Transient transfection of *p16*-specific artificial transcription factor can induce transcription of methylated *p16* alleles in cancer cells, but cannot induce demethylation of its CpG islands [45]. In contrast, most *p16* methylation in gastritis lesions is unstable and *H. pylori*-dependent [28, 30]. The mechanisms contributing to the difference of the stability of *p16* methylation between gastritis and cancer cells remains elusive. Characterization of the natural methylation pattern of *p16* CpG islands in human tissue samples with various pathological lesions may elucidate the mechanisms accounting for the diverse stability of *p16* methylation and could potentially be used to develop a tumor-specific methylation biomarker assay. We demonstrated that in normal gastric tissues, the majority of the samples either did not show CpG methylation or only contained sporadically methylated-CpG sites in the exon-1 coding-nucleosome region. In contrast, the gastritis and GC samples showed various degrees of methylation in the same region. Extensive methylation in both the promoter and the exon-1 regions was observed in the majority of the GC specimens. We propose that a methylation wave progressively extends from the *p16* exon-1 coding- nucleosome to its promoter nucleosome *in vivo*. (Fig. 3) The overall *p16* methylation profiles constructed from a panel of clinical specimens may approximate the natural extension pattern of *de novo* methylation of *p16* CpG islands in gastric carcinogenesis [46].

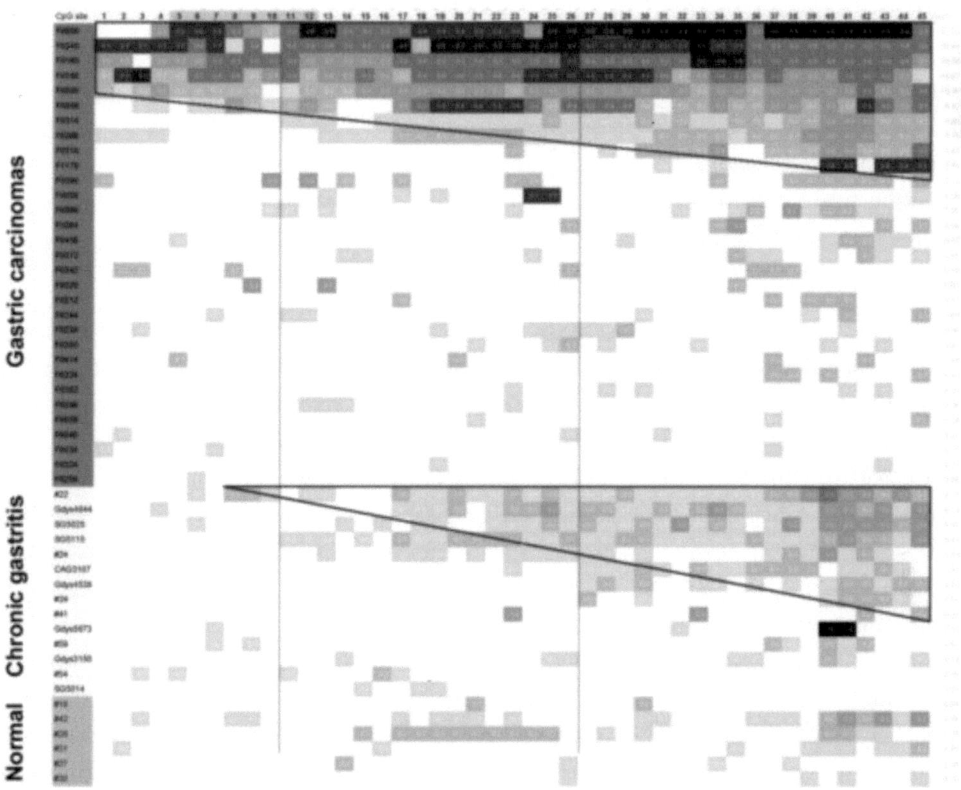

Figure 3. Comparison of methylation status of *p16* CpG island in gastric carcinomas, chromic gastritis, and normal gastric mucosa [46]. A gray-graded representation of the average methylation density at individual CpG sites within the *p16* promoter and exon-1 region

4. DNA methylation as a clinical biomarker for risk assessment, and anticancer drugs target

Epigenetic changes provide a potential explanation for how environmental factors can modify the risk for common diseases among individuals. The growing interest in cancer epigenetics stems from the fact that epigenetic changes are implicated in virtually every step of the development and progression of cancers. This is supported by the studies demonstrating that epigenetic changes including DNA hypermethylation are an early event in carcinogenesis. A distinguishing feature of epigenetic changes in comparison with genetic changes is that epigenetic changes are reversible. Therefore, aberrant DNA methylation, histone acetylation and methylation are attractive targets for cancer prevention and the epigenetic therapy. There are some evidences that methylation-based tests could predict which individuals are at high risk for different types of cancers, so that screening tests and prophylactic treatment can be applied more effectively. A pharmacological modification of the epigenetic status may be a potent strategy for the prevention of gastric cancers, based on the fact that methylation was a frequent event, particularly in *H. pylori*-infected patients. Perhaps methylation in normal gastric mucosa either directly predisposes the tissue to cancer or is associated with some other factors predisposing to cancer. In either case, methylation analysis of normal tissue could help determine the risk of those individuals for future development of the disease. It is reported that the genetic reduction of DNA methylation levels suppressed the incidence, number and size of gastric tumors in gastric tumorigenesis [47].

Aberrant DNA methylation is more frequently present in gastric cancers than mutations [48], so we can take advantage of the frequent presence of aberrant methylation in cancers by using it as a clue to identify tumor markers for cancer screening purposes and carcinogenic risk assessment. One advantage of using aberrant DNA methylation as a biomarker instead of mutations/expression is that it is possible to detect even a single aberrantly methylated DNA molecule embedded in 1000 unmethylated DNA molecules [49]. The high sensitivity and specificity of measurements has particular application when it is well recognized that stem cells in precancerous or cancer tissues should contribute to cancer development, metastasis, recurrence, and formation of drug resistance. In contrast, using regular gene expression assays, such as immunostaining, Western blot, RT-PCR, and Northern blot, detection of alterations of gene expression in limited number of stem cells is very difficult. Additionally, DNA methylation can be remained in various samples stored at wide-range conditions (fresh/frozen or paraffin- embedded tissue blocks, free DNA in plasma, detached cells in gastric juice, sputum, urine, stool samples, and other body fluids). For example, we observed that methylation of *p16*, the G1 ▪ S conversion checkpoint gene in the cell cycle, is a powerful biomarker for prediction malignant transformation of epithelial dysplasia [50,51]. Importantly, we further developed a *p16*-specific probe-based quantitative MethyLight assay for the development of *p16* methylation diagnosis kit [52]. Developments of DNA methylation biomarkers (Septin9, *p16*, MGMT) for cancer screening purposes, carcinogenic risk assessment, and prediction of chemotherapy sensitivity are under clinical trials [3].

Currently, the greatest hopes are associated with clinical applications of several promising epigenetic modification inhibitors target for anticancer therapy, which inhibits DNA methylation and leads to the demethylation of the genome, thereby restoring expression of methylated genes. Such as DNMT inhibitor 5-aza-deoxycytosine and histone deacetylase inhibitors vorinostat or romidepsin, have recently approved by FDA for patients with myelodysplasia syndrome and cutaneous or peripheral T-cell lymphoma, respectively [3,53]. However, the potential pleiotropic effects of such an intervention as a result of induced genome hypomethylation (leading to, e.g., genome instability) need to be carefully considered. Therefore, the basic challenge in designing potential anticancer drugs functioning at the DNA methylation level is the specific recognition of molecular targets.

http://dx.doi.org/10.5772/53147

5. Conclusion

In conclusion, aberrant CpG islands methylation occurs in the early stages of gastric carcinogenesis and tends to increase as the multistep process advances. It is highly plausible that *H. pylori* infection and other environment exposure can lead to the adaptive responses of the host cells to the chronic inflammation triggers the development of these epigenetic changes in the non-cancerous stomach, which eventually lead to neoplastic transformation. The epigenetic profile is highly dynamic and reversible, and varies among cells in the same organism and, in the same cell, between various states, such as health versus disease, or in response to environmental perturbations. Given the plasticity of epigenetic marks in response to cancer-related exposures, such epigenetic marks are attractive candidates for the development of surrogate endpoints which could be used in dietary or lifestyle intervention. In recent years, a lot has been learnt, but much remains to be learnt to combat gastric cancer, one of the most frequent and lethal neoplasias worldwide. The study of epigenetic alterations offers great potential for the identification of biomarkers that can be used to detect and diagnose cancer in its earliest stages, to accurately assess individual risk and as targets for chemotherapeutic strategies.

Author details

Zheming Lu* and Dajun Deng

*Address all correspondence to: zheminglu@163.com

Key Laboratory of Carcinogenesis and Translational Research, Ministry of Education, Division of Cancer Etiology, Beijing University Cancer Hospital and Institute, Beijing, China

References

[1] Esteller M. Epigenetics in cancer. N Engl J Med. 2008; 358: 1148–59.

[2] Jones PA, Baylin SB. The epigenomics of cancer. Cell. 2007;128:683-92.

[3] Deng DJ, Liu ZJ, Du YT. Epigenetic alterations as cancer diagnostic, prognostic, and predictive biomarkers. Adv Genet. 2010; 71: 125-76.

[4] Kang GH. CpG Island Hypermethylation in Gastric Carcinoma and Its Premalignant Lesions. Korean J Pathol. 2012; 46:1-9

[5] Hatakeyama M, Brzozowski T. Pathogenesis of Helicobacter pylori infection. Helicobacter. 2006; 11(Suppl 1): 14-20.

[6] Compare D, Rocco A, Liguori E, D'Armiento FP, Persico G, Masone S, Coppola-Bottazzi E, Suriani R, Romano M, Nardone G. Global DNA hypomethylation is an early

event in Helicobacter pylori-related gastric carcinogenesis. J Clin Pathol. 2011; 64: 677-82.

[7] Kang GH, Shim YH, Jung HY, Kim WH, Ro JY, Rhyu MG. CpG island methylation in premalignant stages of gastric carcinoma. Cancer Res 2001; 61: 2847-51.

[8] Kang GH, Lee S, Kim JS, Jung HY. Profile of aberrant CpG island methylation along multistep gastric carcinogenesis. Lab Invest. 2003a; 83: 519-26.

[9] Park SY, Yoo EJ, Cho NY, Kim N, Kang GH. Comparison of CpG island hypermethylation and repetitive DNA hypomethylation in premalignant stages of gastric cancer, stratified for Helicobacter pylori infection. J Pathol 2009; 219: 410-6.

[10] Kuipers EJ, Perez-Perez GI, Meuwissen SGM, Blaser MJ. Helicobacter pylori and atrophic gastritis: importance of the cagA status. J Natl Cancer Inst. 1995; 87: 1777-80

[11] Chan AO, Lam SK, Wong BC, Wong WM, Yuen MF, Yeung YH, Hui WM, Rashid A, Kwong YL. Promoter methylation of E-cadherin gene in gastric mucosa associated with Helicobacter pylori infection and in gastric cancer. Gut. 2003; 52: 502-6.

[12] Waki T, Tamura G, Tsuchiya T, Sato K, Nishizuka S, Motoyama T. Promoter methylation status of E-cadherin, hMLH1, and p16 genes in nonneoplastic gastric epithelia. Am J Pathol 2002; 161: 399-403.

[13] Kang GH, Lee HJ, Hwang KS, Lee S, Kim JH, Kim JS. Aberrant CpG island hypermethylation of chronic gastritis, in relation to aging, gender, intestinal metaplasia, and chronic inflammation. Am J Pathol 2003b; 163: 1551-6.

[14] Feinberg AP and Vogelstein B. Hypomethylation distinguishes genes of some human cancers from their normal counterparts. Nature. 1983; 301: 89–92.

[15] Rollins RA, Haghighi F, Edwards JR, Das R, Zhang MQ, Ju J, Bestor TH. Large-scale structure of genomic methylation patterns.Genome Res. 2006; 16: 157-63

[16] Xiang S, Liu Z, Zhang B, Zhou J, Zhu B, Ji J, Deng DJ. Methylation status of individual CpG sites within Alu elements in the human genome and Alu hypomethylation in gastric carcinomas. BMC Cancer. 2010; 10:44.

[17] Yoshida T, Yamashita S, Takamura-Enya T, Niwa T, Ando T, Enomoto S, Maekita T, Nakazawa K, Tatematsu M, Ichinose M, Ushijima T. Alu and Sata hypomethylation in Helicobacter pylori-infected gastric mucosae. Int J Cancer. 2011; 128:33-9

[18] Bester AC, Roniger M, Oren YS, Im MM, Sarni D, Chaoat M, Bensimon A, Zamir G, Shewach DS, Kerem B. Nucleotide deficiency promotes genomic instability in early stages of cancer development. Cell. 2011; 145: 435-46.

[19] Gonzalez-Zulueta M, Bender CM, Yang AS, Nguyen T, Beart RW, Van Tornout JM, Jones PA. Methylation of the 59 CpG island of the p16/CDKN2 tumor suppressor gene in normal and transformed human tissues correlates with gene silencing. Cancer Res 1995; 55: 4531-5.

[20] Little M, Wainwright B. Methylation and p16: suppressing the suppressor. Nat Med 1995;1:633-4.

[21] Egger G, Aparicio AM, Escobar SG, Jones PA. Inhibition of histone deacetylation does not block resilencing of p16 after 5-aza-2'-deoxycytidine treatment. Cancer Res, 2007, 67: 346-53

[22] Waterland, R. A. Assessing the effects of high methionine intake on DNA methylation. J. Nutr., 2006;136, 1706S–1710S.

[23] Bai H, Gu L, Zhou J, Deng D. p16 hypermethylation during gastric carcinogenesis of Wistar rats by N-methyl-N'-nitro-N-nitrosoguanidine. Mutat Res. 2003 ; 535: 73-8.

[24] Issa JP, Ottaviano YL, Celano P, Hamilton SR, Davidson NE, Baylin SB. Methylation of the oestrogen receptor CpG island links ageing and neoplasia in human colon. Nat Genet. 1994;7:536– 40.

[25] Peek RM, Blaser MJ. 2002. Helicobacter pylori and gastrointestinal tract adenocarcinomas.Nat Rev Cancer. 2002;2:28-37.

[26] Maekita T, Nakazawa K, Mihara M, Nakajima T, Yanaoka K, Iguchi M, ArII K, Kaneda A, Tsukamoto T, Tatematsu M, Tamura G, Saito D, Sugimura T, Ichinose M, Ushijima T. High levels of aberrant DNA methylation in Helicobacter pylori-infected gastric mucosae and its possible association with gastric cancer risk. Clin Cancer Res. 2006; 12: 989–95.

[27] Ushijima T, Nakajima T, Maekita T. DNA methylation as a marker for the past and future.J Gastroenterol. 2006;41:401-7.

[28] Dong CX, Deng DJ, Pan KF, Zhang L, Zhang Y, Zhou J, You WC. Promoter methylation of p16 associated with Helicobacter pylori infection in precancerous gastric lesions: a population-based study. Int J Cancer. 2009; 124: 434-9.

[29] Leung WK, Man EP, Yu J, Go MY, To KF, Yamaoka Y, Cheng VY, Ng EK, Sung JJ. Effects of Helicobacter pylori eradication on methylation status of E-cadherin gene in noncancerous stomach. Clin Cancer Res. 2006; 12: 3216-21.

[30] Perri F, Cotugno R, Piepoli A, Merla A, Quitadamo M, Gentile A, Pilotto A, Annese V, Andriulli A. Aberrant DNA Methylation in Non-Neoplastic Gastric Mucosa of H. Pylori Infected Patients and Effect of Eradication, Am J Gastroenterol. 2007;102:1361–1371

[31] Nozaki K, Shimizu N, Ikehara Y, Inoue M, Tsukamoto T, Inada K, Tanaka H, Kumagai T, Kaminishi M, Tatematsu M.Effect of early eradication on Helicobacter pylori-related gastric carcinogenesis in Mongolian gerbils. Cancer Sci 2003;94: 235-9.

[32] Niwa, T.T., Tsukamoto, T., Toyoda, T., Mori, A., Tanaka, H., Maekita, T., Ichinose, M., Tatematsu, M., and Ushijima, T. Inflammatory processes triggered by Helicobacter pylori infection cause aberrant DNA methylation in gastric epithelial cells. Cancer Res. 2010; 70, 1430–1440

[33] Niwa T, Ushijima T. Induction of epigenetic alterations by chronic inflammation and its significance on carcinogenesis. Adv Genet 2010;71:41-56

[34] Nakajima T, Enomoto S, Ushijima T. DNA methylation: a marker for carcinogen exposure and cancer risk. Environ Health Prev Med. 2008;13:8-15

[35] Nakajima T, Yamashita S, Maekita T, Niwa T, Nakazawa K, Ushijima T.The presence of a methylation fingerprint of Helicobacter pylori infection in human gastric mucosae. Int J Cancer. 2009; 124: 905-10

[36] Feinberg AP, Ohlsson R, Henikoff S. The epigenetic progenitor origin of human cancer. Nat Rev Genet. 2006; 7: 21–33.

[37] Ushijima T, Hattori N. Molecular Pathways: Involvement of Helicobacter pylori–Triggered Inflammation in the Formation of an Epigenetic Field Defect, and Its Usefulness as Cancer Risk and Exposure Markers. Clin Cancer Res. 2012;18:923-9

[38] El-Omar EM, Carrington M, Chow WH, McColl KE, Bream JH, Young HA, Herrera J, Lissowska J, Yuan CC, Rothman N, Lanyon G, Martin M, Fraumeni JF Jr, Rabkin CS. Interleukin-1β polymorphisms associated with increased risk of gastric cancer. Nature. 2000, 404: 398–402.

[39] Yamaoka Y, Kita M, Kodama T, Sawai N, Kashima K, Imanishi J. Induction of various cytokines and development of severe mucosal inflammation by cagA gene positive Helicobacter pylori strains, Gut.1997, 41442 -451

[40] Hmadcha A, Bedoya FJ, Sobrino F, Pintado E. Methylation-dependent gene silencing induced by interleukin 1beta via nitric oxide production.J Exp Med. 1999; 190: 1595-604.

[41] Fu S, Ramanujam KS, Wong A, Fantry GT, Drachenberg CB, James SP, Meltzer SJ, Wilson KT. Increased expression and cellular localization of inducible nitric oxide synthase and cyclooxygenase 2 in Helicobacter pylori gastritis. Gastroenterology. 1999; 116: 1319-29.

[42] Watanabe S, Takagi A, Koga Y, Kamiya S, Miwa T. Helicobacter pylori induces apoptosis in gastric epithelial cells through inducible nitric oxide. J Gastroenterol Hepatol. 2000;15:168-74.

[43] Rajnakova A, Moochhala S, Goh PM, Ngoi S.Expression of nitric oxide synthase, cyclooxygenase, and p53 in different stages of human gastric cancer. Cancer Lett. 2001;172:177-85.

[44] Qian X, Huang C, Cho CH, Hui WM, Rashid A, Chan AO. E-cadherin promoter hypermethylation induced by interleukin-1beta treatment or H. pylori infection in human gastric cancer cell lines. Cancer Lett. 2008; 263: 107-13.

[45] Zhang B, Xiang S, Zhong Q, Yin Y, Gu L, Deng D. The p16-Specific Reactivation and Inhibition of Cell Migration Through Demethylation of CpG Islands by Engineered Transcription Factors. Human Gene Therapy. 2012; 23: (doi:10.1089/hum.2012.070)

[46] Lu ZM, Zhou J, Wang X, Guan Z, Bai H, Liu ZJ, Su N, Pan K, Ji J, Deng D. Nucleosomes correlate with in vivo progression pattern of de novo methylation of p16 CpG islands in human gastric carcinogenesis. PLoS ONE. 2012; 7(4): E35928.

[47] Tomita H, Hirata A, Yamada Y, Hata K, Oyama T, Mori H, Yamashita S, Ushijima T, Hara A.Suppressive effect of global DNA hypomethylation on gastric carcinogenesis. Carcinogenesis. 2010;31:1627-33.

[48] Ushijima T, Sasako M. Focus on gastric cancer. Cancer Cell 2004;5:121–5

[49] Laird PW. The power and the promise of DNA methylation markers. Nat Rev Cancer. 2003; 3: 253–66

[50] Sun Y, Deng D, You WC, Bai H, Zhang L, Zhou J, Shen L, Ma JL, Xie YQ, Li JY.. Methylation of p16 CpG islands associated with malignant transformation of gastric dysplasia in a population-based study. Clin Cancer Res, 2004, 10: 5087-5093

[51] Cao J, Zhou J, Gao Y, Gu L, Meng H, Liu H, Deng D. Methylation of p16 CpG island associated with malignant progression of oral epithelial dysplasia: a prospective cohort study. Clin Cancer Res. 2009; 15: 5178-83.

[52] Zhou J, Cao J, Lu Z, Liu H, Deng D. A 115-bp MethyLight assay for detection of p16 (CDKN2A) methylation as a diagnostic biomarker in human tissues. BMC Med Genet. 2011, 12: 67

[53] Dawson MA, Kouzarides T. Cancer epigenetics: from mechanism to therapy. Cell. 2012; 150: 12-27.

Chapter 9

Does Eradication of *Helicobacter pylori* Decreases the Expression of p53 and c-Myc oncogenes in the Human Gastric Mucosa?

Hanan AlSaeid Alshenawy and
Amr Mahrous Alshafey

Additional information is available at the end of the chapter

http://dx.doi.org/10.5772/53673

1. Introduction

Helicobacter pylori (*H.pylori*) may cause many gastroduodenal diseases including acute gastritis, atrophic gastritis, intestinal metaplasia, peptic ulcer and others disorders. Although many studies revealed close association between gastric cancer and *H.pylori*, there have been only few studies that report on gastric carcinogenesis associated with chronic *H.pylori* [1,2]

H.pylori is a class 1 gastric carcinogen. However, it remains unclear whether *H.pylori* affects molecular alterations in chronic gastritis. It is well known that only a minority of *H.pylori* positive patients with chronic gastritis develop gastric cancer, and so the link is unclear [2].

Nardone et al [3] had stated that gastric carcinogenesis is a multistep process progressing from chronic gastritis through glandular atrophy, metaplasia, and dysplasia. Acquired genomic instability, generally precedes neoplastic clonal expansion. *H.pylori* damages stimulates gastric cell proliferation, which leads to mucosal repair, but which can also induce cellular DNA damage. The most frequent epiphenomenon of DNA alteration is activation of oncogenes and/or mutation of oncosuppressor genes. The role of these genes has been studied in gastric carcinogenesis, but their interrelation with *H.pylori* infection has yet to be defined. Thus, this study was designed to detect the relation between *H.pylori* and gastric carcinogenesis and to investigate the effect of its eradication on the expression of p53 and c-Myc in *H.pylori* associated chronic gastritis.

As a transcription factor, p53 has roles in regulation of proliferation, apoptosis, genomic repair, controls the onset of cellular senescence and suppresses angiogenesis [4,5]. p53 mutation is among the major episodes in the multi-step process of gastric carcinogenesis, while it has also been reported in pre-malignant lesions of the stomach, such as chronic atrophic gastritis, intestinal metaplasia, and dysplasia [1].

c-Myc is a basic transcriptional factor that regulates several genes involved in cell proliferation, differentiation, apoptosis, and oncogenesis. c-Myc expression was studied in gastric cancer with *H.pylori* infection by many authors [6,7]. Also the relationship between *H.pylori* infection and c-Myc expressions was investigated in a series of diseases and concluded that in gastric carcinogenesis, *H.pylori* might cause the imbalance of proliferation and apoptosis in precancerous lesions, leading to tumor-suppressor system mutation and telomerase reactivation, and finally causes gastric cancer [8].

2. Material and methods

2.1. Patients and tissue collection

A total of 55 chronic gastritis patients (38 male and 17 female with mean age: 57.1) underwent endoscopic examination for evaluation of dyspypsia. *H.pylori*-positive (+) were 45 cases while *H.pylori*-negative (-) were only 10 cases. All *H.pylori*-positive patients had successful eradication therapy (15 days of treatment with omeprazole 20 mg twice a day, clarithromycin 500 mg twice a day, and tinidazole 500 mg twice a day), and underwent biopsies before and six months after eradication.

2.2. Detection of *H. pylori* in gastric biopsy specimens

H.pylori in the stomach was detected by rapid urease test, and histological examination. For the urease test, biopsy specimens were immediately inserted into the rapid urease test solution. *H.pylori* was histologically detected by May-Giemsa stain. *H.pylori* eradication was considered successful when the results of the two tests (both the urase test and Giemsa stain) were found negative.

2.3. Histological evaluation

Biopsy specimens were taken from five points of the stomach, as recommended by the updated Sydney system [9], i.e. the lesser curvature of the antrum, and the greater curvature of the antrum, the smaller curvature of the angle, and the lesser curvature of the middle corpus, and the greater curvature of the upper corpus. All biopsy materials were fixed in buffered formalin for 24 hours and embedded in paraffin. Serial sections were stained with haematoxylin-eosin and May-Giemsa stain. The status of the gastric mucosa was evaluated according to the updated Sydney system. The degree of inflammation (manifested by mild lymphocyte and plasma-cell infiltration), neutrophil activity, atrophy (glandular morphology absent in the mucosa and replaced by connective tissue, inter-glandular space was infiltrated by plasma cells and lymphocytes), dysplasia (nuclear atypia with or without architectural abnormalities in the gastric epithelium, but without invasion) and intestinal metaplasia (presence of goblet cells in gastric mucosa) were classed by four grades, with 0 being for 'normal', 1 for 'mild', 2 for 'moderate', and 3 for 'marked'.

2.4. Immunohistochemical detection of p53and c-Myc

Serial paraffin sections were washed in 1/15 mol/L phosphate buffered saline (pH 7.4) three times for five minutes, and pre-incubated in normal rabbit serum (1:10 in PBS) for 20 min. Next, sections were incubated with primary antibodies for 16 hours at 4C, followed by the avidin-biotin complex method. The sections were immersed in 0.05 mol/L Tris-HCl buffer containing 0.02% 3, 3'-diaminobenzidine tetrahydrochloride and 0.005% H_2O_2, and the nuclei were counterstained with hematoxylin. Control sections incubated with normal mouse IgG instead of the primary antibody showed no non-specific staining. The primary antibodies used in this study for p53, staining the sections were incubated with anti-rabbit or mouse antibody (Envision HRP, Dako Company) for 10 min and anti-c-Myc protein (Oncogene Science, San Diego, California, USA; c-Myc p62, dilution 1:50) After antigen retrieval (for c-Myc in 1mM EDTA (pH 8.0), sections were incubated overnight at 41C with monoclonal mouse antibodies to c-Myc (1:100 dilution, Abcam Inc., Cambridge, MA, USA). Immunoreactivity was detected using the DAB Map Kit (PIERCE, Woburn, MA, USA), based on the avidin–biotin complex immunoperoxidase technique.

2.5. Evaluation of p53 and c-Myc staining

The degree of immunopositivity was evaluated semiquantitatively. A total of 300 cells was counted in random fields from representative areas of the lesions, and the immunoreactive cells were roughly assessed and expressed as percentages. The scoring system for both antibodies tested was: 0–5% (negative -); 5–25% (low positivity +); 25–50% (moderate positivity + +); >50% (high positivity +++) according to Nardone et al [3].

2.6. Statistical analysis

All data were put into SPSS 10.0 statistical computer system. Statistical analysis was performed with *t* test or *chi-square* test, with statistical significance indicated by a value of $P \leq 0.05$.

3. Results

The study included 55 cases, 45 cases of them were *H.pylori* (+). The neutrophilic infiltrate was detected only in *H.pylori* (+) cases and the majority of cases were grade 3, 26 cases were positive for lymphoplasmacytic infiltrate; 20 of them were *H.pylori* (+), 23 cases showing atrophy; 20 of them were *H.pylori* (+) and the remaining 3 cases were *H.pylori* (-); they were grade 1. Intestinal metaplasia were seen in 16 cases; 15 of them were *H.pylori* (+). Glandular dysplasia was detected only in 10 cases; all of them were *H.pylori* (+). The degree of activity of chronic gastritis was summarized in table (1).

	PNLs n=38				Lymphocytes n=26				Atrophy n=23				IM N=16				Dysplasia n=10				Sig.
	0	1	2	3	0	1	2	3	0	1	2	3	0	1	2	3	0	1	2	3	
H.pylori(-) N=10	10 (100%)	0	0	0	4 (40%)	1 (10%)	2 (20%)	3 (30%)	7 (70%)	3 (30%)	0	0	9 (90%)	1 (10%)	0	0	10 (100%)	0	0	0	0.03
H.pylori(+) N=45	7 (15%)	10 (22%)	12 (27%)	16 (36%)	25 (56%)	10 (22%)	7 (15%)	3 (7%)	25 (56%)	11 (24%)	8 (18%)	1 (2%)	30 (67%)	7 (15%)	6 (13%)	2 (5%)	35 (77%)	3 (7%)	4 (9%)	3 (7%)	0.04
Sig	0.001				0.03				0.04				0.01				0.02				

Table 1. The activity of chronic gastritis in the studied cases

Table (2) summarize the correlation study between the histological variables and the studied oncogens. According to p53, the positive cases were 12 and all of them were *H.pylori* (+), 4 of them were +, 5 were ++ and 3 were +++ as in figure (1). There were a significant difference between the staining positivity of p53 and all the studied variables including neutrophilic infiltrate, lymphoplasmacytic infiltrate, gastric glandular atrophy, intestinal metaplasia and dysplasia. According to c-Myc staining, the total positive cases were 10 and all of them were *H.pylori* (+) cases, 4 were +, 3 were ++ as seen in figure (2) and 3 were +++. And again there were a significant correlation between the staining positivity and the grades of the studied variables. As the grade of chronic gastritis activity increases, the expression positivity of both p53 and c-Myc increases, with significant difference between the grades as seen in table (2).

		PNLs				Lymphocytes				Atrophy				IM				Dysplasia				Total
		0	1	2	3	0	1	2	3	0	1	2	3	0	1	2	3	0	1	2	3	
p53 (n=12)	-	7 (16%)	8	7	11	25	6	2	0	25	6	2	0	30	3	0	0	31	2	0	0	33
	+	0	2	2	0	0	3	1	0	0	2	2	0	0	1	3	0	4	0	0	0	4
	++	0	0	3	2	0	1	3	1	0	3	2	0	0	3	1	1	0	1	3	1	5
	+++	0	0	0	3	0	0	1	2	0	0	2	1	0	0	2	1	0	0	1	2	3
Sig		0.003				0.02				0.01				0.02				0.004				55
c-Myc (n=10)	-	7	8	8	12	25	7	3	0	25	5	5	0	30	3	2	0	31	2	0	0	35
	+	0	2	2	0	0	2	2	0	0	4	0	0	0	2	2	0	2	0	2	0	4
	++	0	0	2	1	0	1	2	0	0	1	2	0	0	1	2	0	0	1	1	1	3
	+++	0	0	0	3	0	0	0	3	0	1	1	1	0	0	1	2	0	0	1	2	3
Sig		0.01				0.009				0.03				0.005				0.03				55

Table 2. Correlation between the p53 and c-Myc and the studied histological variables in H.pylori (+) cases

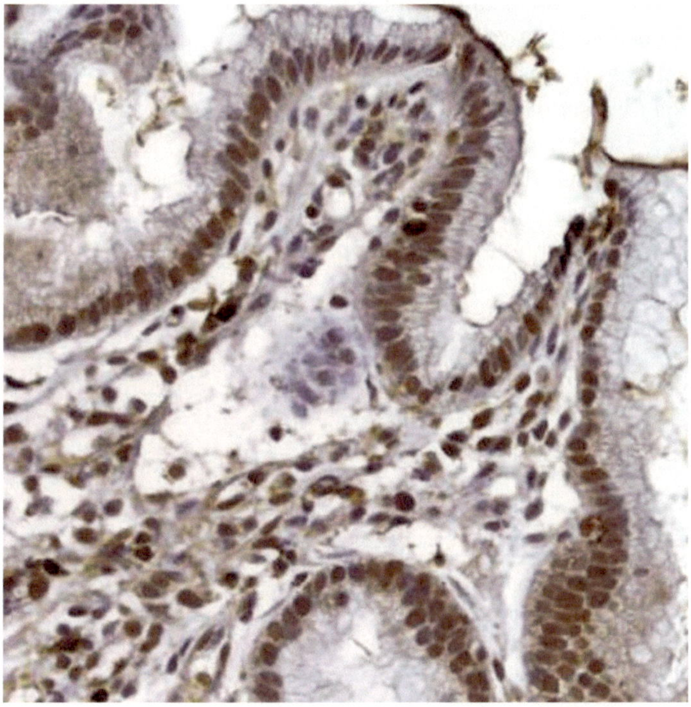

Figure 1. *H.pylori* (+) case showing +++ p53 expression, this case showed moderate intestinal metaplasia, note the intense inflammatory infiltrate. (strept avidin-biotin-DAB, 400x).

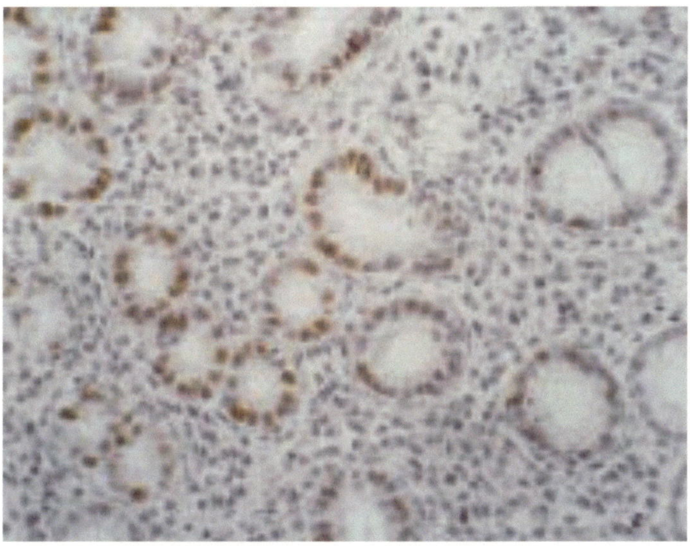

Figure 2. c-Myc moderate expression in a case of H.pylori (+) case, the positivity mainly in intestinal metaplasia portion. (strept avidin-biotin-DAB, 200x).

After treatment and complete resolution of *H.pylori* infection in all the cases, the same histopathological variables and immunohistochemical stainig of the studied oncogenes were evalualed. The activity of chronic gastritis was measured and summarized in table (3). It was found that the number of the cases which were positive for neutrophilic infiltrate, lymphocytic infiltrtate, atrophy, intestinal metaplsia and even the glandular dysplasia were less than the number before the treatment and even the grading of all these parameters become much less as shown in table (3) when compared with table (1) with significant difference between the same cases before and after treatment.

	PNLs				**Lymphocytes**				**Atrophy**				**IM**				**Dysplasia**			
	n=18				**n=8**				**n= 9**				**n=7**				**n=7**			
	0	**1**	**2**	**3**	**0**	**1**	**2**	**3**	**0**	**1**	**2**	**3**	**0**	**1**	**2**	**3**	**0**	**1**	**2**	**3**
Treated cases N=45	27 (60%)	15 (33%)	3 (7%)	0	37 (82%)	4 (9%)	3 (7%)	1 (2%)	36 (80%)	5 (11%)	4 (9%)	0	38 (84%)	3 (7%)	3 (7%)	1 (2%)	38 (84%)	3 (7%)	2 (4%)	2 (4%)
Sig	0.004				0.003				0.005				0.009				0.007			

Table 3. The activity of chronic gastritis in the studied cases after treatment:

As regarding p53 study after treatment, the number of positive cases become only 7 instead of 12, 3 cases were +, 3 cases were ++ as seen in figure (3) and only one case was +++. as regarding the correlative study between p53 and the histological variables, there still positive correlation between the p53 and all the variables of chronic gastritis as summarized in table (4).

		PNLs				**Lymphocytes**				**Atrophy**				**IM**				**Dysplasia**				**Total**
		0	1	2	3	0	1	2	3	0	1	2	3	0	1	2	3	0	1	2	3	
P53 (n=7)	-	27	11	0	0	37	1	0	0	36	2	0	0	38	0	0	0	38	0	0	0	38
	+	0	3	0	0	0	2	1	0	0	2	1	0	0	2	2	0	0	2	1	0	3
	++	0	1	2	0	0	1	2	0	0	1	2	0	0	1	1	0	0	1	1	1	3
	+++	0	0	1	0	0	0	0	1	0	0	1	0	0	0	0	1	0	0	0	1	1
Sig		0.01				0.01				0.03				0.02				0.01				45
c-Myc(n=6)	-	27	11	1	0	37	1	1	0	36	3	0	0	37	1	1	0	38	1	0	0	39
	+	0	2	1	0	0	3	0	0	0	2	1	0	1	1	1	0	0	2	1	0	3
	++	0	1	1	0	0	0	2	0	0	0	2	0	0	1	1	0	0	0	1	1	2
	+++	0	1	0	0	0	0	0	1	0	0	1	0	0	0	0	1	0	0	0	1	1
Sig		0.03				0.04				0.04				0.02				0.01				45

Table 4. Correlation between p53 and c-Myc and the studied histological variables after treatment

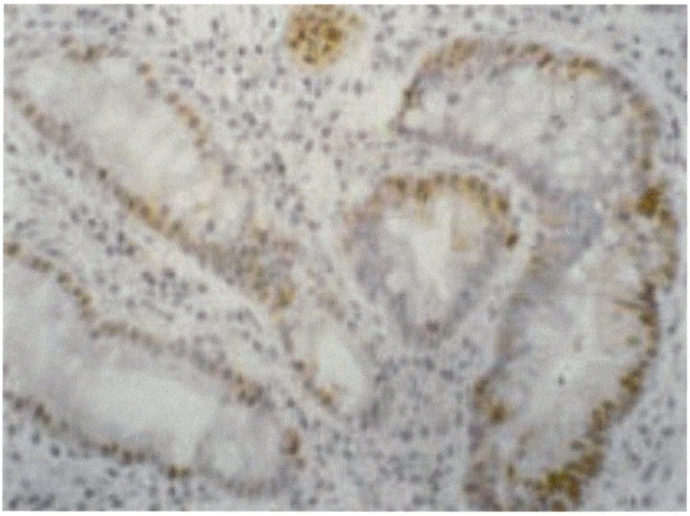

Figure 3. p53 expression after treatment in a case of chronic gastritis was +++ and become ++ confined to the area of intestinal metasplasia (strept avidin-biotin-DAB, 400x).

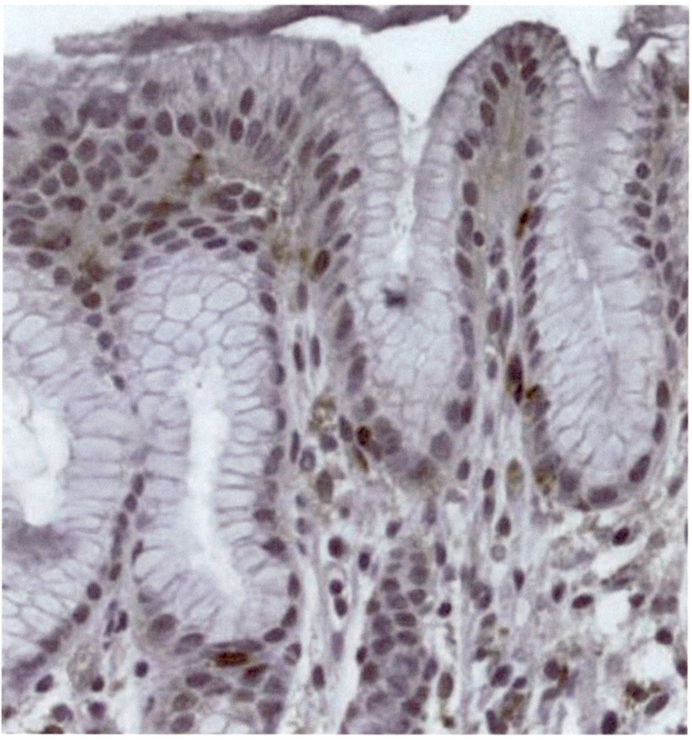

Figure 4. c-Myc expression after treatment was ++ and become + expression only. (strept avidin-biotin-DAB, 400x).

On the other hand, as regarding c-Myc study after treatment, the number of positive cases become only 6 instead of 10, 3 cases were + as seen in figure (4), 2 cases were ++ and only one case was +++. as regarding the correlative study between c-Myc positivity and the histological variables, there still positive correlation between the c-Myc and all the variables of chronic gastritis as summarized in table (4).

4. Discussion

In the present study, it was found that large number of chronic gastritis cases were associated with *H.pylori*. In *H.pylori* (+) cases, the majority showed active neutrophilic infiltrate, lymphocytic infiltrate with occasional lymphoid follicles, atrophy, intestinal metaplasia and dysplasia.

c-Myc and p53 expression are the most widely used markers of genomic instability [10]. Interestingly, in this work, c-Myc and p53 expression were not detected in *H.pylori* (-) cases and this was similar to Van Der et al study [11].

In this work, with the lesions changed between the studied cases from active chronic gastritis to atrophic gastritis to intestinal metaplasia to dysplasia, the positive immunostaining grades of p53 expression increased significantly, the increasing tendency for p53 had a good linear correlation with lesions progression toword the more dangerous precancerous lesions. It is indicated that increased p53 expression may be important molecular events involved in the early stage of gastric carcinogenesis. Thus, this accumulation may be useful biomarkers to assess risk for the development of gastric carcinoma. This was similar to other authors [1,4,12] who have reported that *H.pylori*-positive gastritis especially that accompanied with intestinal metaplasia showed a higher p53 expression. But unlike Anagnostopoulos et al [13] who reported that p53 was expressed only in cases with high grade dysplasia and not in pre-dysplastic stages and concluded that p53 mutation is a late event during the development of gastric cancer. Our results confirm the relationship between atrophic and/or metaplastic gastric mucosa with *H.pylori* infection and p53 expression.

Marinone et al [14] data indicated that irreversible genetic changes in the p53 protein has not yet occurred in non-neoplastic gastric mucosa with metaplasia and *H.pylori* related chronic gastritis and they concluded that the increase in p53 levels is due to an increased production of the wild-type protein probably related to an inflammatory response induced by *H.pylori* infection.

In this work, *H.pylori* (-) cases were completely negative for c-Myc expression while *H.pylori* infection was associated with positive expression of c-Myc unlike others [15] who found that no evidence of expression of c-Myc in any gastritis sample. c-Myc has been reported to be increased in *H.pylori*-associated gastritis, is associated with increased cell proliferation.

The results of this study may be explained by other studies [6,7] who found that in *H.pylori*-associated gastritis, there is downregulation of p27 and increased c-Myc, the net result of which is increased cell proliferation and also *H.pylori* may influence both telomerase activity and c-Myc expression in chronic atrophic gastritis.

Again in Zhan et al [16] study, expression of c-Myc was significantly higher in carcinoma than that in dysplasia than in metaplasia. Also the expression of c-Myc in metaplastic cases and dysplasia with *H.pylori* infection was significantly higher than that without infection; in this work, c-Myc was completely negative in cases without *H.pylori* infection. So this study support the others who concluded that *H.pylori* infection can cause serious imbalance between cell proliferation and apoptosis in the precancerous lesions, giving chances for gastric carcinogenesis.

After eradication treatment, it was found that there were decrease in the cases showed neutrophilic and lymphocytic infiltration and even in the same case there was decrease in the grade of the inflammatory infiltrate. Also the number and the grade of atrophy, intestinal metaplasia and dysplasia were also significantly decreased.

The effects of *H.pylori* eradication on atrophy and intestinal metaplasia are controversial in the previous studies. Some authors [17,18] have reported similar results with the present work. The patchy nature of the lesions and the subjective nature of the interpretation may account for these controversial findings. Our finding of disappearance or regression of atrophy after *H.pylori* eradication suggests that inflammatory infiltration plays a role in this controversial histological finding. On the other hand, some studies [11] revealed no changes in intestinal metaplasia and atrophy were detected after *H.pylori* eradication. While others [19] reported that *H.pylori* eradication does not reduce the histologic metaplasia score, but changes the cellular phenotype of metaplasia. This change of phenotype may be an important factor in the reduction of cancer incidence after eradication of *H.pylori*.

In the present study, *H.pylori* eradication led to a significant reduction in the expression of p53. The number of p53-positive patients was significantly decreased and the grade of positivity was also deceased significantly. Masaaki et al [1] also described a reduction in the expression of p53 after eradication. They reported that *H.pylori* eradication reduced gastritis activity, atrophy, and complete metaplasia, accompanied by the disappearance of genomic instability markers.

After eradication therapy, the number of cases and the grade of positive c-Myc expression was significantly deceased. This results was the same of others [7] who concuded that *H.pylori* downregulates p27 and this is reversed following *H.pylori* eradication.

Finally we can conclude that, *H.pylori* infection in the gastric mucosa may be implicated in the pathway of gastric carcinogenesis. it seems to be responsible for genomic instability and its eradication can reverse inflammation and related atrophy, metaplasia, and genomic instability. So, we recommend that *H.pylori* patients especially those with precancerous lesions should receive intense eradication therapy and closely monitored. Because this study confirm that eradication reverses the atrophic changes in the gastric mucosa and the genetic instability, thus may prevent the development of gastric cancer

Author details

Hanan AlSaeid Alshenawy[1*] and Amr Mahrous Alshafey[2]

*Address all correspondence to: hanan_alshenawy@yahoo.com

1 Department of Pathology, Faculty of Medicine, Tanta University, Tanta, Egypt

2 Department of Internal Medicine, Faculty of Medicine, Tanta University, Tanta, Egypt

References

[1] Masaaki K, Kazunari M, Tadayoshi O, et al., Expression of mutant type-p53 products in H pylori-associated chronic gastritis. World J Gastroenterol, 2007, 14;13(10): 1541-1546.

[2] Zhu Y, Shu X, Chen J, et al., Effect of Helicobacter pylori eradication on oncogenes and cell proliferation. Eur J Clin Invest. 2008 ;38 (9):628-633.

[3] Nardone G, Staibano S, Rocco A, et al., Effect of Helicobacter pylori infection and its eradication on cell proliferation, DNA status, and oncogene expression in patients with chronic gastritis. Gut 1999;44:789–799

[4] Chang W, Li Dong W, Lian Hua J, et al., Expression of p53, inducible nitric oxide synthase and vascular endothelial growth factor in gastric precancerous and cancerous lesions: correlation with clinical features. BMC Cancer. 2002; 2-8.

[5] James G., Barbara J, Charles A. et al., Germ-Line p53-targeted Disruption Inhibits Helicobacter-induced Premalignant. Lesions and Invasive Gastric Carcinoma through Down-Regulation of Th1 Proinflammatory Responses. Cancer Research. 2002,(1), 62, 696–702.

[6] Zhang G, Gu Y, Zhao Z, et al., Coordinate increase of telomerase activity and c-Myc expression in Helicobacter pylori-associated gastric diseases. World J Gastroenterol. 2004,15;10(12):1759-1762.

[7] Kim S S, Meitner P, Konkin T, et al., Altered expression of Skp2, c-Myc and p27 proteins but not mRNA after H. pylori eradication in chronic gastritis. Modern Pathology. 2006, 19, 49–58.

[8] Lan J, Xiong Y, Lin Y, et al., Helicobacter pylori infection generated gastric cancer through p53-Rb tumor-suppressor system mutation and telomerase reactivation. World J Gastroenterol. 2003; 9 (1):54-58.

[9] Dixon M, Genta R, Yardley J, et al., Classification and grading of gastritis. The updated Sydney System. International Workshop on the Histopathology of Gastritis, Houston 1994. Am J Surg Pathol. 1996; 20: 1161-1181.

[10] Liang-jing W, Shu-jie C, Zhe C, et al, Morphological and pathologic changes of experimental chronic atrophic gastritis (CAG) and the regulating mechanism of protein expression in rats. J Zhejiang Univ Sci B. 2006; 7(8): 634–640.

[11] Van Der H, Van Der E, Dekker F, et al. Effect of Helicobacter pylori eradication on gastritis in relation to CagA: a prospective 1-year follow-up study. Gastroenterology 1997;113:25–30.

[12] Unger Z, Molnar B, Pronai L, et al., Mutant p53 expression and apoptotic activity of Helicobacter pylori positive and negative gastritis in correlation with the presence of intestinal metaplasia. Eur J Gastroenterol Hepatol 2003; 15: 389-393.

[13] Anagnostopoulos G, Stefanou D, Arkoumani E, et al., Immunohistochemical expression of cell-cycle proteins in gastric precancerous lesions. 2008;23 (4):626-631.

[14] Marinone C, Martinetti A, Mestriner M, et al., p53 evaluation in gastric mucosa of patients with chronic Helicobacter pylori infection. Anticancer Res. 2001;21(2A): 1115-1118.

[15] Wang J, Chi D, Kalin G, et al., Helicobacter pylori infection and oncogene expressions in gastric carcinoma and its precursor lesions. Dig Dis Sci. 2002;47(1):107-113.

[16] Zhan N, Xiong Y, Lan J, et al., Relationship between Helicobacter pylori infection and expression of c-Myc, Bcl-2, and Bax protein in different gastric mucosa lesions. Ai Zheng. 2003;22(10):1034-1037.

[17] Pasztorova I, Chinyama C, Filipe M, et al., Regression of gastric intestinal metaplasia after eradication of Helicobacter pylori: a prospective study [abstract]. Gut 1996; 39(suppl 2):A55.

[18] Murakami K, Kodama M, Sato R, et al., Helicobacter pylori eradication and associated changes in the gastric mucosa. Expert Rev Anti Infect Ther 2005; 3: 757-764.

[19] Watari J, Das K, Amenta P, et al., Effect of eradication of Helicobacter pylori on the histology and cellular phenotype of gastric intestinal metaplasia. Clin Gastroenterol Hepatol. 2008;6(4):409-417.

Chapter 10

Gastric Cancer Risk Diagnosis Using Molecular Biological and Serological Markers Based on *Helicobacter pylori*-Related Chronic Gastritis

Shotaro Enomoto, Takao Maekita,
Kazuyuki Nakazawa, Takeichi Yoshida,
Mika Watanabe, Chizu Mukoubayashi,
Hiroshi Ohata, Mikitaka Iguchi, Kimihiko Yanaoka,
Hideyuki Tamai, Jun Kato, Masashi Oka,
Osamu Mohara and Masao Ichinose

Additional information is available at the end of the chapter

http://dx.doi.org/10.5772/53116

1. Introduction

Helicobacter pylori (*H. pylori*) infection causes chronic infection of the gastric mucosae and is a major risk factor for the onset of gastric cancer via a series of steps comprising gastritis, atrophy, metaplasia, dysplasia and cancer [1--20]. However, in Japan and other countries with a high rate of *H. pylori* infection, the presence or absence of *H. pylori* infection alone in diagnosing gastric cancer risk is not appropriate in terms of specificity. Thus, it is necessary to clarify the groups at high risk of gastric cancer based on the natural history of gastric cancer development, and the evaluation of gastric cancer risk through the use of serological and molecular biological evaluation for chronic gastritis accompanying *H. pylori* infection is important [21-23]. This may contribute to both gastric cancer screening and various measures to prevent gastric cancer, such as the formulation of follow-up plans for metachronous gastric cancer [24] after endoscopic resection [25, 26], procedures developed in Japan that have recently been applied in the treatment of early gastric cancer.

This article describes the diagnosis of gastric cancer risk with DNA methylation as an indicator, using gastric mucosa tissue from endoscopic biopsy, which has been studied by the authors as a molecular biological gastric cancer risk marker. Also discussed is the significance of serum pepsinogen (PG) as a marker of gastric cancer risk, as recently reported by the authors, and discusses the groups at high risk for gastric cancer based on more detailed evaluation of *H. pylori* -related chronic gastritis.

2. Aberrant DNA methylation in chronic gastritis and application of gastric cancer risk diagnosis

2.1. Concept of DNA methylation

Genetic defects in cancer include both abnormalities in genetic makeup, such as mutations or chromosomal deletions, and epigenetic abnormalities. Deoxyribonucleic acid (DNA) methylation is one type of epigenetic process. DNA methylation occurs physiologically, and is observed in CpG sites where guanine (G) follows cytosine (C) in the gene sequence. CpG sites exist with a low frequency in the genome, but there are exceptional regions where CpG sites are clustered, called CpG islands (CGI). When a CGI is in a gene promoter region, transcription to messenger ribonucleic acid (mRNA) of downstream genes is strongly inhibited (silencing) if that entire CGI is methylated. DNA methylation, along with mutations and chromosomal deletions, is a major factor in the gene inactivation in many cancers [27-29].

Cancer cells show lower methylation of the entire genome and more localized high methylation than normal cells. Low methylation of the entire genome contributes to carcinogenesis through elicitation of genomic instability [30]. Localized high methylation means abnormal methylation in certain CGIs among CGIs that are not normally methylated. Elicitation of high methylation in promoter region CGIs of tumor suppressor genes causes inactivation of that gene. This elicits cell cycle or proliferation signal abnormalities and accumulation of mutations, and contributes to the onset and progression of cancer.

In gastric cancer and other gastrointestinal cancers, silencing of many important tumor suppressor genes has been reported. In gastric cancer in particular, cadherin 1 (*CDH1*), mutL homolog 1 (*MLH1*) and cyclin-dependent kinase inhibitor 2A (*CDKN2A*) are more often inactivated from methylation than from mutations or chromosomal deletion [31].

2.2. Contribution of aberrant DNA methylation in carcinogenesis

Mutations in tumor suppressor genes are a genetic abnormality, and are a cause (driver) of the onset and progression of cancer. In addition, it has been found that many secondary mutations (passengers) are also present in cancer cells with monoclonal proliferation of these cancer cells [32]. Epigenetic abnormalities in DNA methylation play a large role in gastric cancer, and similarly to genetic abnormalities, DNA methylation of tumor suppressor genes can also be a driver (driver methylation) of carcinogenesis. In addition, it has been shown that aberrant methylation in cancer cells also occurs in numerous genes other than tumor suppressor genes (passenger methylation) [33]. Many genes with passenger methylation are genes that originally have low levels of transcription or no transcription and are thought to be an accompanying phenomenon to cancer development. Such aberrant DNA methylation in genes is seen in cancer cells, and it has also been shown to be elicited in non-cancerous tissue as well. Numerous studies have thus been conducted on this topic.

2.3. Induction of aberrant DNA methylation in *H. pylori*-related chronic gastritis

In gastrointestinal organs, precancerous conditions are closely related to chronic infection from viral or bacterial infections [34]. Chronic inflammation has also been shown to be an important inducing factor for aberrant DNA methylation [35]. For example, greater accumulation of aberrant DNA methylation is seen in liver tissue of patients with chronic hepatitis C, which is a background factor for hepatocellular carcinoma, than in normal liver tissue [36]. High-level aberrant DNA methylation exists in colon mucosa tissue of patients with ulcerative colitis, which is a background factor for colon cancer [37]. In the pancreas as well, analysis of endoscopically collected pancreatic juice showed accumulation of aberrant DNA methylation associated with the level of abnormality on pancreatic duct images [38].

When evaluating aberrant DNA methylation in non-cancerous regions, it is extremely important to be mindful of the differences between cancerous and non-cancerous tissue [39]. In non-cancerous tissue, which is polyclonal, quantitative evaluation that asks the question "What is the proportion of the existence of aberrant DNA methylation in specific genes?" is important. In other words, measuring the proportion of molecules with aberrant DNA methylation in non-cancerous specimens (DNA methylation level) and estimating the proportion of cells in which aberrant DNA methylation has been induced will lead to accurate evaluation of aberrant DNA methylation in non-cancerous regions. Therefore, quantitative analysis of methylation levels is necessary to evaluate aberrant DNA methylation in the gastric mucosae, a non-cancerous region. Quantitative methylation-specific polymerase chain reaction (MSP) is a very effective means of resolving such problems [40].

The authors conducted a detailed investigation with quantitative MSP to evaluate aberrant DNA methylation in *H. pylori* -infected gastric mucosae, a background factor for gastric cancer [40]. Using gastric mucosae specimens collected endoscopically from healthy individuals positive and negative for *H. pylori* infection, the DNA methylation level was measured in CpG islands in eight regions of seven genes (Lysyl Oxidase (*LOX*), heart and neural crest derivatives expressed 1 (*HAND1*), thrombomodulin (*THBD*), *p41ARC*, *CDKN2A*, filamin C (*FLNc*), HRAS-like suppressor (*HRASLS*)), in which DNA methylation is seen with high frequency in gastric cancer [41]. The level of DNA methylation was 5.4– to 303- fold higher in the gastric mucosae of individuals positive for *H. pylori* infection than in those who were negative. *THBD* and other passenger methylation showed particularly high DNA methylation levels when compared with driver methylation such as in *CDKN2A*, which is a tumor suppressor gene (Fig. 1). Certain characteristics are seen in genes with aberrant DNA methylation in *H. pylori*-infected gastric mucosae. Low gene expression levels in gastric mucosae are thought to be a possible predisposing factor (methylation susceptibility) in the elicitation of DNA methylation [42]. This strongly suggests that high levels of aberrant DNA methylation are seen in *H. pylori* -infected gastric mucosae and that *H. pylori* infection induces aberrant DNA methylation. It has been shown in animal experiments that *H. pylori* infection induces aberrant DNA methylation and inflammation of gastric mucosae evoked by infection is important in inducing aberrant DNA methylation [43].

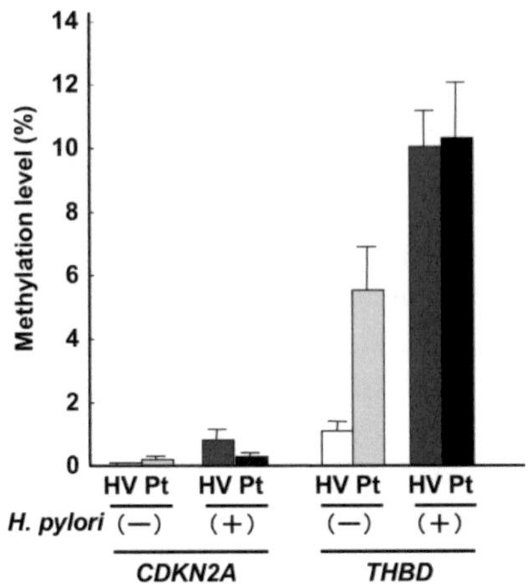

Figure 1. Relationship between *H. pylori* infection, presence or absence of gastric cancer, and gastric mucosae methylation level (citation changed from Reference 40)

Mean methylation level of cyclin-dependent kinase inhibitor 2A (*CDKN2A*) and thrombomodulin (*THBD*) genes in gastric mucosae endoscopic specimens measured using the quantitative methylation-specific polymerase chain reaction (MSP) method. In cases when there is no current *H. pylori* infection, non-cancerous gastric mucosae of gastric cancer patients (Pt) shows a higher methylation level than the gastric mucosae of healthy volunteers (HV). In the case of *H. pylori* infection, the methylation level was high, irrespective of whether the person had gastric cancer. High levels of aberrant DNA methylation are seen in *H. pylori* -infected gastric mucosae and that *H. pylori* infection induces aberrant DNA methylation. Ease of methylation differs depending on CpG islands (CGI), and the induction of methylation is much lower in *CDKN2A* than in *THBD*. Error bars indicate standard error.

2.4. Hypomethylation of repetitive elements in *H. pylori*-infected gastric mucosae

Global hypomethylation during gastric carcinogenesis remains unclear, not only when but also where in the genome it takes place. Repetitive elements such as LINE, Alu, and Satα, which occupy some 40% of the entire genome, have abundant CpG and a physiologically high DNA methylation state in normal cells. In cancer cells, however, all of these repetitive elements have a low methylation state. As a result, the overall genome has low methylation (low total amount of 5-methylcytosine), which is thought to lead to genome instability. In *H. pylori* -infected gastric mucosae, it has been shown that low methylation similar to that in cancer is already seen in repetitive elements of Alu and Satα [44]. In enlarged-fold gastritis, for which a relationship with poorly differentiated gastric cancer has been indicated, the DNA methylation level of LINE-1 is reported to be lower than in normal gastric mucosae or chronic gastritis without an enlarged fold [45]. There is a strong possibility that hypomethylation of repetitive elements is induced partially in *H. pylori* infected gastric mucosae. Further investigation will be necessary in the future with regard to the role of chronic inflammation associated with *H. pylori* infection in inducing hypomethylation of repetitive elements.

2.5. Accumulation of aberrant DNA methylation in gastric mucosae and gastric cancer risk

The DNA methylation levels of gastric mucosae of healthy individuals and non-cancerous gastric mucosae of gastric cancer patients were investigated with respect to the relationship between aberrant DNA methylation and gastric cancer risk (Fig. 1). The results showed that while the methylation levels were high and there were no significant differences between those who were positive for *H. pylori* infection, methylation levels were low and inhibited in those who were negative for current HP infection, and were 2- to 32- fold higher in the non-cancerous gastric mucosae of gastric cancer patients than in the gastric mucosae of healthy indivudals [40]. In other groups, DNA methylation levels were also investigated in the non-cancerous gastric mucosae of multiple gastric cancer patients, non-cancerous gastric mucosae of single gastric cancer patients, and gastric mucosae of healthy individuals, and it was found that in individuals negative for current *H. pylori* infection the DNA methylation level of *FLNc, HAND1* and *THBD* in particular was correlated with gastric cancer risk [46]. These are known as passenger methylations, but DNA methylation levels were high as a whole, and so quantitative measurement was simple and application as a cancer risk marker is thought to be possible. Mean DNA methylation of tumor suppressor genes *CDKN2A* and *MLH1* was very low, and it would be difficult to use these as cancer risk markers. However, among microRNA genes that function as tumor suppressor genes, some have high DNA methylation levels, as well as correlations with gastric cancer risk [47].

As shown above, passenger genes and microRNA genes are methylated in many cells in gastric mucosae by *H. pylori* infection, and tumor suppressor genes are thought to be methylated in a proportionately smaller number of cells. A high cancer risk state (epigenetic field for cancerization) is thought to be formed by this accumulation [48]. In gastric cancers, an epigenetic field for cancerization is likely to be present and can be detected using appropriate marker genes.

2.6. Progress of gastric mucosae DNA methylation level and gastric cancer risk diagnosis

H. pylori infection potently induces aberrant DNA methylation in gastric mucosae, and its accumulation is associated with gastric cancer risk. To clarify the temporal profiles of aberrant DNA methylation in gastric mucosae, we analyzed time trends of *FLNc* and *THBD* methylation levels in gastric mucosae before, and six weeks and 1 year after *H. pylori* eradication by Quantitative MSP. With respect to the relationship between aberrant DNA methylation in gastric mucosae and *H. pylori* eradication therapy, the authors investigated the trend in DNA methylation before and after *H. pylori* eradication therapy. After bacterial elimination, the DNA methylation levels decreased after six weeks and one year together with the improvement in chronic inflammation associated with *H. pylori* infection, and a certain level of DNA methylation remained [49].

A model such as in Fig. 2 is assumed if the DNA methylation that disappeared with *H. pylori* eradication is temporarily methylated and the DNA methylation that remained after bacterial elimination is permanently methylated. In other words, in cases of existing *H. pylori* infection, DNA methylation is strongly induced in cells of the entire gland, but if chronic inflammation resolves with *H. pylori* eradication therapy or spontaneous *H. pylori* elimination from the progression of gastric mucosal atrophy, the elicitation of new DNA methylation is decreased. Perhaps the DNA methylation that occurred in differentiated ductal epithelial cells disappears with cell turnover, and the aberrant DNA methylation that occurs in ductal stem cells or progenitor cells remains, even with resolution of chronic inflammation, reflecting the gastric cancer risk. It is possible that individuals with low levels of this permanent methylation also have a low risk of gastric cancer, and conversely, that those with high levels also have a high risk of gastric cancer. A prospective clinical trial is currently underway to test this.

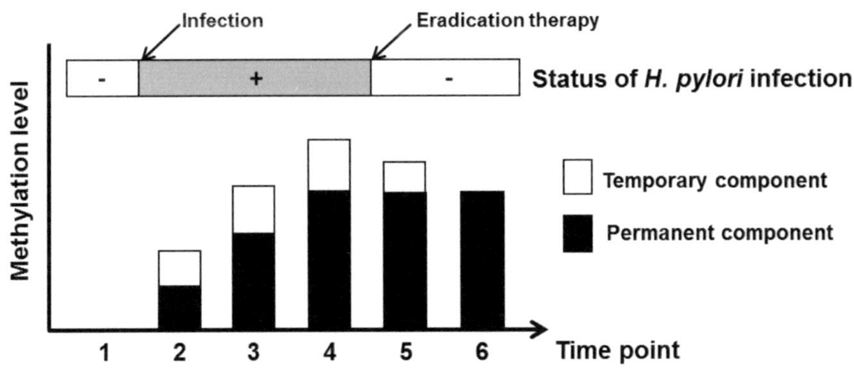

Figure 2. Model of the course of DNA methylation in *H. pylori*-infected gastric mucosae

DNA methylation is assumed to include temporary methylation, which is induced only during the time *H. pylori* infection is present, and permanent methylation that persists even after *H. pylori* infection has been eliminated with eradication therapy. Time point 1: Without *H. pylori* infection, the methylation is initially. Time points: 2–4, *H. pylori* infection induces both permanent and temporary components of methylation, and the total methylation level fluctuates due to fluctuation of the temporary component. Time points 5–6: after *H. pylori* infection discontinues, the temporary component disappears, and the increase in the permanent component stops. Permanent methylation very likely reflects gastric cancer risk.

3. Identification of gastric cancer risk group by serum PG test

3.1. Evaluation of *H. pylori*-related chronic gastritis by PG test

H. pylori -related chronic gastritis normally spreads from the gastric antrum to the gastric corpus [50, 51], and the progression of chronic atrophic gastritis (CAG) increases the risk for cancer [52-56]. An accurate and reliable evaluation of the extent of CAG is considered to be important for identifying high-risk individuals for cancer; however, it is difficult to accurately diagnose the extent of CAG based on a few biopsy samples, as CAG and intestinal metaplasia represent a multifocal process. Furthermore, histological diagnosis of gastric atrophy depends on subjective judgment without a gold standard [57, 58]. A more convenient and economical test for CAG progression, free of discomfort or risk and based on objective parameters, is necessary.

PG is an inactive precursor of the digestive enzyme pepsin produced exclusively in the stomach. Immunologically, there are two isoenzymes [59]. PG I is produced by chief cells and mucous neck cells of the fundic gland region. PG II, in addition to chief cells and mucous neck cells, is produced in the cardiac glands, pyloric glands and Brunner's glands, with producing cells located over a wide range from the stomach through the duodenum. The majority of PG produced (about 99%) is secreted in the gastric lumen and acts as a digestive enzyme, but a very small amount of PG (about 1%) is also located in the blood and can be measured and evaluated as serum PG. There is general agreement that serum PG levels reflect the morphological and functional status of the stomach mucosa [60, 61].

When the gland margin elevates with the progression of gastric mucosal atrophy diagnosed with chromoendoscopy using Congo red, a high correlation is seen in the incremental decrease in serum PG I levels and PG I/II ratio [62]. Thus, by measuring serum PG I levels and PG I/II ratio, it is possible to objectively evaluate the progress of CAG, which is the bed where gastric cancer develops [63]. In addition, elevated serum PG I and PG II levels and decreased PG I/II ratio are observed at the time of *H. pylori* infection, and have been shown to improve after eradication therapy [64], making them useful as inflammation markers of gastric mucosae.

Various criteria are used in the serum PG test. As criteria for the purpose of gastric cancer screening, a combination of PG I ≤70 ng/ml and PG I/II of ≤3.0, the reference value by Miki et al., has generally been adopted (PG index 1+) [63, 65]. When levels below the reference value are observed, the PG test is judged to be positive. In addition to this reference value, criteria such as PG I ≤50 ng/ml and PG I/II ratio ≤3.0 (PG index 2+), or PG I ≤30 ng/ml and PG I/II ratio ≤2.0 (PG index 3+), are the main criteria used to identify more highly advanced CAG. Since 1992, when PG assay kits became commercially available, a number of screening services provided by workplace or community health services adopted this serum test as a filter test [21, 66-71]. However, the long-term prognosis of subjects with extensive CAG identified by PG filter test is not fully known.

3.2. Accuracy of detecting gastric cancer using the serum PG test

Using a cohort of healthy middle-aged males, the authors conducted a 10-year follow-up survey of gastric cancer development [72-74]. Based on the results, the accuracy of each criterion for the serum PG test for gastric cancer with onset in the observation period was investigated [73]. With the best reference value (PG index 1+), sensitivity was 58.7%, specificity was 73.4%, and the positive predictive value was 2.6%. The low value for the overall sensitivity was conspicuous. Compared with a report from a meta-analysis of the accuracy of the PG test [75], these results were obviously poorer, with the low value for sensitivity in particular standing out.

One reason for this low sensitivity is thought to be that the patients in past reports of the above-mentioned meta-analysis were groups in which analysis had been performed soon after the start of the PG test and conventional stomach examinations by barium stomach x-ray. In other words, the subjects were groups with gastric cancer prevalence that did not fit well with conventional methods. The low sensitivity in the authors' investigation was thought to be because patients who developed gastric cancer soon after the start of the PG test were excluded, and the observations were of individuals who developed cancer over a longer period of 10 years. From the results of this study, even when performed with the PG test criteria having the best sensitivity, barium stomach x-ray test or some other type of stomach examination was thought to be essential, even for PG test-negative patients, to avoid overlooking gastric cancer, as about 40% of developed gastric cancer was excluded from the subjects of the accuracy test.

3.3. Gastric cancer risk in serum PG test-positive group

As one part of an investigation of the natural history of gastric cancer development, the authors investigated the gastric cancer risk in cohorts identified using each of the serum PG tests [73]. When the subjects were healthy middle-aged males, the annual gastric cancer incidence from the atrophy-negative group was 0.07%, when compared with 0.28% in the PG index 1+ group, 0.32% in the PG index 2+ group, and 0.42% in the PG index 3+ group. The gastric cancer incidence rose incrementally and significantly with the progression of CAG (Fig. 3). The above results thus show that the PG test-positive group is a high risk group for gastric cancer, and even if the development of gastric cancer is not seen at this time, the possibility that they will be affected with gastric cancer in the future is high, and therefore these subjects should continue to undergo detailed examinations and be carefully observed. Thus, the results show again that the PG test is useful as a marker for high risk of gastric cancer.

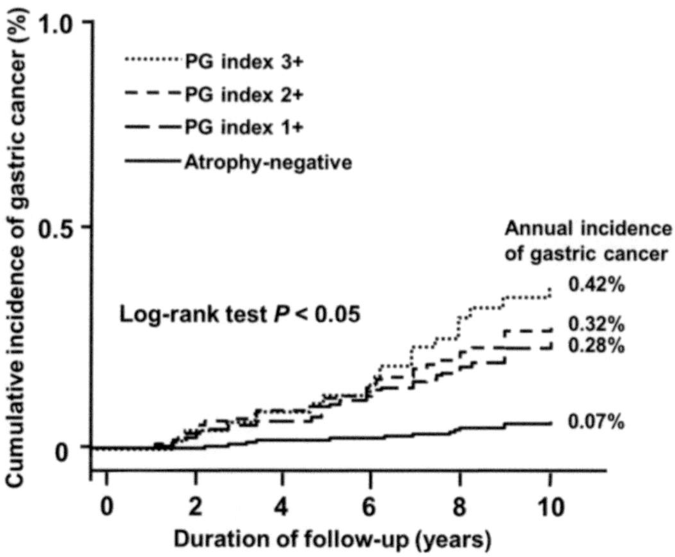

Figure 3. Kaplan-Meier analysis of gastric cancer development in subjects classified using the criteria of the serum PG test

The annual incidence of gastric cancer in cohorts identified using each serum PG test cut-off value (PG I ≤70 ng/ml and PG I/II of ≤3.0 (PG index 1+), PG I ≤50 ng/ml and PG I/II ratio ≤3.0 (PG index 2+), or PG I ≤30 ng/ml and PG I/II ratio ≤2.0 (PG index 3+)) in healthy middle-aged males is shown. Gastric cancer incidence increases in a stepwise fashion and significantly with the progression of chronic atrophic gastritis.

3.4. Identification of high risk for gastric cancer based on staging of *H. pylori*-related chronic gastritis

The relationship between the risk of developing gastric cancer and *H. pylori*-related chronic gastritis staging was also investigated in these same groups [72, 74]. In diagnosing *H. pylori* infection, anti- *H. pylori* antibody titer that can be easily performed with blood tests, similarly to serum PG levels, was used. *H. pylori* -related chronic gastritis stage, including the course from establishment of *H. pylori* infection to establishment of atrophic gastritis, was classified as follows based on a combination of both blood tests. The natural history of *H. pylori* -related chronic gastritis from the establishment of *H. pylori* infection can be expressed as a progression of A → B → C → D in each group. Thus, it is classified into four stages: Group A [*H. pylori* (-) & PG(-)], Group B [*H. pylori* (+) & PG(-)], Group C [*H. pylori* (+) & PG(+)] and Group D [*H. pylori* (-) & PG(+)]. Group A comprised *H. pylori* non-infected healthy men. Group B showed established *H. pylori* infection, but without CAG. Group C had CAG, and Group D had severe intestinal metaplasia due to progression of CAG. However, *H. pylori* in Group D had been spontaneously eliminated, representing so-called metaplastic gastritis.

The results of a 10-year follow-up survey showed that the annual gastric cancer incidence in each group with this staging was 0% in Group A (no occurrence of gastric cancer in 10 years in this group), 0.11% in Group B (1 in 1,000 individuals developed gastric cancer each year), 0.24% in Group C (1 in 400 individuals developed gastric cancer each year) and 1.31% in Group D (1 in about 80 individuals developed gastric cancer each year). Similar results were observed in a study by Watabe et al.[76]. The above shows that gastric cancer incidence rises incrementally together with the stage progression of *H. pylori*-related chronic gastritis (Fig. 4). In the 10-year follow-up survey, all of those who developed gastric cancer were positive for *H. pylori* infection. This shows that nearly all cases of gastric cancer in Japan derive from *H. pylori*-related chronic gastritis. Based on this fact, it is theoretically possible to identify both high- and low-risk groups (Group A). Using blood test results in this way, the evaluation of the gastric cancer risk in individuals is possible and expected to be useful in grouping individuals for appropriate gastric cancer screening.

H. pylori-related chronic gastritis stage	Group A HP(-), PG(-)	Group B HP(+), PG(-)	Group C HP(+), PG(+)	Group D HP(-), PG(+)
	Non-HP infection	Established HP infection	Extensive CAG	Metaplastic gastritis
Annual incidence of gastric cancer	0%	Approximately 0.1%	Approximately 0.25%	Approximately 1%

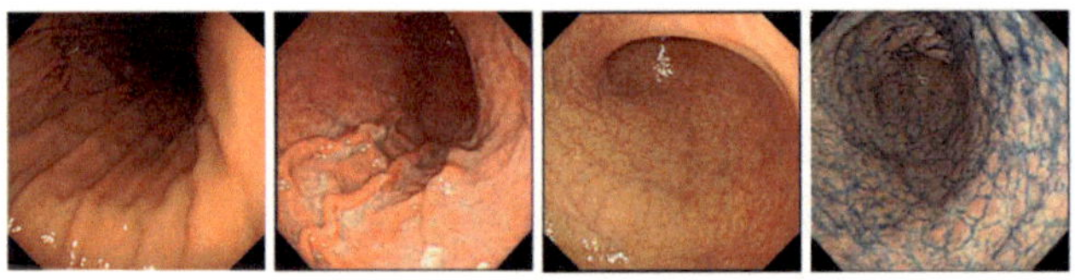

Figure 4. Gastric cancer risk based on *H. pylori*-related chronic gastritis stage classification

H. pylori-related chronic gastritis stage classified based on a combination of both Serum PG test and *H. pylori* antibody is shown. The gastric cancer incidence in healthy middle-aged males increases incrementally and significantly from Group A to Group D in accordance with stage progression.

3.5. Gastric cancer risk in serum PG test-negative group

Even though the serum PG test was shown to be a very useful test as a marker of gastric cancer risk, gastric cancer (particularly diffuse type gastric cancer) was seen in the PG test-negative group. In the authors' investigation, about 40% of gastric cancers were found to be PG test-negative gastric cancers, even using the PG test criteria (PG index 1+) that are thought to have the best balance for test accuracy. This needs to be kept fully in mind when diagnosing gastric cancer risk with the serum PG test. Even in the PG test-negative group, there is thought to be one group in which gastric cancer occurs with a high frequency in Group B of the *H. pylori* -related chronic gastritis staging. Serum PG levels are specific risk markers of gastric cancer development. The risk of developing cancer has been confirmed to increase incrementally with lower PG I levels and I/II ratio in particular [74].

Reviewing the PG-negative group based on this result, it was found to consist of three groups with different risks. Specifically, the PG test-negative group was further divided into three groups: Group α (serum PG I ≤70 ng/ml and PG I/II >3); Group β (serum PG I >70 ng/ml and PG I/II >3); and Group γ (serum PG I >70 ng/ml and PG I/II ≤3). The gastric cancer incidence in Group γ, which showed high serum PG II levels and is thought to have strong inflammation in the gastric mucosae, reached 0.2%, meaning this was a new high-risk group, in which mainly undifferentiated gastric cancer occurs (Fig. 5) [73]. Although the percentage in Group γ was not particularly high in the PG test-negative group, it is a subgroup that should be kept fully in mind. Furthermore, similarly to serum PG II levels, the group with high anti- *H. pylori* antibody titer, which is thought to be an indicator reflecting the level of inflammation, was shown to have a higher incidence of gastric cancer than the low group [74]. In addition, it was shown recently that in Group γ in particular, there are many cases of undifferentiated gastric cancer in individuals with high *H. pylori* antibody titer and endoscopic rugal hyperplastic gastritis[77]. The possibility of gastric cancer inhibition effects from *H. pylori* eradication therapy in such groups has also been demonstrated [78].

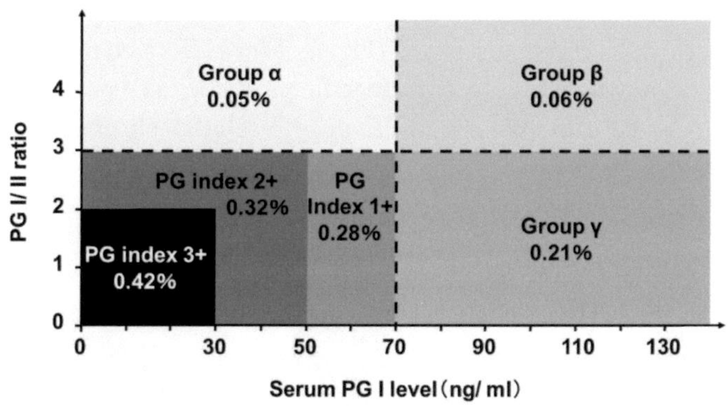

Figure 5. Group determination based on serum PG test and gastric cancer incidence

Schematic presentation of the atrophy-positive criterion and pepsinogen index, which are widely used for the PG filter test in Japan. PG index is used to detect subjects with severe gastric atrophy by subdividing the atrophy-positive criterion identified by PG I of ≤70 ng/mL and PG I/II ratio of ≤3.0 into three groups (PG index 1+ to 3+). Gastric cancer incidence increases in a stepwise fashion and significantly with the progression of chronic atrophic gastritis. In addition, the figure illustrates three subgroups, groups α, β, and γ, in the atrophy-negative criterion. The gastric cancer incidence in Group γ reached 0.2%, meaning this was a new high-risk group, in which mainly undifferentiated gastric cancer occurs.

3.6. Points to bear in mind in diagnosing gastric cancer risk from serum PG test

In the PG test-negative group, the development of cancer in Group A in the *H. pylori*-related chronic gastritis staging (PG test-negative and *H. pylori* judgment-negative) was not seen in a single case in the 10-year follow-up survey by the authors, but there are points to be mindful of in terms of the definitive diagnosis of a patient being in Group A. First is that when *H. pylori* antibody titer measurement kits have low sensitivity, the antibody titer may be negative despite existing HP infection. Second is the need for attention in patients who have undergone *H. pylori* eradication (they are negative for *H. pylori* but the risk of developing gastric cancer is not zero). Third is that, with regard to judging risk from serum PG levels, it cannot be applied in kidney failure patients or patients taking proton pump inhibitors (PPI) following gastrectomy. In addition, the authors have reported that individuals with PG I/II ratio ≤3.0, serum PG I ≤30 ng/ml, or serum PG II >30 ng/ml have a significantly higher risk of gastric cancer [74]. Thus, when the PG I/II ratio is ≤3.0 or serum PG I is ≤30 ng/ml, even in Group A, endoscopic examination should be performed and CAG should be evaluated.

4. Conclusion

Diagnosis of gastric cancer risk using the accumulation of aberrant DNA methylation in the gastric mucosae in endoscopic biopsy tissue and identification of high-risk gastric cancer groups based on serum PG test is discussed (Fig. 6). More effective measures for the prevention of gastric cancer may be possible with specific predictions of gastric cancer risk in individuals based on the natural history of *H. pylori* -related chronic gastritis, and future research results are anticipated.

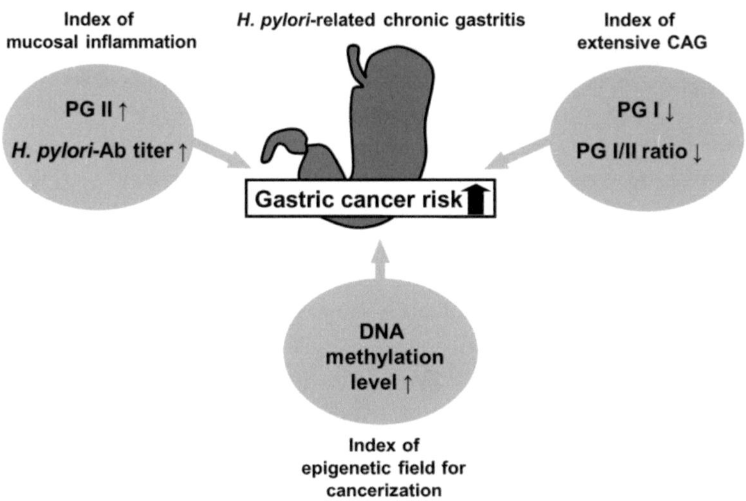

Figure 6. Schematic presentation of gastric cancer risk diagnosis based on *H. pylori* -related chronic gastritis. This article indicated that DNA methylation level of certain genes was associated with *H. pylori* infection and involved in the formation of epigenetic field for cancerization. The serum PG and/or *H. pylori* antibody levels provide an index of gastric cancer development, and that based on these markers the risk for gastric cancer can be objectively determined in each individual with *H. pylori* related chronic gastritis.

http://dx.doi.org/10.5772/53116

Author details

Shotaro Enomoto[1], Takao Maekita[1], Kazuyuki Nakazawa[1], Takeichi Yoshida[1], Mika Watanabe[1], Chizu Mukoubayashi[1], Hiroshi Ohata[1], Mikitaka Iguchi[1], Kimihiko Yanaoka[1], Hideyuki Tamai[1], Jun Kato[1], Masashi Oka[1], Osamu Mohara[2] and Masao Ichinose[1]

1 Second Department of Internal Medicine, Wakayama Medical University, Japan

2 Wakayama Wellness FoundationJapan,

References

[1] Marshall BJ, Warren JR. Unidentified curved bacilli in the stomach of patients with gastritis and peptic ulceration. Lancet. 1984; 1: 1311-5.

[2] Dooley CP, Cohen H, Fitzgibbons PL, et al. Prevalence of Helicobacter pylori infection and histologic gastritis in asymptomatic persons. N Engl J Med. 1989; 321: 1562-6.

[3] International Agency for Research on Cancer (IARC). Schistosomes,liver flukes, and Helicobacter pylori Working group on the evaluation of carcinogenic risks to humans. IARC Monogr Eval Carcinog Risks Hum. 1994; 61: 177-241.

[4] Correa P. Human gastric carcinogenesis: a multistep and multifactorial process--First American Cancer Society Award Lecture on Cancer Epidemiology and Prevention. Cancer Res. 1992; 52: 6735-40.

[5] Forman D, Newell DG, Fullerton F, et al. Association between infection with Helicobacter pylori and risk of gastric cancer: evidence from a prospective investigation. BMJ. 1991; 302: 1302-5.

[6] Parsonnet J, Friedman GD, Vandersteen DP, et al. Helicobacter pylori infection and the risk of gastric carcinoma. N Engl J Med. 1991; 325: 1127-31.

[7] Nomura A, Stemmermann GN, Chyou PH, Kato I, Perez-Perez GI, Blaser MJ. Helicobacter pylori infection and gastric carcinoma among Japanese Americans in Hawaii. N Engl J Med. 1991; 325: 1132-6.

[8] Talley NJ, Zinsmeister AR, Weaver A, et al. Gastric adenocarcinoma and Helicobacter pylori infection. J Natl Cancer Inst. 1991; 83: 1734-9.

[9] Sipponen P, Kosunen TU, Valle J, Riihela M, Seppala K. Helicobacter pylori infection and chronic gastritis in gastric cancer. J Clin Pathol. 1992; 45: 319-23.

[10] EUROGAST Study Group. An international association between Helicobacter pylori infection and gastric cancer.. Lancet. 1993; 341: 1359-62.

[11] Blaser MJ, Perez-Perez GI, Kleanthous H, et al. Infection with Helicobacter pylori strains possessing cagA is associated with an increased risk of developing adenocarcinoma of the stomach. Cancer Res. 1995; 55: 2111-5.

[12] Huang JQ, Sridhar S, Chen Y, Hunt RH. Meta-analysis of the relationship between Helicobacter pylori seropositivity and gastric cancer. Gastroenterology. 1998; 114: 1169-79.

[13] Uemura N, Okamoto S, Yamamoto S, et al. Helicobacter pylori infection and the development of gastric cancer. N Engl J Med. 2001; 345: 784-9.

[14] Watanabe T, Tada M, Nagai H, Sasaki S, Nakao M. Helicobacter pylori infection induces gastric cancer in mongolian gerbils. Gastroenterology. 1998; 115: 642-8.

[15] Honda S, Fujioka T, Tokieda M, Satoh R, Nishizono A, Nasu M. Development of Helicobacter pylori-induced gastric carcinoma in Mongolian gerbils. Cancer Res. 1998; 58: 4255-9.

[16] Hirayama F, Takagi S, Iwao E, Yokoyama Y, Haga K, Hanada S. Development of poorly differentiated adenocarcinoma and carcinoid due to long-term Helicobacter pylori colonization in Mongolian gerbils. J Gastroenterol. 1999; 34: 450-4.

[17] Zheng Q, Chen XY, Shi Y, Xiao SD. Development of gastric adenocarcinoma in Mongolian gerbils after long-term infection with Helicobacter pylori. J Gastroenterol Hepatol. 2004; 19: 1192-8.

[18] Sugiyama A, Maruta F, Ikeno T, et al. Helicobacter pylori infection enhances N-methyl-N-nitrosourea-induced stomach carcinogenesis in the Mongolian gerbil. Cancer Res. 1998; 58: 2067-9.

[19] Tokieda M, Honda S, Fujioka T, Nasu M. Effect of Helicobacter pylori infection on the N-methyl-N'-nitro-N-nitrosoguanidine-induced gastric carcinogenesis in mongolian gerbils. Carcinogenesis. 1999; 20: 1261-6.

[20] Shimizu N, Inada K, Nakanishi H, et al. Helicobacter pylori infection enhances glandular stomach carcinogenesis in Mongolian gerbils treated with chemical carcinogens. Carcinogenesis. 1999; 20: 669-76.

[21] Ohata H, Oka M, Yanaoka K, et al. Gastric cancer screening of a high-risk population in Japan using serum pepsinogen and barium digital radiography. Cancer Sci. 2005; 96: 713-20.

[22] Mukoubayashi C, Yanaoka K, Ohata H, et al. Serum pepsinogen and gastric cancer screening. Intern Med. 2007; 46: 261-6.

[23] Enomoto S, Maekita T, Ohata H, Yanaoka K, Oka M, Ichinose M. Novel risk markers for gastric cancer screening: Present status and future prospects. World J Gastrointest Endosc. 2010; 2: 381-7.

[24] Nakajima T, Oda I, Gotoda T, et al. Metachronous gastric cancers after endoscopic resection: how effective is annual endoscopic surveillance? Gastric Cancer. 2006; 9: 93-8.

[25] Gotoda T. Endoscopic resection of early gastric cancer. Gastric Cancer. 2007; 10: 1-11.

[26] Kakushima N, Fujishiro M. Endoscopic submucosal dissection for gastrointestinal neoplasms. World J Gastroenterol. 2008; 14: 2962-7.

[27] Esteller M. Epigenetics in cancer. N Engl J Med. 2008; 358: 1148-59.

[28] Jones PA, Baylin SB. The epigenomics of cancer. Cell. 2007; 128: 683-92.

[29] Ushijima T. Detection and interpretation of altered methylation patterns in cancer cells. Nat Rev Cancer. 2005; 5: 223-31.

[30] Gaudet F, Hodgson JG, Eden A, et al. Induction of tumors in mice by genomic hypomethylation. Science. 2003; 300: 489-92.

[31] Ushijima T, Sasako M. Focus on gastric cancer. Cancer Cell. 2004; 5: 121-5.

[32] Greenman C, Stephens P, Smith R, et al. Patterns of somatic mutation in human cancer genomes. Nature. 2007; 446: 153-8.

[33] Ushijima T, Asada K. Aberrant DNA methylation in contrast with mutations. Cancer Sci. 2010; 101: 300-5.

[34] Hussain SP, Harris CC. Inflammation and cancer: an ancient link with novel potentials. Int J Cancer. 2007; 121: 2373-80.

[35] Ushijima T, Okochi-Takada E. Aberrant methylations in cancer cells: where do they come from? Cancer Sci. 2005; 96: 206-11.

[36] Nishida N, Nagasaka T, Nishimura T, Ikai I, Boland CR, Goel A. Aberrant methylation of multiple tumor suppressor genes in aging liver, chronic hepatitis, and hepatocellular carcinoma. Hepatology. 2008; 47: 908-18.

[37] Issa JP, Ahuja N, Toyota M, Bronner MP, Brentnall TA. Accelerated age-related CpG island methylation in ulcerative colitis. Cancer Res. 2001; 61: 3573-7.

[38] Matsubayashi H, Canto M, Sato N, et al. DNA methylation alterations in the pancreatic juice of patients with suspected pancreatic disease. Cancer Res. 2006; 66: 1208-17.

[39] Enomoto S, Maekita T, Tsukamoto T, et al. Lack of association between CpG island methylator phenotype in human gastric cancers and methylation in their background non-cancerous gastric mucosae. Cancer Sci. 2007; 98: 1853-61.

[40] Maekita T, Nakazawa K, Mihara M, et al. High levels of aberrant DNA methylation in Helicobacter pylori-infected gastric mucosae and its possible association with gastric cancer risk. Clin Cancer Res. 2006; 12: 989-95.

[41] Kaneda A, Kaminishi M, Yanagihara K, Sugimura T, Ushijima T. Identification of silencing of nine genes in human gastric cancers. Cancer Res. 2002; 62: 6645-50.

[42] Nakajima T, Yamashita S, Maekita T, Niwa T, Nakazawa K, Ushijima T. The presence of a methylation fingerprint of Helicobacter pylori infection in human gastric mucosae. Int J Cancer. 2009; 124: 905-10.

[43] Niwa T, Tsukamoto T, Toyoda T, et al. Inflammatory processes triggered by Helicobacter pylori infection cause aberrant DNA methylation in gastric epithelial cells. Cancer Res. 2010; 70: 1430-40.

[44] Yoshida T, Yamashita S, Takamura-Enya T, et al. Alu and Sata Hypomethylation in Helicobacter pylori-Infected Gastric Mucosae Int J Cancer. 2011; 128: 33-9.

[45] Yamamoto E, Toyota M, Suzuki H, et al. LINE-1 hypomethylation is associated with increased CpG island methylation in Helicobacter pylori-related enlarged-fold gastritis. Cancer Epidemiol Biomarkers Prev. 2008; 17: 2555-64.

[46] Nakajima T, Maekita T, Oda I, et al. Higher methylation levels in gastric mucosae significantly correlate with higher risk of gastric cancers. Cancer Epidemiol Biomarkers Prev. 2006; 15: 2317-21.

[47] Ando T, Yoshida T, Enomoto S, et al. DNA methylation of microRNA genes in gastric mucosae of gastric cancer patients: its possible involvement in the formation of epigenetic field defect. Int J Cancer. 2009; 124: 2367-74.

[48] Ushijima T. Epigenetic field for cancerization. J Biochem Mol Biol. 2007; 40: 142-50.

[49] Nakajima T, Enomoto S, Yamashita S, et al. Persistence of a component of DNA methylation in gastric mucosae after Helicobacter pylori eradication. J Gastroenterol. 2010; 45: 37-44.

[50] Kimura K. Chronological transition of the fundic-pyloric border determined by stepwise biopsy of the lesser and greater curvatures of the stomach. Gastroenterology. 1972; 63: 584-92.

[51] Tatsuta M, Saegusa T, Okuda S. Studies on Gastritis in the Upper Portion of Stomach by Endoscopic Congo Red Test Endoscopy. 1973; 5: 61-9.

[52] Siurala M, Varis K, Wiljasalo M. Studies of patients with atrophic gastritis: a 10-15-year follow-up. Scand J Gastroenterol. 1966; 1: 40-8.

[53] Meister H, Holubarsch C, Haferkamp O, Schlag P, Herfarth C. Gastritis, intestinal metaplasia and dysplasia versus benign ulcer in stomach and duodenum and gastric carcinoma -- a histotopographical study. Pathol Res Pract. 1979; 164: 259-69.

[54] Sipponen P, Kekki M, Haapakoski J, Ihamaki T, Siurala M. Gastric cancer risk in chronic atrophic gastritis: statistical calculations of cross-sectional data. Int J Cancer. 1985; 35: 173-7.

[55] Testoni PA, Masci E, Marchi R, Guslandi M, Ronchi G, Tittobello A. Gastric cancer in chronic atrophic gastritis. Associated gastric ulcer adds no further risk. J Clin Gastroenterol. 1987; 9: 298-302.

[56] Tatsuta M, Iishi H, Nakaizumi A, et al. Fundal atrophic gastritis as a risk factor for gastric cancer. Int J Cancer. 1993; 53: 70-4.

[57] Plummer M, Buiatti E, Lopez G, et al. Histological diagnosis of precancerous lesions of the stomach: a reliability study. Int J Epidemiol. 1997; 26: 716-20.

[58] Guarner J, Herrera-Goepfert R, Mohar A, et al. Interobserver variability in application of the revised Sydney classification for gastritis. Hum Pathol. 1999; 30: 1431-4.

[59] Kageyama T, Ichinose M. Diversity of structure and function of pepsinogens and pepsins Rescent Research Developments and Biophysics and Biochemistry. 2003; 3: 159-78.

[60] Hirschowitz BI. Pepsinogen: its origins, secretion and excretion. Physiol Rev. 1957; 37: 475-511.

[61] Samloff IM, Varis K, Ihamaki T, Siurala M, Rotter JI. Relationships among serum pepsinogen I, serum pepsinogen II, and gastric mucosal histology. A study in relatives of patients with pernicious anemia. Gastroenterology. 1982; 83: 204-9.

[62] Miki K, Ichinose M, Shimizu A, et al. Serum pepsinogens as a screening test of extensive chronic gastritis. Gastroenterol Jpn. 1987; 22: 133-41.

[63] Ichinose M, Yahagi N, Oka M, et al. Screening for gastric cancer in Japan. Totowa, New Jersey: Humana Press, 2001; 87-102

[64] Furuta T, Kaneko E, Baba S, Arai H, Futami H. Percentage changes in serum pepsinogens are useful as indices of eradication of Helicobacter pylori. Am J Gastroenterol. 1997; 92: 84-8.

[65] Watanabe Y, Kurata JH, Mizuno S, et al. Helicobacter pylori infection and gastric cancer. A nested case-control study in a rural area of Japan. Dig Dis Sci. 1997; 42: 1383-7.

[66] Miki K, Ichinose M, Ishikawa KB, et al. Clinical application of serum pepsinogen I and II levels for mass screening to detect gastric cancer. Jpn J Cancer Res. 1993; 84: 1086-90.

[67] Kodoi A, Yoshihara M, Sumii K, Haruma K, Kajiyama G. Serum pepsinogen in screening for gastric cancer. J Gastroenterol. 1995; 30: 452-60.

[68] Hattori Y, Tashiro H, Kawamoto T, Kodama Y. Sensitivity and specificity of mass screening for gastric cancer using the measurment of serum pepsinogens. Jpn J Cancer Res. 1995; 86: 1210-5.

[69] Yoshihara M, Sumii K, Haruma K, et al. The usefulness of gastric mass screening using serum pepsinogen levels compared with photofluorography. Hiroshima J Med Sci. 1997; 46: 81-6.

[70] Kitahara F, Kobayashi K, Sato T, Kojima Y, Araki T, Fujino MA. Accuracy of screening for gastric cancer using serum pepsinogen concentrations. Gut. 1999; 44: 693-7.

[71] Miki K, Morita M, Sasajima M, Hoshina R, Kanda E, Urita Y. Usefulness of gastric cancer screening using the serum pepsinogen test method. Am J Gastroenterol. 2003; 98: 735-9.

[72] Ohata H, Kitauchi S, Yoshimura N, et al. Progression of chronic atrophic gastritis associated with Helicobacter pylori infection increases risk of gastric cancer. Int J Cancer. 2004; 109: 138-43.

[73] Yanaoka K, Oka M, Mukoubayashi C, et al. Cancer high-risk subjects identified by serum pepsinogen tests: outcomes after 10-year follow-up in asymptomatic middle-aged males. Cancer Epidemiol Biomarkers Prev. 2008; 17: 838-45.

[74] Yanaoka K, Oka M, Yoshimura N, et al. Risk of gastric cancer in asymptomatic, middle-aged Japanese subjects based on serum pepsinogen and Helicobacter pylori antibody levels. Int J Cancer. 2008; 123: 917-26.

[75] Dinis-Ribeiro M, Yamaki G, Miki K, Costa-Pereira A, Matsukawa M, Kurihara M. Meta-analysis on the validity of pepsinogen test for gastric carcinoma, dysplasia or chronic atrophic gastritis screening. J Med Screen. 2004; 11: 141-7.

[76] Watabe H, Mitsushima T, Yamaji Y, et al. Predicting the development of gastric cancer from combining Helicobacter pylori antibodies and serum pepsinogen status: a prospective endoscopic cohort study. Gut. 2005; 54: 764-8.

[77] Watanabe M, Kato J, Inoue I, et al. Development of gastric cancer in nonatrophic stomach with highly active inflammation identified by serum levels of pepsinogen and Helicobacter pylori antibody together with endoscopic rugal hyperplastic gastritis. Int J Cancer. 2012 in press

[78] Yanaoka K, Oka M, Ohata H, et al. Eradication of Helicobacter pylori prevents cancer development in subjects with mild gastric atrophy identified by serum pepsinogen levels. Int J Cancer. 2009; 125: 2697-703.

Section 6

Molecular Phathology, Biochemistry and Genetics in Pathways from H. Pylori Infection to Gastric Cancer

The Role of CagA Protein Signaling in Gastric Carcinogenesis — CagA Signaling in Gastric Carcinogenesis

Stephanie E. Morales-Guerrero,
Eduardo Mucito-Varela,
Germán Rubén Aguilar-Gutiérrez,
Yolanda Lopez-Vidal and Gonzalo Castillo-Rojas

Additional information is available at the end of the chapter

http://dx.doi.org/10.5772/53136

1. Introduction

Even though chronic gastritis was well established as a risk factor for the development of several gastric pathologies, such as peptic ulceration, gastric carcinoma, and lymphoma, before the discovery of *Helicobacter pylori* by Warren and Marshall in 1983 (Warren, 1983), the development of chronic gastritis was thought to be due to a plethora of possible causes such as stress, excessive alcohol consumption, ingestion of hot beverages and spicy food, among others (Mobley et al., 2001). With the association of *Helicobacter pylori* as the cause of chronic gastritis, the understanding of bacterial pathogenicity and the host response against the bacterium take enormous importance to understand the pathophysiology of the infection.

It is estimated that almost half of the world's population is infected with *Helicobacter pylori* and although the majority of colonized individuals remain asymptomatic, the infection represents the primary cause of chronic gastritis and it is a risk factor for the development of gastric cancer; it was the first bacterium classified as a type 1 carcinogen by the IARC in 1994 (IARC, 1994). Gastric cancer, despite its declining incidence rate, it remains as the fourth most common cancer and the second cause of cancer-related death worldwide (Ferlay J, 2010) and epidemiological studies have determined that attributable risk for gastric cancer conferred by *H. pylori* infection is approximately 75% (Peek & Blaser, 2002).

The development of gastritis associated with the infection is a multifactorial process, where the bacterium and host factors influence the pathogenesis of the disease. Colonization by *H. pylori* causes chronic gastritis, that can remain asymptomatic, produces gastric epithelial damage (Ricci et al., 2011). In the initial phase of infection, the bacteria penetrate through the mucous layer to multiply in the proximity of epithelial cells. The gastric epithelium responds to the infection by mucin depletion and cellular regenerative changes (Mobley et al., 2001); it also occurs the infiltration of polymorphonuclear cells into surface epithelium and hypochlorhydria and a deficient ascorbic acid secretion are also observed (Sobala et al., 1993). Later, bacterial components penetrate through the damaged epithelium and stimulates the production of IL-8 and IL-1 by macrophages, the activation and degranulation of mast cells and the release of inflammatory mediators that increase vascular permeability and up-regulate the expression of leukocyte adhesion molecules (Mobley et al., 2001). As the immune response fails to eliminate the bacteria, it occurs a gradual accumulation of inflammatory cells, which represents an active chronic phase of gastritis.

2. *Helicobacter pylori* virulence factors in gastritis and gastric cancer

Researchers have studied *H. pylori*'s virulence factors, to elucidate their role in the development of gastritis and gastric cancer, the most studied are the pathogenicity island (*cag*-PAI) and its effector, the cytotoxin associated protein (CagA) and the vacuolating cytotoxin (VacA). However, there are other virulence factors (Figure 1), including the urease, lipopolysaccharide, peptidoglycan, several adhesins, such as outer inflammatory protein (OipA), sialic acid-binding adhesin (SabA), blood group antigen-binding adhesin (BabA/B), that contribute to the damage in the gastric epithelium (Backert et al., 2010).

3. Urease

To colonize the stomach, *H. pylori* has to survive in the presence of acid produced in the stomach. To counteract this acidic environment, *H. pylori* produces an important enzyme, urease, which hydrolyses urea into NH_3 and CO_2. This enzyme has an essential role in the *H. pylori* infection as observed in urease-defective bacteria mutants which cannot colonize the stomach (Montecucco & Rappuoli, 2001). Urease causes damage to the epithelium through the production of ammonia, that in conjunction with neutrophil metabolites (Megraud et al., 1992), form carcinogenic agents that might participate in the development of gastric malignances (Suzuki et al., 1992). Ammonia is capable of cause different cell alterations, including swelling of intracellular acidic compartments, alterations of vesicular membrane transport, repression of protein synthesis and ATP production, and cell-cycle arrest (Montecucco & Rappuoli, 2001). Urease might also help to the recruitment of neutrophils and monocytes in the mucosa and to the production of proinflammatory cytokines (Harris et al., 1996).

http://dx.doi.org/10.5772/53136

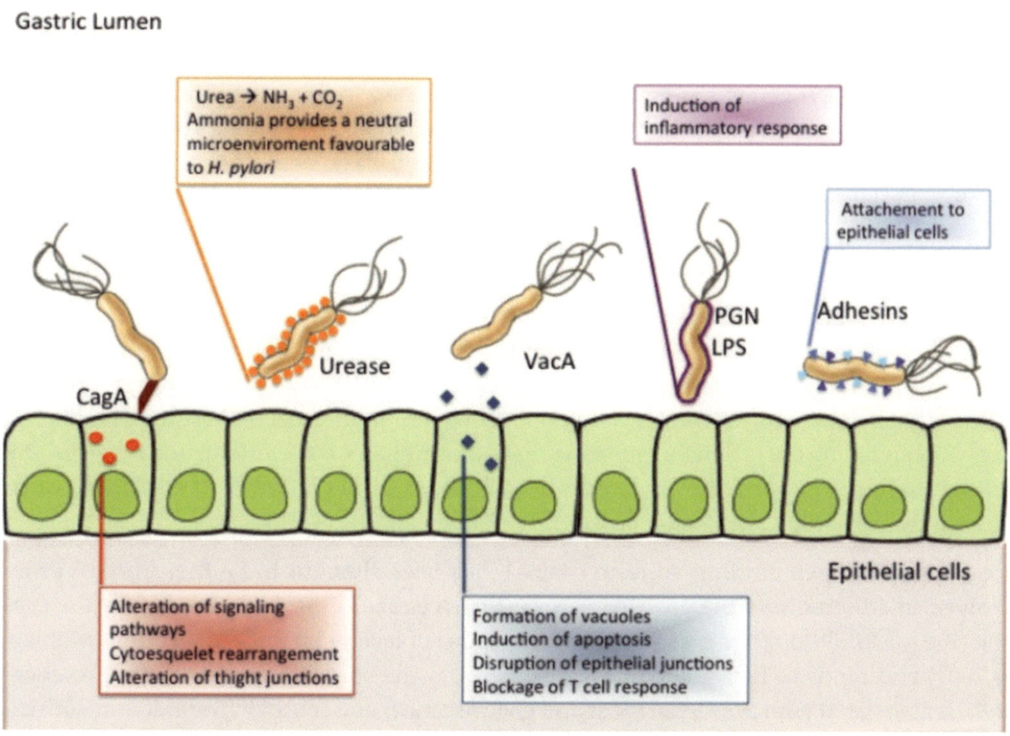

Figure 1. *Helicobacter pylori* virulence factors activities. Although CagA and VacA are the most studied virulence factors, there are more bacterial proteins that promote damage to the host cells.

4. Lipopolysaccharides (LPS) and peptidoglycan

H. pylori LPS are essential components of the bacterial outer membrane that induces a low immunological response in contrary to other bacteria (Moran, 1995). However, despite the low immunological activity of LPS, *H. pylori* colonization is associated with an inflammatory response, because *H. pylori* has the ability of activate mononuclear cells by LPS-independent mechanisms as well as other bacterial surface molecules (Mai et al., 1991, Moran, 1998). Another important component of the cell wall of *H. pylori*, peptidoglycan, interacts with the intracellular pattern recognition receptor Nod1 (an intracellular sensor for peptidoglycan from Gram-negative bacteria), this interaction leads to activation of NF-κB signaling, whit the subsequent secretion of the inflammatory molecules IL-8 (Viala et al., 2004) and β-defensin-2 (Boughan et al., 2006). On the other hand, peptidoglycan translocation of *H. pylori*, leads to enhanced PI3K-AKT signaling, which mediates protection from apoptosis and cell migration, both phenotypes related to carcinogenesis (Nagy et al., 2009).

5. Adhesins

Approximately 4% of the *H. pylori* genome is predicted to encode outer membrane proteins (OMPs) many of which serve as adhesins (Wroblewski et al., 2010), epithelial adhesion provides to *H. pylori* better access to epithelial surface and in this way contributes to deliver bacterial toxins such as CagA (Yamaoka, 2010). Fucosylated ABO blood group antigens and sialyl-Lewis^x and sialyl-Lewis^a antigens (sLe^x and sLe^a) have been identified as functional receptors for *H. pylori* (Boren et al., 1993).

The outer membrane inflammatory protein (OipA), identified in 2000 (Yamaoka et al., 2000), is involved in the attachment of *H. pylori* to gastric epithelial cells *in vitro* (Yamaoka, 2010). OipA is also involved in up-regulation of matrix metalloproteinase 1 (MMP-1), in inhibition of glycogen synthase kinase 3β (GSK-3β) and in β-catenin translocation to the nucleus, this protein also induces an inflammatory response and actin rearrangement through phosphorylation signaling pathways (Wroblewski et al., 2010), although, most of these are also involved in *cag*-PAI signaling alterations, suggesting that there might be some interaction between OipA and *cag*-PAI, it is important to note that it has been found a correlation coefficient of 0.82 between the *oipA* and *cagA* positivity in some virulent strains (Yamaoka et al., 2002).

Blood group antigen binding adhesin (BabA), has been thought to be the primary protein involved in adherence to the gastric mucosa (Boren et al., 1993). It is encoded by the *babA2* gene (the *babA1* although is present, is silent because of lack of an initiation codon (Mobley et al., 2001) and binds to fucosylated Lewis^b antigen. Some studies report that the presence of *babA2* is associated with duodenal ulcer and gastric cancer and found in conjunction with *cagA* and *vacA* s1 allele, provides a greater risk of develop a severe gastric disease (Gerhard et al., 1999).

Sialic acid-binding adhesin (SabA) is responsible of *H. pylori* binding to syalylated Le^x and Le^a in epithelial cells. Infiltration of neutrophils into the gastric mucosa is a characteristic feature of chronic gastritis caused by *H. pylori* and SabA binds to neutrophils through this sialylated carbohydrates and induces oxidative burst in these cells, which has a consequence of produce oxidative damage in gastric epithelium. It has been proposed that SabA-positive status is associated with gastric cancer, intestinal metaplasia, and corpus atrophy and negatively associated with duodenal ulcer and neutrophil infiltration (Yamaoka, 2008).

6. Vacuolating cytotoxin (VacA)

VacA is a pore-forming cytotoxin identified in supernatants of *H. pylori* broth cultures that cause aberrant vacuolation of cultured cells (Leunk et al., 1988). This cytotoxin is secreted from the bacteria as a large 140-kilodalton polypeptide and latter trimmed at both ends to finally deliver it in an active form to host cells, where it exerts its activity.

VacA induces multiple cellular activities, the best studied is the alteration on endosomal maturation which consequently leads to vacuolation of epithelial cells, VacA is also capable of induce membrane-channel formation, cytochrome c release from mitochondria, and binding to cell-membrane receptors activating a proinflammatory response (Amieva & El-Omar, 2008). VacA has the ability to cause leakage of ions and small molecules, by disrupting the barrier function of tight junctions (Papini et al., 1998) and also inhibit T-cell activation and proliferation (Gebert et al., 2003).

All strains of *H. pylori* contain the *vacA* gene, although, there is considerable genetic diversity among them, and consequently the cytotoxicity activity of the toxin varies between strains (Amieva & El-Omar, 2008). The diversity observed is attributed to variations in *vacA* gene structure within the signal (s) region, the middle (m) region, and the intermediate (i) region (Wroblewski et al., 2010).

The amino terminus contains the signal sequence that shows allelic variability and has been classified into different types. Strains with s1 allele secrete an active toxin and are also highly associated with ulcers and gastric cancer (Atherton et al., 1995), however, s1/s2 combination or s2 genotypes are found in patients with gastric cancer (Lopez-Vidal et al., 2008). The middle region of the gene also shows allelic variation, with m1 subtype having stronger vacuolating activity and it is associated with an increased risk for development of gastric epithelial injury and gastric cancer (Yamaoka, 2010).

The clinical isolates of *H. pylori* have been grouped into two broad families defined as type I and type II on the basis of whether they have a functional pathogenicity island (*cag*-PAI), and secrete an active vacuolating cytotoxin (VacA). Type I strains are positive for all these characteristics. In contrast, type II strains do not have a functional *cag*-PAI and possess the *vacA* gene that encodes for non-toxic protein (Censini et al., 1996, Tomb et al., 1997).

7. Cytotoxin associated gen-Pathogenicity Island (*cag*-PAI)

Colonization of the human stomach by *H. pylori* virulent strains is associated with a significantly increased risk for the development of several gastric diseases, such as gastric cancer. These highly virulent *H. pylori* strains harbor a (cytotoxin-associated genes) pathogenicity island (*cag*-PAI) that encode proteins that are components of a type IV secretion system (T4SS) apparatus and the CagA effector protein into host target cells (Castillo-Rojas et al., 2004). T4SS translocates the bacterial oncoprotein CagA and peptidoglycan that induces proinflammatory chemokine and cytokine secretion, including interleukin-8 (IL-8) in gastric epithelial cells (Figueiredo et al., 2005). The hallmark of *H. pylori* virulent strains is the presence of *cag*-PAI that induce of gastric mucosal inflammation, which is a risk factor for developing severe gastric pathologies (Antonio-Rincon et al., 2011).

The presence of flanking direct repeated sequences 605 (IS605) in the *cag*-PAI have been reported to cause rearrangements and partial or total deletions of it. This has generated *H. pylori* strains with varying virulence, and consequently, the clinical outcome of the infection (Censini et al., 1996).

T4SSs are a large group of highly versatile secretion machineries in many Gram-negative pathogenic bacteria that are evolutionarily related to bacterial conjugative systems (Fronzes et al., 2009). Although the *H. pylori cag*-PAI has been evolutionarily related to others T4SSs based on their common features like structural and sequence similarities, only a few *cag* PAI proteins (also termed as HP o VirB/D) show clear sequence similarities to the prototypical system of *A. tumefaciens* and other bacterial species.

A systematic mutagenesis study with isogenic mutants in each of the *cag*-PAI genes, reported that 14 genes out of 27 of *cag*-PAI are essential for CagA translocation and induction of IL-8 secretion in gastric epithelial cells (Aguilar et al., 2001).

Twelve genes out of 27 of *cag*-PAI encoded proteins share sequence similarities with components of the prototypical T4SS system VirB/D4 of *Agrobacterium tumefaciens*, which contains 11 essential proteins of the secretion apparatus (VirB1–VirB11) encoded by the operon *virB* and a coupling protein (VirD4) that mediates substrate recognition (Fronzes et al., 2009). The majority of these proteins are conserved among the known T4SSs of other bacteria (Alvarez-Martinez & Christie, 2009).

The prototypical (macromolecular complex) T4SS of *A. tumefaciens*, is among the best-studied T4SS and is composed of two major structural complexes: the T-pilus and a membrane-associated complex responsible for the translocation of substrates crosss the inner and the outer membrane (Fronzes et al., 2009, Alvarez-Martinez & Christie, 2009). The membrane-associated complex includes the energetic components VirB4, VirB11 and VirD4, which are conserved among the known T4SSs of other bacteria. These proteins contain Walker nucleotide binding, and hydrolysis motifs and are known to energize T4SS for its function. The membrane-associated complex also includes the proteins VirB1, VirB3, VirB6, VirB7, VirB8, VirB9 and VirB10 that form the substrate translocation channel that spans both bacterial membranes. VirB6, VirB8, and VirB10 are part of the subcomplex of proteins attached to the inner membrane with domains spanning the periplasm, while VirB7 and VirB9 are part of the outer membrane subcomplex. The T4SS-determined T-pilus is an extracellular appendage that is thought to initiate cell–cell contact with plant target cells before the initiation of T-DNA transfer. This structure includes the proteins VirB2 and VirB5 as major and minor components, respectively (Backert et al., 2008).

H. pylori and *A. tumefaciens* share similarity in several components of their T4SSs and probably function in a similar manner (Backert & Meyer, 2006). Nevertheless, the molecular mechanisms responsible for assembly, activity and specific recognition of host target cells of these macromolecular complexes remains unclear. It has been suggested that after the induction by cell contact, *H. pylori* forms T4SS pili located at one bacterial pole for the injection of virulence factors into target cells such as the oncoprotein CagA.

8. Cytotoxin-associated protein (CagA)

CagA protein is the only known effector protein translocated to the host cell by the T4SS (Backert et al., 2010). It was firstly described as a very immunogenic protein in humans infected with cytotoxin-producing strains (Covacci et al., 1993). After that, its association with gastric cancer and peptic ulcer was well established.

Recent reports suggest that CagA is able to down regulate the vacuolation effects of VacA on host cells, and conversely, VacA is able to down regulates CagA activity (Oldani et al., 2009, Tegtmeyer et al., 2009). Clinical isolates that contain the *cag*-PAI generally are *babA, oipA* and *vacA* s1 positive, Yamaoka proposes that these virulence factors may interact with each other with a certain biological significance; therefore, these factors interact synergistically with each other to induce gastric diseases (Yamaoka, 2010).

CagA is encoded by the *cag*A gene, located at one end of the *cag*-PAI (Censini et al., 1996). One copy per genome is present in most of the strains whose genome has been sequenced but strains with two gene copies might exist, as revealed by the genome sequence of the Amerindian strains *H. pylori* Shi470 and V225d, although functionality of both copies in these strains is unknown (Kersulyte et al., Mane et al., 2010). It has been estimated that 60-95% of strains worldwide carry the *cag*A gene, which is different between geographic regions (Hatakeyama, 2004). However, the complete *cag*-PAI is important for the translocation of this protein and the completeness of the island may impact on the association of CagA presence and the outcome of the disease.

Other main feature of CagA protein is its high variable size, which range from 120-145 kDa (Covacci et al., 1993, Tummuru et al., 1993). This variation is due to the presence of polymorphism at the carboxy-terminal region given by the presence of repeat sequences called EPIYA motifs, which are present in a copy number varying from one to seven (Xia et al., 2009). Four major types of EPIYA motifs (A, B, C, and D) have been described based on the specific amino acid sequence that flanks the Glu-Pro-Ile-Tyr-Ala motif at both sides (Hatakeyama, 2004).

The EPIYA-repeat region of CagA is made of tandem alignment of the four distinct EPIYA segments (A, B, C, D) in various combinations (Hatakeyama, 2011). CagA molecules containing the EPIYA-A, EPIYA-B and EPIYA-C segments in tandem are denoted as "western type", and are found in many *H. pylori* isolates from Europe, North America, and Australia. On the other hand, CagA carrying EPIYA-A, EPIYA-B and EPIYA-D segments are called "East Asian type" and have been isolated in East Asian countries such as Japan, Korea and China (Furuta et al., 2011).

The EPIYA-C segment in "Western type" isolates can be present in up to five copies which might be due to recombination mediated by a 16 amino acid sequence designated CagA multimerization sequence that is present at both sides of EPIYA-C motif. The CagA multimerization sequence is also present in EPIYA-D but only at one end, therefore cannot duplicate by this mechanism (Furuta et al., 2011). Other implications of CagA multimerization sequence in the bacterial pathogenicity will be discussed later in the text.

It has been proposed that EPIYA motifs of CagA act as "master keys" that can potentially be tyrosine-phosphorylated by host kinases and are capable to interact with a wide range of different host cell proteins (Backert et al., 2010). In the same way, the observation that the EPIYA-region is unstructured and can adopt multiple conformations mimicking host substrates of kinase families, thus manipulating eukaryotic cellular biochemistry during infection, provides further support for this "master key" hypothesis (Nesic et al., 2010).

In contrast to the polymorphic C-terminal EPIYA region of CagA, N-terminal region is well conserved among CagA proteins (Hatakeyama, 2011). The N-terminal CagA region is required for the membrane association of CagA in polarized epithelial cells (Bagnoli et al., 2005) and is important for its translocation into host cells (Murata-Kamiya et al., 2010), the first 200 amino acids at the N-terminus of CagA form a membrane-binding domain in *H. pylori*, mediating proper translocation of the CagA protein via the T4SS (Steininger et al., 2011).

9. CagA tridimensional structure and membrane localization

It has been shown that CagA targeting to the epithelial cell membrane is important for host signaling (Higashi et al., 2002, Bagnoli et al., 2005, Higashi et al., 2005) and there is evidence that membrane binding of CagA is important for its translocation into host cells (Murata-Kamiya et al., 2010, Steininger et al., 2011).

Recently, it has been proposed that interaction of CagA with host cell proteins depends on the localization of CagA into distinct compartments in host cells (Pelz et al., 2011). The model proposed states that membrane localization is mediated by two membrane domains, one composed by residues 1-200 (N-terminal domain) and the other from 200-1216 (C-terminal domain), detailed description of the function of these domains are described in the Figure 2. In addition, C-terminal domain is comprised of two regions that interact with each other and are located in the membrane together when linked to N terminal domain, the first region is from amino acids 200-800 containing phosphatidyl serine binding domain and the second from 800-1216 containing EPIYA and CagA multimerization motifs. The region from 800-1216 when expressed alone localizes in cytosol and produces a strong alteration in cell morphology (Steininger et al., 2011).

According with the above-mentioned model, CagA spatial conformation may play an important role for the proper translocation and compartmentalization, so a tridimentional structure prediction of CagA was made using I-TASSER, which has been ranked as the best method for the automated protein structure prediction in the last two community-wide critical assessment of protein structure prediction (CASP) experiments (Roy et al., 2010). The best predicted model for both East-Asia and Western type of CagA consists of a sinuous super helical structure in which N-terminal region protrudes at one side and C-terminal region forms a loop (Figure 3). These predicted structural models agree with the model proposed of Steininger et al., in which amino acids 200-1216 forms two domains that interact with each other (Steininger et al., 2011). According to the results obtained with I-TASSER the most similar structure available in the PDB database (www.rcsb.org/pdb/home/home.do) is from Cand1 protein, however the only function similarity shared with CagA is the capacity of protein binding.

Interestingly, it is also proposed that N-terminal membrane-binding domain functions as an inhibitory domain of the C-terminal region effects, and that region from 800-1216 when expressed alone induces the highest percentage of epithelial cell elongation (Pelz et al., 2011). Also it has been proposed that CagA is cleaved by proteases in human cells yielding two fragments of about 100-105 kDa and 35-40 kDa (Moese et al., 2001), the last would correspond to the region from amino acid 800-1216. This leads to the question if some structural variants of CagA are better cleaved inside the host cell so that can not be totally inhibited by the N-terminal membrane-binding domain, but this requires investigation.

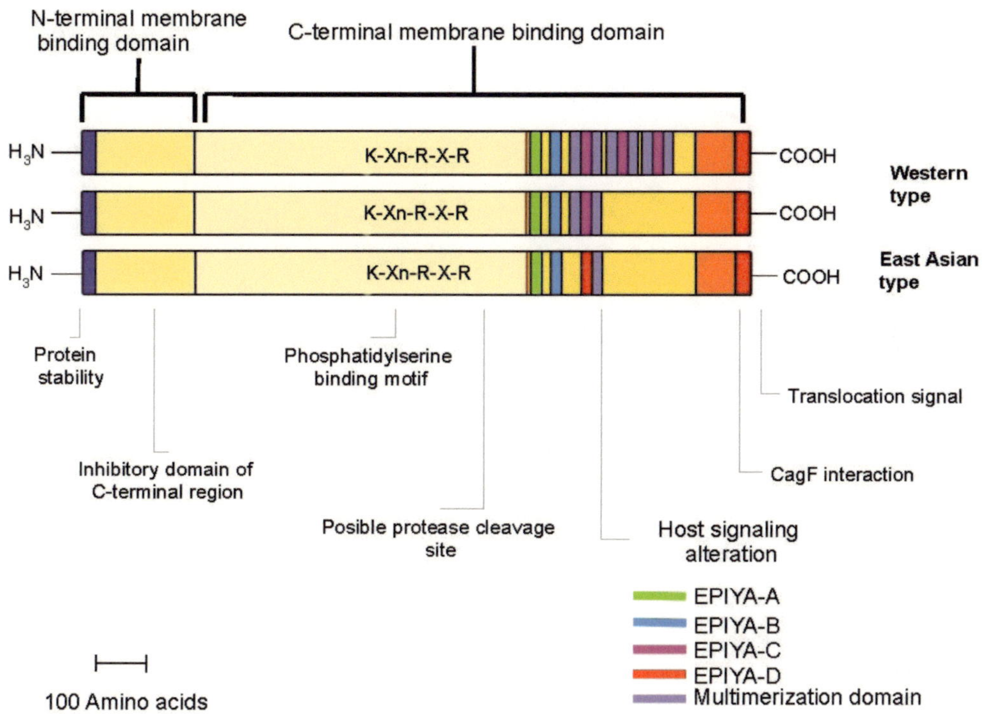

Figure 2. CagA structure in schematic representation. The most common variants of western and East Asian type are depicted. CagA possess at least two membrane-binding domains (Steininger et al., 2011), which are marked with quotation. Main known functions of certain regions are mentioned.

10. Phosphorylation-dependent cell signaling of CagA

Phosphorylation of CagA deregulates several signaling pathways leading to modification in host cell shape and adhesion, contributing to the transformation of cells (Hatakeyama, 2011, Jones et al., 2010). All of the EPIYA motifs in the four distinct EPIYA segments serve as tyrosine phosphorylation sites of CagA in host cells (Hatakeyama, 2011). Enzymes that can phosphorylate CagA *in vitro* and during infection *in vivo* are members of the Src and Abl families, which have been, recognized as oncogenic tyrosine kinases (Selbach et al., 2002, Stein et al., 2002,

Poppe et al., 2007, Tammer et al., 2007). The phosphorylation is a hierarchic regulated process in which c-Src phosphorylates EPIYA-C or EPIYA-D early in infection, while c-Abl phosphorylates either EPIYA-A, EPIYA-B, EPIYA-C, or EPIYA-D later in infection but only 2 EPIYA sites can be simultaneously phosphorylated per CagA molecule (Mueller et al., 2012). Furthermore, simultaneous phosphorylation of EPIYA-AC or EPIYA-BD confers strongest elongation phenotype in an AGS cellular model, even in a single CagA protein with both of the phosphorylatable EPIYA motifs (preferably EPIYA-AC), or in 2 independent CagA proteins, each with a single phosphorylatable EPIYA motif, which may form dimers to trigger this response (Mueller et al., 2012).

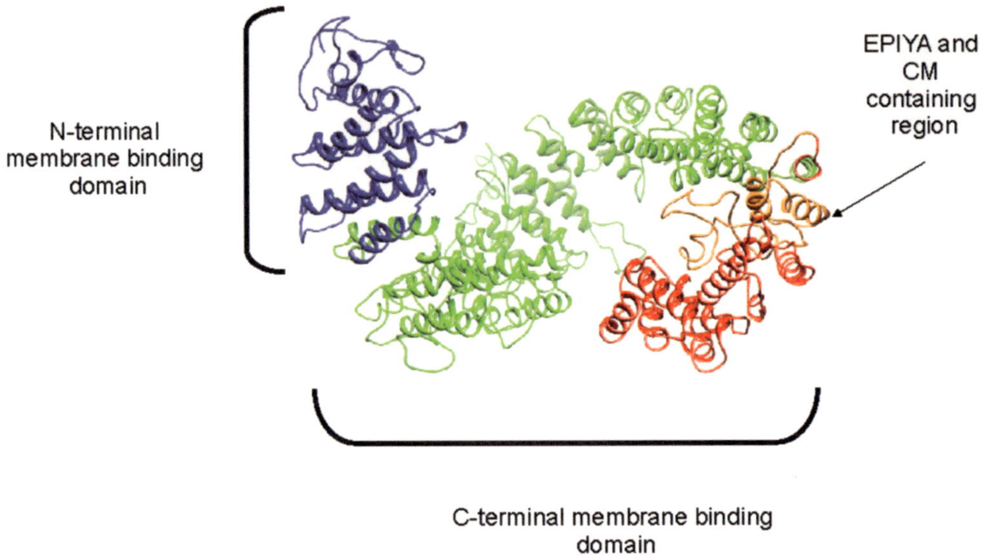

Figure 3. Tridimensional structure of CagA. The model was predicted using I-TASSER, image was obtained using UCSF CHIMERA software (Pettersen et al., 2004).

Once tyrosine phosphorylated, EPIYA-C or -D can bind to SHP-2 phosphatase (Hatakeyama, 2011) and activates the phosphatase activity of Shp2 producing an extremely elongated cell shape known as the hummingbird phenotype and altered cell motility (Backert et al., 2010, Higashi et al., 2004, Tsutsumi et al., 2006). SHP2 is required for full activation of the MAPK/ERK pathway, which conveys a potent mitogenic signal (Matozaki et al., 2009) and for direct dephosphorylation and inactivation of focal adhesion kinase, FAK, that deregulates integrin signaling (Tsutsumi et al., 2006).

Carrying the type EPIYA-D or multiple EPIYA-C repeats is associated with increased SHP-2 phosphatase activity induced by CagA, increasing the risk of precancerous and cancer lesions. This is because East-specific D segment shows higher binding affinity to SHP2 than the West-specific C segment but the C-type motif is variable in copy number and sequence, which can provide more sites for SHP2 binding.

On the other hand, phosphorylated EPIYA-A and EPIYA-B have been shown ability to bind to Csk (Tsutsumi et al., 2003). Interaction of CagA with Csk stimulates the kinase activity of Csk, which in turn inhibits Src in a negative feedback loop that constrains the phosphorylation-dependent CagA activity below a certain threshold to ensure long-term colonization of *H. pylori* in the stomach without causing fatal damages (Hatakeyama, 2011). In addition, phosphorylated EPIYA-B can interact with phosphatidylinositol 3-kinase (PI3K) that regulates diverse cellular functions including proliferation and survival via AKT pathway (Nagy et al., 2009).

11. Phosphorylation-independent cell signaling of CagA

Recent studies have shown that not all cellular interactions exerted by CagA depend on its tyrosine phosphorylation so far more than 13 cellular interaction partners of non-phosphorylated CagA have been identified (Backert et al., 2010, Tegtmeyer et al., 2009, Mimuro et al., 2002). It has been shown that these interactions exert effects such as pro-inflammatory and mitogenic responses, disruption of cell-to-cell junctions or loss of cell polarity.

The first cellular interaction partner described of non-phosphorylated CagA was the adapter protein Gbr2 (Mimuro et al., 2002). Recently, it was reported that Gbr2 is the only host factor that interacts with both phosphorylated and non-phosphorylated EPIYA motifs (Selbach et al., 2009). Non-phosphorylated CagA was shown to interact with Gbr2 *both in vitro* and *in vivo*, which provides a mechanism by which Gbr2-associated SOS (son of sevenless) is recruited to the plasma membrane, this complex (CagA-Gbr2-SOS) can promote Ras-GTP formation, leading to cell scattering by stimulation of the MAPK/ERK signaling pathway as well as activation of nuclear transcription factors involved in cell proliferation and expression of the anti-apoptotic myeloid cell leukemia sequence-1 protein (Mimuro et al., 2007).

On the other hand, Chang YJ, et al., 2006, reported that *cagA*-positive *H. pylori* strains affect the cell cycle during infection by stimulating cyclin D1 expression, G1-S phase progression and host cell survival, suggesting the presence of distinct functional domains within CagA that play essential roles in protein targeting and alteration of host-cell transcription signaling pathways (Chang et al., 2006).

Yokoyama et al., 2005, found that CagA can stimulate the calcium-dependent serine/threonine phosphatase calcineurin in gastric epithelial cells, inducing translocation of the nuclear factor of activated T cells (NFAT) from the cytoplasm to the nucleus, where activates NFAT-dependent genes (Yokoyama et al., 2005). It is possible that the reported CagA-PLC interaction triggers Ca^{2+} mobilization and subsequent activation of calcineurin.

One of the NFAT-dependent genes activated by CagA in gastric epithelial cells is p21Cip1, a cyclin-dependent kinase inhibitor. Accordingly, although CagA activates a growth-promoting signal via the SHP-2-MAP kinase pathway or the Grb2-Ras-MAP kinase pathway, it simultaneously inhibits cell proliferation through NFAT-dependent p21Cip1 induction. Intriguingly, the *H. pylori*-vacuolating toxin *vac*A counteracts the activity of CagA to stimulate NFAT. Thus,

VacA has a role in determining the magnitude of NFAT deregulation in gastric epithelial cells expressing CagA. Such a functional interplay between CagA and VacA has already been suggested from the observation that secretion of VacA protein is associated with the presence of CagA despite the presence of vacA gene in all *H. pylori* strains (Yokoyama et al., 2005).

The CagA multimerization sequence mediates a stable binding with SHP-2 protein potentiating CagA virulence and is also responsible of the phosphorylation-independent activity of CagA (Ren et al., 2006, Nagase et al., 2011). Furthermore, it has been shown that CagA binds and inhibits the polarity-regulating kinase partitioning-defective 1 (PAR1)/ microtubule affinity-regulating kinase (MARK) through CagA multimerization sequence (Nagase et al., 2011). Kurashima et al., showed that CagA multimerization sequence destabilizes the E-cadherin/beta-catenin complex to trigger aberrant activation of the beta-catenin signal that underlies intestinal metaplasia (Kurashima et al., 2008). Recently, it was shown that the diversity in the structure and number of CagA multimerization sequences influence the strength of pathological activities of individual CagA with its cellular targets (PAR1b and SHP-2), emphasising its importance as a determinant of the degree of virulence of CagA (Lu et al., 2008) for development of gastric cancer.

A recent study shows that CagA can also interact with runt-related transcription factor gene 3 (RUNX3, a tumor suppressor that is frequently inactivated in gastric cancer) by a novel identified WW domain in the amino-terminal region of CagA (Tsang et al., 2010). In particular, CagA induces the ubiquitination and degradation of RUNX3, thereby extinguishing its ability to inhibit the transcriptional activation of RUNX3; currently, functional inactivation of RUNX3 can be caused by mutation, epigenetic gene silencing (promoter methylation) or cytoplasmic protein mislocalization (Ito, 2011). Recent evidence shows a strong association between methylation of the RUNX3 promoter and gastric cancer (Fan et al., 2011, Li et al., 2011). Recently, Lin et al., found that loss of RUNX3 in gastric cancer prevents G1 phase arrest and promotes tumorigenesis through Akt1/ß-catenin/cyclin D1 signaling pathway (Lin et al., 2012).

A consequence of non-phosphorylated CagA interactions in polarized epithelial cells is the disruption of cell junctions. In particular, tight and adherence junctions are essential for the integrity of the gastric epithelium (Wessler & Backert, 2008). CagA interferes with these intercellular junctions via several pathways. 1) Injected CagA associates with the epithelial tight-junction scaffolding protein, zone occludens-1 (ZO-1), and the transmembrane protein, junction adhesion molecule (JAM2), causing an ectopic assembly of tight-junction components at sites of bacterial attachment (Amieva & El-Omar, 2008), leading to alterations of cell polarity. 2) Non-phosphorylated CagA can interact with the transmembrane cell-cell junction protein E-cadherin (Hatakeyama, 2008). Subsequently, it was found that CagA forms a complex with c-Met recruiting E-cadherin and the Armadillo-domain protein, catenin delta, indicating that the interaction between CagA and E-cadherin is not direct (Oliveira et al., 2009). Baek et al., in 2007, reported that the interaction of alpha-Pix (PAK-interactive exchange factor) with CagA activates PAK1, ERK and NF-κB, which induces IL-8 expression (Baek et al., 2007, Lim et al., 2009); beta 1 integrin (integrin ß1) is another CagA-independent signaling that promotes cell motility (Snider et al., 2008), although the functional importance of this interaction needs to be investigated.

12. Concluding remarks

Studies host interactions with *H. pylori* virulence factors, such as CagA and the T4SS, have provided us many fundamental insights into the processes leading to *H. pylori* pathogenesis. The current hypothesis implies a model with translocated CagA as an "eukaryotic" signaling mimetic molecule either present in a large multiprotein complex or simultaneously in separated locations whitin infected target cells, which may have an important impact on the multistep pathogenesis of *H. pylori*. In the future, it will be important to search for additional injected proteins because it is rather unlikely that *cag*-PAI acquisition during evolution was intended to inject few effectors like CagA and peptidoglycan. Future studies are required to uncover the complex mechanisms that explain how *H. pylori* interacts whit host cells at the molecular level to accomplish its persistence through host life.

Author details

Stephanie E. Morales-Guerrero[1], Eduardo Mucito-Varela[1], Germán Rubén Aguilar-Gutiérrez[2], Yolanda Lopez-Vidal[1] and Gonzalo Castillo-Rojas[1]

1 Programa de Inmunología Molecular Microbiana, Departamento de Microbiología y Parasitología, Facultad de Medicina, Universidad Nacional Autónoma de México (UNAM), México City, México

2 Centro de Investigación Sobre Enfermedades Infecciosas (CISEI), Instituto Nacional de Salud Pública (INSP). Cuernavaca, Morelos, México

References

[1] Aguilar, G. R., G. Ayala & G. Fierros-Zarate, (2001) *Helicobacter pylori*: recent advances in the study of its pathogenicity and prevention. *Salud Publica Mex* 43: 237-247.

[2] Alvarez-Martinez, C. E. & P. J. Christie, (2009) Biological diversity of prokaryotic type IV secretion systems. *Microbiol Mol Biol Rev* 73: 775-808.

[3] Amieva, M. R. & E. M. El-Omar, (2008) Host-bacterial interactions in *Helicobacter pylori* infection. *Gastroenterology* 134: 306-323.

[4] Antonio-Rincon, F., Y. Lopez-Vidal, G. Castillo-Rojas, E. C. Lazcano-Ponce, S. Ponce-de-Leon, M. L. Tabche-Barrera & G. R. Aguilar-Gutierrez, (2011) Pathogenicity island

cag, vacA and IS605 genotypes in Mexican strains of *Helicobacter pylori* associated with peptic ulcers. *Ann Clin Microbiol Antimicrob* 10: 18.

[5] Atherton, J. C., P. Cao, R. M. Peek, Jr., M. K. Tummuru, M. J. Blaser & T. L. Cover, (1995) Mosaicism in vacuolating cytotoxin alleles of *Helicobacter pylori*. Association of specific *vacA* types with cytotoxin production and peptic ulceration. *J Biol Chem* 270: 17771-17777.

[6] Backert, S., R. Fronzes & G. Waksman, (2008) VirB2 and VirB5 proteins: specialized adhesins in bacterial type-IV secretion systems? *Trends Microbiol* 16: 409-413.

[7] Backert, S. & T. F. Meyer, (2006) Type IV secretion systems and their effectors in bacterial pathogenesis. *Curr Opin Microbiol* 9: 207-217.

[8] Backert, S., N. Tegtmeyer & M. Selbach, (2010) The versatility of *Helicobacter pylori* CagA effector protein functions: The master key hypothesis. *Helicobacter* 15: 163-176.

[9] Baek, H. Y., J. W. Lim & H. Kim, (2007) Interaction between the *Helicobacter pylori* CagA and alpha-Pix in gastric epithelial AGS cells. *Ann N Y Acad Sci* 1096: 18-23.

[10] Bagnoli, F., L. Buti, L. Tompkins, A. Covacci & M. R. Amieva, (2005) *Helicobacter pylori* CagA induces a transition from polarized to invasive phenotypes in MDCK cells. *Proc Natl Acad Sci U S A* 102: 16339-16344.

[11] Boren, T., P. Falk, K. A. Roth, G. Larson & S. Normark, (1993) Attachment of *Helicobacter pylori* to human gastric epithelium mediated by blood group antigens. *Science* 262: 1892-1895.

[12] Boughan, P. K., R. H. Argent, M. Body-Malapel, J. H. Park, K. E. Ewings, A. G. Bowie, S. J. Ong, S. J. Cook, O. E. Sorensen, B. A. Manzo, N. Inohara, N. J. Klein, G. Nunez, J. C. Atherton & M. Bajaj-Elliott, (2006) Nucleotide-binding oligomerization domain-1 and epidermal growth factor receptor: critical regulators of beta-defensins during *Helicobacter pylori* infection. *J Biol Chem* 281: 11637-11648.

[13] Castillo-Rojas, G., M. Mazari-Hiriart & Y. Lopez-Vidal, (2004) [*Helicobacter pylori*: focus on CagA and VacA major virulence factors]. *Salud Publica Mex* 46: 538-548.

[14] Censini, S., C. Lange, Z. Xiang, J. E. Crabtree, P. Ghiara, M. Borodovsky, R. Rappuoli & A. Covacci, (1996) *cag*, a pathogenicity island of *Helicobacter pylori*, encodes type I-specific and disease-associated virulence factors. *Proc Natl Acad Sci U S A* 93: 14648-14653.

[15] Chang, Y. J., M. S. Wu, J. T. Lin, R. G. Pestell, M. J. Blaser & C. C. Chen, (2006) Mechanisms for *Helicobacter pylori* CagA-induced cyclin D1 expression that affect cell cycle. *Cell Microbiol* 8: 1740-1752.

[16] Covacci, A., S. Censini, M. Bugnoli, R. Petracca, D. Burroni, G. Macchia, A. Massone, E. Papini, Z. Xiang, N. Figura & et al., (1993) Molecular characterization of the 128-kDa immunodominant antigen of *Helicobacter pylori* associated with cytotoxicity and duodenal ulcer. *Proc Natl Acad Sci U S A* 90: 5791-5795.

[17] Fan, X. Y., X. L. Hu, T. M. Han, N. N. Wang, Y. M. Zhu, W. Hu, Z. H. Ma, C. J. Zhang, X. Xu, Z. Y. Ye, C. M. Han & W. S. Pan, (2011) Association between RUNX3 promoter methylation and gastric cancer: a meta-analysis. *BMC Gastroenterol* 11: 92.

[18] Ferlay J, S. H., Bray F, Forman D, Mathers C and Parkin DM, (2010) GLOBOCAN 2008, Cancer Incidence and Mortality Worldwide: IARC CancerBase No. 10. In: Lyon, France: International Agency for Research on Cancer. pp.

[19] Figueiredo, C., J. C. Machado & Y. Yamaoka, (2005) Pathogenesis of *Helicobacter pylori* Infection. *Helicobacter* 10 Suppl 1: 14-20.

[20] Fronzes, R., P. J. Christie & G. Waksman, (2009) The structural biology of type IV secretion systems. *Nat Rev Microbiol* 7: 703-714.

[21] Furuta, Y., K. Yahara, M. Hatakeyama & I. Kobayashi, (2011) Evolution of *cagA* oncogene of *Helicobacter pylori* through recombination. *PLoS One* 6: e23499.

[22] Gebert, B., W. Fischer, E. Weiss, R. Hoffmann & R. Haas, (2003) *Helicobacter pylori* vacuolating cytotoxin inhibits T lymphocyte activation. *Science* 301: 1099-1102.

[23] Gerhard, M., N. Lehn, N. Neumayer, T. Boren, R. Rad, W. Schepp, S. Miehlke, M. Classen & C. Prinz, (1999) Clinical relevance of the *Helicobacter pylori* gene for blood-group antigen-binding adhesin. *Proc Natl Acad Sci U S A* 96: 12778-12783.

[24] Harris, P. R., H. L. Mobley, G. I. Perez-Perez, M. J. Blaser & P. D. Smith, (1996) *Helicobacter pylori* urease is a potent stimulus of mononuclear phagocyte activation and inflammatory cytokine production. *Gastroenterology* 111: 419-425.

[25] Hatakeyama, M., (2004) Oncogenic mechanisms of the *Helicobacter pylori* CagA protein. *Nat Rev Cancer* 4: 688-694.

[26] Hatakeyama, M., (2008) SagA of CagA in *Helicobacter pylori* pathogenesis. *Curr Opin Microbiol* 11: 30-37.

[27] Hatakeyama, M., (2011) Anthropological and clinical implications for the structural diversity of the *Helicobacter pylori* CagA oncoprotein. *Cancer Sci* 102: 36-43.

[28] Higashi, H., A. Nakaya, R. Tsutsumi, K. Yokoyama, Y. Fujii, S. Ishikawa, M. Higuchi, A. Takahashi, Y. Kurashima, Y. Teishikata, S. Tanaka, T. Azuma & M. Hatakeyama, (2004) *Helicobacter pylori* CagA induces Ras-independent morphogenetic response through SHP-2 recruitment and activation. *J Biol Chem* 279: 17205-17216.

[29] Higashi, H., R. Tsutsumi, S. Muto, T. Sugiyama, T. Azuma, M. Asaka & M. Hatakeyama, (2002) SHP-2 tyrosine phosphatase as an intracellular target of *Helicobacter pylori* CagA protein. *Science* 295: 683-686.

[30] Higashi, H., K. Yokoyama, Y. Fujii, S. Ren, H. Yuasa, I. Saadat, N. Murata-Kamiya, T. Azuma & M. Hatakeyama, (2005) EPIYA motif is a membrane-targeting signal of *Helicobacter pylori* virulence factor CagA in mammalian cells. *J Biol Chem* 280: 23130-23137.

[31] IARC, (1994) Schistosomes, liver flukes and *Helicobacter pylori*. IARC Working Group on the Evaluation of Carcinogenic Risks to Humans. Lyon, 7-14 June 1994. *IARC Monogr Eval Carcinog Risks Hum* 61: 1-241.

[32] Ito, K., (2011) RUNX3 in oncogenic and anti-oncogenic signaling in gastrointestinal cancers. *J Cell Biochem* 112: 1243-1249.

[33] Jones, K. R., J. M. Whitmire & D. S. Merrell, (2010) A tale of two toxins: *Helicobacter pylori* CagA and VacA modulate host pathways that impact disease. *Frontiers in Microbiology* 1: 1-17.

[34] Kersulyte, D., A. Kalia, R. H. Gilman, M. Mendez, P. Herrera, L. Cabrera, B. Velapatino, J. Balqui, F. Paredes Puente de la Vega, C. A. Rodriguez Ulloa, J. Cok, C. C. Hooper, G. Dailide, S. Tamma & D. E. Berg, (2010) *Helicobacter pylori* from Peruvian amerindians: traces of human migrations in strains from remote Amazon, and genome sequence of an Amerind strain. *PLoS One* 5(11): e15076.

[35] Kurashima, Y., N. Murata-Kamiya, K. Kikuchi, H. Higashi, T. Azuma, S. Kondo & M. Hatakeyama, (2008) Deregulation of beta-catenin signal by *Helicobacter pylori* CagA requires the CagA-multimerization sequence. *Int J Cancer* 122: 823-831.

[36] Leunk, R. D., P. T. Johnson, B. C. David, W. G. Kraft & D. R. Morgan, (1988) Cytotoxic activity in broth-culture filtrates of *Campylobacter pylori*. *J Med Microbiol* 26: 93-99.

[37] Li, W. Q., K. F. Pan, Y. Zhang, C. X. Dong, L. Zhang, J. L. Ma, T. Zhou, J. Y. Li & W. C. You, (2011) RUNX3 methylation and expression associated with advanced precancerous gastric lesions in a Chinese population. *Carcinogenesis* 32: 406-410.

[38] Lim, J. W., K. H. Kim & H. Kim, (2009) alphaPix interacts with *Helicobacter pylori* CagA to induce IL-8 expression in gastric epithelial cells. *Scand J Gastroenterol* 44: 1166-1172.

[39] Lin, F. C., Y. P. Liu, C. H. Lai, Y. S. Shan, H. C. Cheng, P. I. Hsu, C. H. Lee, Y. C. Lee, H. Y. Wang, C. H. Wang, J. Q. Cheng, M. Hsiao & P. J. Lu, (2012) RUNX3-mediated transcriptional inhibition of Akt suppresses tumorigenesis of human gastric cancer cells. *Oncogene*.

[40] Lopez-Vidal, Y., S. Ponce-de-Leon, G. Castillo-Rojas, R. Barreto-Zuniga & A. Torre-Delgadillo, (2008) High diversity of *vacA* and *cagA Helicobacter pylori* genotypes in patients with and without gastric cancer. *PLoS One* 3: e3849.

[41] Lu, H. S., Y. Saito, M. Umeda, N. Murata-Kamiya, H. M. Zhang, H. Higashi & M. Hatakeyama, (2008) Structural and functional diversity in the PAR1b/MARK2-binding region of *Helicobacter pylori* CagA. *Cancer Sci* 99: 2004-2011.

[42] Mai, U. E., G. I. Perez-Perez, L. M. Wahl, S. M. Wahl, M. J. Blaser & P. D. Smith, (1991) Soluble surface proteins from *Helicobacter pylori* activate monocytes/macrophages by lipopolysaccharide-independent mechanism. *J Clin Invest* 87: 894-900.

[43] Mane, S. P., M. G. Dominguez-Bello, M. J. Blaser, B. W. Sobral, R. Hontecillas, J. Skoneczka, S. K. Mohapatra, O. R. Crasta, C. Evans, T. Modise, S. Shallom, M. Shukla,

C. Varon, F. Megraud, A. L. Maldonado-Contreras, K. P. Williams & J. Bassaganya-Riera, (2010) Host-interactive genes in Amerindian *Helicobacter pylori* diverge from their Old World homologs and mediate inflammatory responses. *J Bacteriol* 192: 3078-3092.

[44] Matozaki, T., Y. Murata, Y. Saito, H. Okazawa & H. Ohnishi, (2009) Protein tyrosine phosphatase SHP-2: a proto-oncogene product that promotes Ras activation. *Cancer Sci* 100: 1786-1793.

[45] Megraud, F., V. Neman-Simha & D. Brugmann, (1992) Further evidence of the toxic effect of ammonia produced by *Helicobacter pylori* urease on human epithelial cells. *Infect Immun* 60: 1858-1863.

[46] Mimuro, H., T. Suzuki, S. Nagai, G. Rieder, M. Suzuki, T. Nagai, Y. Fujita, K. Nagamatsu, N. Ishijima, S. Koyasu, R. Haas & C. Sasakawa, (2007) *Helicobacter pylori* dampens gut epithelial self-renewal by inhibiting apoptosis, a bacterial strategy to enhance colonization of the stomach. *Cell Host Microbe* 2: 250-263.

[47] Mimuro, H., T. Suzuki, J. Tanaka, M. Asahi, R. Haas & C. Sasakawa, (2002) Grb2 is a key mediator of *Helicobacter pylori* CagA protein activities. *Mol Cell* 10: 745-755.

[48] Mobley, H. L., G. L. Mendz & S. L. Hazell, (2001) *Helicobacter pylori: physiology and genetics*, p. 626. ASM Press, Washington DC.

[49] Moese, S., M. Selbach, U. Zimny-Arndt, P. R. Jungblut, T. F. Meyer & S. Backert, (2001) Identification of a tyrosine-phosphorylated 35 kDa carboxy-terminal fragment (p35CagA) of the *Helicobacter pylori* CagA protein in phagocytic cells: processing or breakage? *Proteomics* 1: 618-629.

[50] Montecucco, C. & R. Rappuoli, (2001) Living dangerously: how *Helicobacter pylori* survives in the human stomach. *Nat Rev Mol Cell Biol* 2: 457-466.

[51] Moran, A., (1998) The products of *Helicobacter pylori* that induce inflammation. *Eur. J. Gastroenterol. Hepatol.* 10 Suppl 1: S3–S8.

[52] Moran, A. P., (1995) Cell surface characteristics of *Helicobacter pylori*. *FEMS Immunol Med Microbiol* 10: 271-280.

[53] Mueller, D., N. Tegtmeyer, S. Brandt, Y. Yamaoka, E. De Poire, D. Sgouras, S. Wessler, J. Torres, A. Smolka & S. Backert, (2012) c-Src and c-Abl kinases control hierarchic phosphorylation and function of the CagA effector protein in Western and East Asian *Helicobacter pylori* strains. *J Clin Invest* 122: 1553-1566.

[54] Murata-Kamiya, N., K. Kikuchi, T. Hayashi, H. Higashi & M. Hatakeyama, (2010) *Helicobacter pylori* exploits host membrane phosphatidylserine for delivery, localization, and pathophysiological action of the CagA oncoprotein. *Cell Host Microbe* 7: 399-411.

[55] Nagase, L., N. Murata-Kamiya & M. Hatakeyama, (2011) Potentiation of *Helicobacter pylori* CagA protein virulence through homodimerization. *J Biol Chem* 286: 33622-33631.

[56] Nagy, T. A., M. R. Frey, F. Yan, D. A. Israel, D. B. Polk & R. M. Peek, Jr., (2009) *Helicobacter pylori* regulates cellular migration and apoptosis by activation of phosphatidylinositol 3-kinase signaling. *J Infect Dis* 199: 641-651.

[57] Nesic, D., M. C. Miller, Z. T. Quinkert, M. Stein, B. T. Chait & C. E. Stebbins, (2010) *Helicobacter pylori* CagA inhibits PAR1-MARK family kinases by mimicking host substrates. *Nat Struct Mol Biol* 17: 130-132.

[58] Oldani, A., M. Cormont, V. Hofman, V. Chiozzi, O. Oregioni, A. Canonici, A. Sciullo, P. Sommi, A. Fabbri, V. Ricci & P. Boquet, (2009) *Helicobacter pylori* counteracts the apoptotic action of its VacA toxin by injecting the CagA protein into gastric epithelial cells. *PLoS Pathog* 5: e1000603.

[59] Oliveira, M. J., A. M. Costa, A. C. Costa, R. M. Ferreira, P. Sampaio, J. C. Machado, R. Seruca, M. Mareel & C. Figueiredo, (2009) CagA associates with c-Met, E-cadherin, and p120-catenin in a multiproteic complex that suppresses *Helicobacter pylori*-induced cell-invasive phenotype. *J Infect Dis* 200: 745-755.

[60] Papini, E., B. Satin, N. Norais, M. de Bernard, J. L. Telford, R. Rappuoli & C. Montecucco, (1998) Selective increase of the permeability of polarized epithelial cell monolayers by *Helicobacter pylori* vacuolating toxin. *J Clin Invest* 102: 813-820.

[61] Peek, R. M., Jr. & M. J. Blaser, (2002) *Helicobacter pylori* and gastrointestinal tract adenocarcinomas. *Nat Rev Cancer* 2: 28-37.

[62] Pelz, C., S. Steininger, C. Weiss, F. Coscia & R. Vogelmann, (2011) A novel inhibitory domain of *Helicobacter pylori* protein CagA reduces CagA effects on host cell biology. *J Biol Chem* 286: 8999-9008.

[63] Pettersen, E. F., T. D. Goddard, C. C. Huang, G. S. Couch, D. M. Greenblatt, E. C. Meng & T. E. Ferrin, (2004) UCSF Chimera--a visualization system for exploratory research and analysis. *J Comput Chem* 25: 1605-1612.

[64] Poppe, M., S. M. Feller, G. Romer & S. Wessler, (2007) Phosphorylation of *Helicobacter pylori* CagA by c-Abl leads to cell motility. *Oncogene* 26: 3462-3472.

[65] Ren, S., H. Higashi, H. Lu, T. Azuma & M. Hatakeyama, (2006) Structural basis and functional consequence of *Helicobacter pylori* CagA multimerization in cells. *J Biol Chem* 281: 32344-32352.

[66] Ricci, V., M. Romano & P. Boquet, (2011) Molecular cross-talk between *Helicobacter pylori* and human gastric mucosa. *World J Gastroenterol* 17: 1383-1399.

[67] Roy, A., A. Kucukural & Y. Zhang, (2010) I-TASSER: a unified platform for automated protein structure and function prediction. *Nat Protoc* 5: 725-738.

[68] Selbach, M., S. Moese, C. R. Hauck, T. F. Meyer & S. Backert, (2002) Src is the kinase of the *Helicobacter pylori* CagA protein in vitro and in vivo. *J Biol Chem* 277: 6775-6778.

[69] Selbach, M., F. E. Paul, S. Brandt, P. Guye, O. Daumke, S. Backert, C. Dehio & M. Mann, (2009) Host cell interactome of tyrosine-phosphorylated bacterial proteins. *Cell Host Microbe* 5: 397-403.

[70] Snider, J. L., C. Allison, B. H. Bellaire, R. L. Ferrero & J. A. Cardelli, (2008) The beta1 integrin activates JNK independent of CagA, and JNK activation is required for *Helicobacter pylori* CagA+-induced motility of gastric cancer cells. *J Biol Chem* 283: 13952-13963.

[71] Sobala, G. M., C. J. Schorah, S. Shires, D. A. Lynch, B. Gallacher, M. F. Dixon & A. T. Axon, (1993) Effect of eradication of *Helicobacter pylori* on gastric juice ascorbic acid concentrations. *Gut* 34: 1038-1041.

[72] Stein, M., F. Bagnoli, R. Halenbeck, R. Rappuoli, W. J. Fantl & A. Covacci, (2002) c-Src/Lyn kinases activate *Helicobacter pylori* CagA through tyrosine phosphorylation of the EPIYA motifs. *Mol Microbiol* 43: 971-980.

[73] Steininger, S., C. Pelz & R. Vogelmann, (2011) Purpose of recently detected inhibitory domain of the *Helicobacter pylori* protein CagA. *Gut Microbes* 2: 167-172.

[74] Suzuki, M., S. Miura, M. Suematsu, D. Fukumura, I. Kurose, H. Suzuki, A. Kai, Y. Kudoh, M. Ohashi & M. Tsuchiya, (1992) *Helicobacter pylori*-associated ammonia production enhances neutrophil-dependent gastric mucosal cell injury. *Am J Physiol* 263: G719-725.

[75] Tammer, I., S. Brandt, R. Hartig, W. Konig & S. Backert, (2007) Activation of Abl by *Helicobacter pylori*: a novel kinase for CagA and crucial mediator of host cell scattering. *Gastroenterology* 132: 1309-1319.

[76] Tegtmeyer, N., D. Zabler, D. Schmidt, R. Hartig, S. Brandt & S. Backert, (2009) Importance of EGF receptor, HER2/Neu and Erk1/2 kinase signalling for host cell elongation and scattering induced by the *Helicobacter pylori* CagA protein: antagonistic effects of the vacuolating cytotoxin VacA. *Cell Microbiol* 11: 488-505.

[77] Tomb, J. F., O. White, A. R. Kerlavage, R. A. Clayton, G. G. Sutton, R. D. Fleischmann, K. A. Ketchum, H. P. Klenk, S. Gill, B. A. Dougherty, K. Nelson, J. Quackenbush, L. Zhou, E. F. Kirkness, S. Peterson, B. Loftus, D. Richardson, R. Dodson, H. G. Khalak, A. Glodek, K. McKenney, L. M. Fitzegerald, N. Lee, M. D. Adams, E. K. Hickey, D. E. Berg, J. D. Gocayne, T. R. Utterback, J. D. Peterson, J. M. Kelley, M. D. Cotton, J. M. Weidman, C. Fujii, C. Bowman, L. Watthey, E. Wallin, W. S. Hayes, M. Borodovsky, P. D. Karp, H. O. Smith, C. M. Fraser & J. C. Venter, (1997) The complete genome sequence of the gastric pathogen *Helicobacter pylori*. *Nature* 388: 539-547.

[78] Tsang, Y. H., A. Lamb, J. Romero-Gallo, B. Huang, K. Ito, R. M. Peek, Jr., Y. Ito & L. F. Chen, (2010) *Helicobacter pylori* CagA targets gastric tumor suppressor RUNX3 for proteasome-mediated degradation. *Oncogene* 29: 5643-5650.

[79] Tsutsumi, R., H. Higashi, M. Higuchi, M. Okada & M. Hatakeyama, (2003) Attenuation of *Helicobacter pylori* CagA x SHP-2 signaling by interaction between CagA and C-terminal Src kinase. *J Biol Chem* 278: 3664-3670.

[80] Tsutsumi, R., A. Takahashi, T. Azuma, H. Higashi & M. Hatakeyama, (2006) Focal adhesion kinase is a substrate and downstream effector of SHP-2 complexed with *Helicobacter pylori* CagA. *Mol Cell Biol* 26: 261-276.

[81] Tummuru, M. K., T. L. Cover & M. J. Blaser, (1993) Cloning and expression of a high-molecular-mass major antigen of *Helicobacter pylori*: evidence of linkage to cytotoxin production. *Infect Immun* 61: 1799-1809.

[82] Viala, J., C. Chaput, I. G. Boneca, A. Cardona, S. E. Girardin, A. P. Moran, R. Athman, S. Memet, M. R. Huerre, A. J. Coyle, P. S. DiStefano, P. J. Sansonetti, A. Labigne, J. Bertin, D. J. Philpott & R. L. Ferrero, (2004) Nod1 responds to peptidoglycan delivered by the *Helicobacter pylori cag* pathogenicity island. *Nature immunology* 5: 1166-1174.

[83] Warren, J. R. M., B, (1983) Unidentified curved bacilli on gastric epithelium in active chronic gastritis. *Lancet* 1: 1273-1275.

[84] Wessler, S. & S. Backert, (2008) Molecular mechanisms of epithelial-barrier disruption by *Helicobacter pylori*. *Trends Microbiol* 16: 397-405.

[85] Wroblewski, L. E., R. M. Peek, Jr. & K. T. Wilson, (2010) *Helicobacter pylori* and gastric cancer: factors that modulate disease risk. *Clin Microbiol Rev* 23: 713-739.

[86] Xia, Y., Y. Yamaoka, Q. Zhu, I. Matha & X. Gao, (2009) A comprehensive sequence and disease correlation analyses for the C-terminal region of CagA protein of *Helicobacter pylori*. *PLoS One* 4: e7736.

[87] Yamaoka, Y., (2008) Increasing evidence of the role of *Helicobacter pylori* SabA in the pathogenesis of gastroduodenal disease. *J Infect Dev Ctries* 2: 174-181.

[88] Yamaoka, Y., (2010) Mechanisms of disease: *Helicobacter pylori* virulence factors. *Nat Rev Gastroenterol Hepatol* 7: 629-641.

[89] Yamaoka, Y., S. Kikuchi, H. M. el-Zimaity, O. Gutierrez, M. S. Osato & D. Y. Graham, (2002) Importance of *Helicobacter pylori oipA* in clinical presentation, gastric inflammation, and mucosal interleukin 8 production. *Gastroenterology* 123: 414-424.

[90] Yamaoka, Y., D. H. Kwon & D. Y. Graham, (2000) A M(r) 34,000 proinflammatory outer membrane protein (oipA) of *Helicobacter pylori*. *Proc Natl Acad Sci U S A* 97: 7533-7538.

[91] Yokoyama, K., H. Higashi, S. Ishikawa, Y. Fujii, S. Kondo, H. Kato, T. Azuma, A. Wada, T. Hirayama, H. Aburatani & M. Hatakeyama, (2005) Functional antagonism between *Helicobacter pylori* CagA and vacuolating toxin VacA in control of the NFAT signaling pathway in gastric epithelial cells. *Proc Natl Acad Sci U S A* 102: 9661-9666.

Chapter 12

From Gastritis to Gastric Cancer: The Importance of CagPAI of *Helicobacter Pylori* on the Development of Early and Advanced Gastric Adenocarcinoma

Bruna Maria Roesler and
José Murilo Robilotta Zeitune

Additional information is available at the end of the chapter

http://dx.doi.org/10.5772/53208

1. Introduction

The genus *Helicobacter* belongs to the ε subdivision of the *Proteobacteria*, order *Campylobacterales*, family *Helicobacteraceae*. Members of this genus are all microaerophilic organisms and in most cases are catalase and oxidase positive, and many but not all species are also urease positive [1].

In 1984, Warren and Marshall isolated a bacterium from human stomachs in some patients with gastrointestinal disorders [2]. The organism was initially named "*Campylobacter-like organism*", "*Campylobacter pyloridis*" and "*Campylobacter pylori*", and, after more studies, it is named *Helicobacter pylori* (*H. pylori*) in recognition of the fact that this organism is distinct from members of the genus *Campylobacter* [3].

H. pylori is a spiral-shaped Gram-negative flagellate bacterium that colonizes the human stomach and can establish a long-term infection of the gastric mucosa. Since its isolation, its infection has been associated to the development of various gastrointestinal diseases, such as chronic gastritis, peptic ulcer disease, gastric MALT lymphoma and gastric cancer [1, 4-6]. Nowadays, it has also been related to some extradigestive diseases [7, 8], such as idiopathic thrombocytopenic purpura [9], iron deficiency anemia [10], and hepatobiliary diseases [11, 12], and amongst others.

The prevalence of *H. pylori* infection varies widely by geographical area, age, race, and socioeconomic status [13]. Because it is not possible to ascertain when infection occurs clinically, most of the information on the rates of *H. pylori* in geographically and demographically diverse populations comes from seroprevalence studies [14]. There have been numerous reports of a strong correlation between socioeconomic status and prevalence of infection. Generally, low prevalence occurs in industrialized countries and higher prevalence rates have been observed in underdeveloped and developing countries, possibly due to crowded households, habits and lack of sanitary facilities [15-17].

Even though its transmission pathways are not completely clarified [18], the infection appears to be usually acquired during childhood and is characterized as being chronic [19]. Routes of *H. pylori* transmission described include fecal-oral, oral-oral and gastric-oral. *H. pylori* appears to be transmitted most readily within families, possibly from parent to child and among siblings [20]. Evidence also supports child-to-child transmission among those in crowded school or in some living conditions, while transmission among adults is considered rare [21].

After colonization, all patients with *H. pylori* infection develop histological gastritis, which corresponds to classical chronic gastritis and is characterized by the infiltration of neutrophils and other inflammatory cells. However, most patients are asymptomatic for life, while only some will come to develop a digestive disease [22].

Colonization with *H. pylori* virtually leads to infiltration of the gastric mucosa in both antrum and corpus with neutrophilic and mononuclear cells. Gastritis can be classified as an acute or chronic gastritis and it can involve all parts of the stomach or just the fundus, corpus or antrum. The chronic active gastritis is the primary condition related to *H. pylori* colonization, and other *H. pylori*-associated disorders, in particular, resulting from this chronic inflammatory process [1], as atrophic gastritis (Figure 1) and intestinal metaplasia (Figure 2), causing an elevated risk of gastric adenocarcinoma, both intestinal type and diffuse type [23].

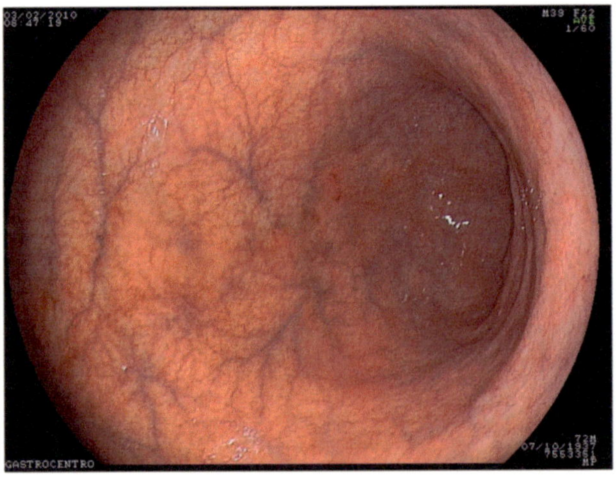

Figure 1. Atrophic gastritis(Copyright © Center of Diagnosis of Digestive Diseases, State University of Campinas, SP, Brazil. All rights reserved)

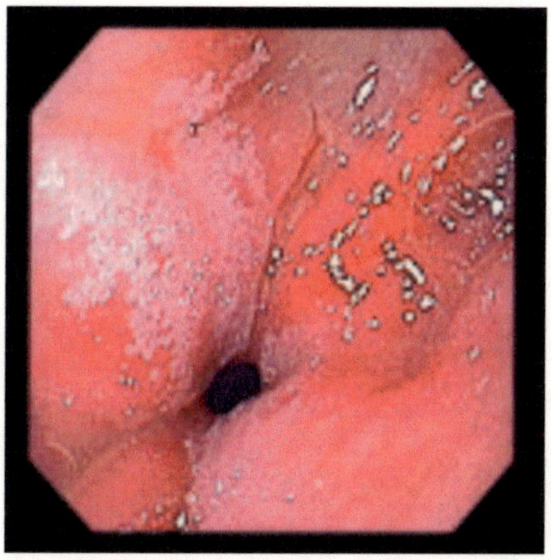

Figure 2. – Intestinal metaplasia, prepyloric antrum(Copyright© Atlanta South Gastroenterology, P.C. All rights reserved)

However, the propensity to develop disease is an aspect that remains unclear, but may depend on host characteristics, particular bacterial factors (virulence of the infecting strains), or to the specific interactions between host and microbe, besides the environmental factors [24].

In fact, the interest in *H. pylori* as a cause of gastric cancer began after the pioneering discoveries of Marshall and Warren [2]. Prior to the isolation of the organism, it was know that gastric adenocarcinomas typically arose in areas of gastritis. When the relationship between *H. pylori* and chronic gastritis was established, investigators began to take interest in the causal role of the bacterium in gastric cancer. Consequently, in 1994, the bacterium was classified as a group I carcinogen by the International Agency for Research on Cancer and is regarded as a primary factor for gastric cancer development [25].

The vast majority of gastric cancers are adenocarcinomas, which can be prevalently divided into two types, the intestinal and the diffuse [26], which corresponds, respectively, to the well-differentiated type and to the poorly-differentiated type, in the Japanese classification [22]. In contrast to the diffuse type often associated with familial distribution and developed in the stomach following chronic inflammation, especially in the cardia [27], intestinal type adenocarcinomas are generally thought to be preceded by a sequence of precursor lesions [28]. The basic components of this process are chronic inflammation of the gastric mucosa, which slowly progresses through the premalignant stages of atrophic gastritis, intestinal metaplasia and dysplasia to gastric cancer [29] that are most frequently localized in the antrum [30].

Patients diagnosed in an early stage of the cancer (Figure 3) present an excellent prognosis, with a five-year survival rate greater than 90%. In cases with advanced lesions, gastric cancer carries a poor prognosis, with an overall five-year survival rate of less than 20% [31].

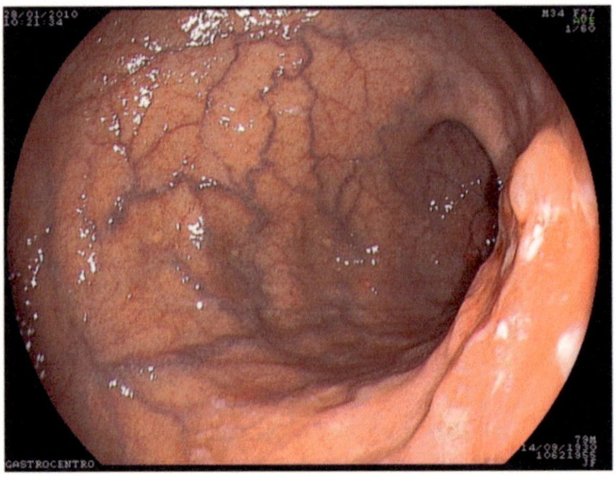

Figure 3. – Early gastric adenocarcinoma(Copyright © Center of Diagnosis of Digestive Diseases, State University of Campinas, SP, Brazil. All rights reserved)

With respect specifically to the bacterium strains, *H. pylori* has a high level of genetic diversity that represents an important factor in its adaptation to the host stomach and also for the clinical outcome of the infection [32,33]. Virulence factors of *Helicobacter pylori* are essential players in modulating the immune response involved in the initiation of carcinogenesis in the stomach. One category of the genes that are responsible for produce virulence factors is the strain-specific ones, which are present in only some *H. pylori* strains [34]. Among then, the best studied is the *cytotoxin-associated gene pathogenicity island* (cagPAI).

The cagPAI is a 40 kb region of chromosomal DNA encoding approximately 31 genes that forms a type IV secretion system and can be divided into two regions, cag I and cag II, according to a novel insertion sequence [35]. This secretion system forms a pilus that delivers CagA, an oncoprotein, into the cytosol of gastric epithelial cells through a rigid needle structure covered by CagY, a VirB10-homologous protein and CagT, a Virb7-homologous protein, at the base [36-38].

Upon delivery into host cells by the *cag* secretion system, the product of the terminal gene in the island, CagA, undergoes Src-dependent tyrosine phosphorylation and activates an eukaryotic phosphatase (SHP-2), leading to dephosphorylation of host cell proteins and cellular morphologic changes [39,40]. CagA has also been shown to dysregulate β-catenin signaling [41,42] and apical-junctional complexes [43], events that have been linked to increased cell motility and oncogenic transformation in a variety of models [44,45]. In addition, some studies have been reported that the cagPAI appears to be involved in the induction of gastric interleukin-8 (IL-8) production, a potent neutrophil-activating chemokine [46].

Consequently, the presence of the cagA gene has been associated with higher grades of inflammation, which may lead to the development of the most severe gastrointestinal diseases, such as peptic ulcer [47-49] and gastric cancer [50-54]. In Western countries, it has been reported that individuals infected with cagA-positive strains of *H. pylori* are at a higher risk of peptic ulcer or gastric cancer than those infected with cagA-negative strains [34,55]. However, in East Asia, most strains of *H. pylori* have the cagA gene irrespective of the disease [56].

Furthermore, cagA is a polymorphic gene that presents different numbers of repeat sequences located in its 3′ region. Each repeat region of the CagA protein contains Glu-Pro-Ile-Tyr-Ala (EPIYA) motifs, including a tyrosine phosphorylation site. The first repeat region is commonly named as EPIYA-A and EPIYA-B segments and the second repeat region is named EPIYA-C or EPIYA-D segments, for Western and East Asian strains, respectively [57]. Despite the know variability in the N-terminal cagA gene and other cagPAI genes, there has been limited information concerning clinical relevance of genetic variants outside the EPIYAs [58].

Together with cagA gene, cagT gene is found at the base of the outgrowing pilus of the type IV secretion system and is supposed to be responsible for binding to a cellular receptor to induce interleukine-8 secretion and eject CagA [37]. The cagT gene has also been associated with higher degrees of inflammation, being encountered in *H. pylori* strains from patients with early and advanced gastric adenocarcinoma [54].

Thus, considering each gene, there are two types of clinical *H. pylori* isolate, CagA-producing (cagA positive) strains and CagA-nonproducing (cagA negative) strains, and CagT-producing (cagT positive) strains and CagT-nonproducing (cagT negative) strains, genotypes that were considered in this study.

As gastric cancer still ranks as a leading cause of cancer-related deaths in many parts of the world, the aims of the present study were to investigate the presence of cagA and cagT genes in Brazilian patients with early and advanced distal type intestinal adenocarcinoma, in order to determine the general incidence of this gene in gastric cancer and to compare the results obtained between the two stages of the disease, trying to understand if the cagA and the cagT genes and/or the genotype cagAcagT could be important to the development of one or other stage of distal intestinal type gastric adenocarcinoma in Brazil.

2. Clinical samples, methods and results

2.1. Clinical Samples

The present study was carried out utilizing clinical samples of *H. pylori* obtained from 2005 January to 2009 January from the Laboratory of Pathology of the Center of Diagnosis of Digestive Diseases, Faculty of Medical Sciences, State University of Campinas (UNICAMP), São Paulo, Brazil. Eighty nine paraffin wax-embedded specimens of gastric tissue were analysed from a total of 89 patients, 31 from patients diagnosed with early distal type intestinal gastric adenocarcinoma (group one) and 58 from patients with advanced distal type intestinal gastric adenocarcinoma (group two). The mean ages of group one was 61.0 years, with 20 male cases (64.5%) and 11 female cases (35.5%). For group two the mean ages was 64.5 years, with 40 male cases (69.0%) and 18 female cases (31.0%). All the gastric tissue samples were obtained from endoscopic biopsy and had positive results for *H. pylori* by histological analysis. *H. pylori* positive strains for cagA and cagT genes were used as a control for all the reactions performed in this study. All the stages of this study were approved by the Ethics Committee of the Faculty of Medical Sciences, State University of Campinas (UNICAMP), São Paulo, Brazil.

2.2. Methods

2.2.1. DNA extraction

Paraffin wax-embedded tissue DNA extraction was performed by carrying out the pre-extraction treatment of fixed tissues, using xylene and ethanol washes for paraffin removal. Subsequently, successive steps using proteinase K, phenol, chloroform and isoamyl alcohol were carried out, in order to isolate and purify the DNA [59]. Quantification of the extracted DNA and polymerase chain reaction (PCR) for human betaglobin gene [60] were carried out in order to guarantee the quality of this research.

2.2.2. PCR for urease C gene, cagA gene and cagT gene

Primers pairs for all the genes are described in Table 1, as well as the length of the fragments amplified for each reaction, urease C [61], cagA [62], and cagT [63]. PCR for urease C gene was performed with the aim to identify the bacterium DNA in samples.

After amplification, each PCR product was submitted to eletrophoresis on a 2.0% agarose gel stained by ethidium bromide with a 0.5X tris-acetate-EDTA buffer. A 100-bp ladder was used as standard.

Then, for each specific reaction, after being tested positive for urease C gene, products obtained were classified in cagA positive or negative and cagT positive or negative.

Gene	Strand	Primer sequence (5´-3´)	Length (bp)
betaglobin	+	ACA CAA CTG TGT TCA CTA GC	110
	-	CAA CTT CAT CCA CGT TTC ACC	
urease C	+	AAG CTT TTA GGG GTG TTA GGG GTT T	294
	-	AAG CTT ACT TTC TAA CAC TAA CGC	
cagA	+	GAT AAC AGG CAA GCT TTT GAG G	349
	-	CTG CAA AAG ATT GTT TGG CAG A	
cagT	+	CCA TGT TTA TAC GCC TGT GT	301
	-	CAT CAC CAC ACC CTT TTG AT	

Table 1. Sequence of synthetic oligonucleotide primers used to characterize *H. pylori* strains.

2.2.3. Statistical Analysis

After the amplification reactions, the results were analysed by a chi-square test at the Statistical Service of the Faculty of Medical Sciences, State University of Campinas (UNICAMP), with the *Statistical Analysis for Windows* ® (*SAS*) 9.1.3 (SAS Institute Inc, 2002-2003, Cary, NC, USA). Results were then related to the diseases in study, observing possible differences among H. pylori strains encountered in early and in advanced distal type intestinal gastric adenocarcinoma. Values of $p<0.05$ were considered to be statistically significant. The results as a whole, after comparison between the two groups, were depicted. Odd ratios with a confidence interval of 95% were also observed. Tables with absolute frequencies (n) and percentages (%) were made in order to determine genotypes combinations. Finally, Exact Fisher's Test was used to compare the genotypes combinations between early and advanced gastric adenocarcinoma groups. Values of $p<0.05$ were considered to be statistically significant.

2.3. Results

PCR for the urease C gene of *H. pylori* was positive in all 89 samples, identifying the bacterium DNA (Table 2). Analyzing the results obtained for cagA gene, from patients with early gastric cancer, 61.3% (19 cases) were positive and from patients with advanced gastric cancer, 82.8% (48 cases) were positive, with a p = 0.025 (OR = 3.032; 95% CI = 1.123-8.185) (Table 2; Figure 4). In the group as a whole, there were 67 positive cases (75.3%) for the cagA gene.

As regards to cagT gene of *H. pylori*, from patients with early gastric adenocarcinoma, 54.8% (17 cases) were positive and, in patients with advanced gastric cancer, 65.5% (38 cases) were positive, with a p = 0.323 (OR = 1.565; 95% CI = 0.642-3.813). (Table 3; Figure 5) In the group as a whole, there were 55 positive cases (61.8%) for the cagT gene.

Classification	Early gastric cancer	Advanced gastric cancer	Total	p value
urease C	31 (100.0%)	58 (100.0%)	89 (100.0%)	
cagA positive	19 (61.3%)	48 (82.8%)	89 (100.0%)	0.025*
cagA negative	12 (38.7%)	10 (17.2%)		
cagT positive	17 (54.8%)	38 (65.5%)	89 (100.0%)	0.323
cagT negative	14 (45.2%)	20 (34.5%)		
Total	31 (100.0%)	58 (100.0%)	89 (100.0%)	

Table 2. General results obtained after PCRs for urease C, cagA and cagT genes of *H. pylori*. * cagA gene (p=0.025) OR=3.032, 95% CI = 1.123-8.185)

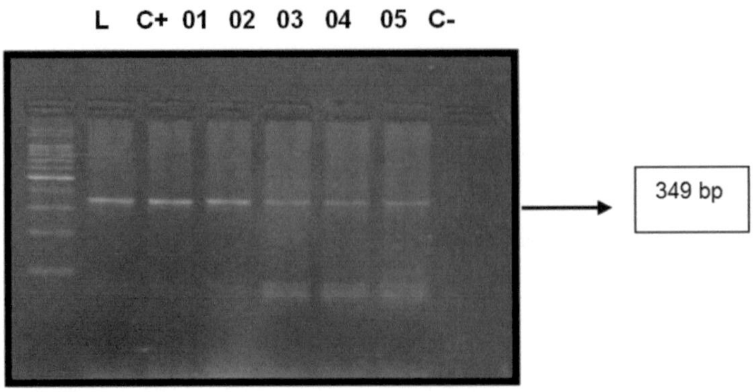

Figure 4. Amplification of cagA gene of *H. pylori* (349 bp). L, ladder 100 bp; C+, positive control; 01-05, positive samples for cagA gene; C-, negative control.

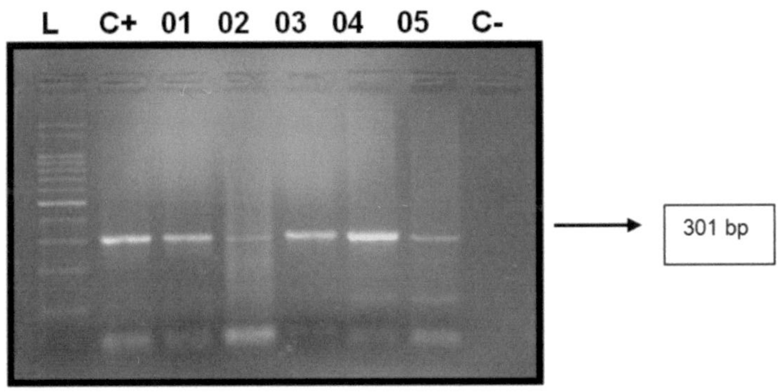

Figure 5. Amplification of cagT gene of *H. pylori* (301 bp). L, ladder 100 bp; C+, positive control; 01-05, positive samples for cagT gene; C-, negative control.

After the individual analysis, a table with absolute frequencies (n) and percentages (%) was made in order to compare the results individually for each gene and the genotypes combinations (Table 3; Table 4, respectively). There were 75.28% of positive cases for cagA gene and 61.80% of positive cases for cagT gene (table 3). As regards to cagAcagT, the most frequent genotype was cagA+cagT+, that was presented in 52.81% of the samples (table 4). The second most frequent genotype was cagA+cagT-, presented in 22.47% of the samples (table 4).

Subsequently, the combinations of genotypes were made and then compared between the two groups of patients, with early and advanced gastric adenocarcinoma. Although the most frequent genotype (cagA+cagT+) was the same in both groups of patiens, there was found a statistically significant difference between the groups, with cagA+cagT+ in advanced gastric cancer group (62.07%, 36 cases) and with cagA-cagT+ in early gastric cancer group (19.35%, 6 cases), p=0.027 (table 5).

Genes	Frequency (n)	Percentage (%)
cagA negative	22	24.72
cagA positive	67	75.28
cagT negative	34	38.20
cagT positive	55	61.80

Table 3. Descriptive analysis of categorical variables for total samples

cagA cagT combination	Frequency (n)	Percentage (%)
cagA cagT		
negative negative	14	15.73
negative positive	8	8.99
positive negative	20	22.47
positive positive	47	52.81

Table 4. Descriptive analysis of categorical variables for total samples according to genotype (cagAcagT)

cagAcagT	Advanced gastric cancer	Early Gastric cancer	Total
negative negative	8	6	14
	13.79	19.35	
negative positive	2	6	8
	3.45	**19.35**	
positive negative	12	8	20
	20.69	25.81	
positive positive	36	11	47
	62.07	35.48	
Total	58	31	89

Table 5. - Genotypes comparison between the two groups of patients, advanced and early gastric cancerp = 0.027

3. Conclusion

Gastritis is the most common illness associated to the stomach and can be considered as the beginning of different complication that may led to peptic ulcers disease and gastric adenocarcinoma. Specifically concerning to gastric cancer, the understanding of the development of this disease has advanced considerably in recent decades, especially as regards to the role of *H. pylori* (the principal etiologic agent) in the progression of chronic gastritis in precancerous lesions and cancer, changes that occur in the gastric mucosa in the development of the intestinal type gastric adenocarcinoma [30].

The risk of development of this disease is also related to genetic characteristics of the host and environmental factors, which, associated with specific bacterium strain characteristics, influence the severity of the chronic inflammatory response [64]. Thus, although infection with *H. pylori* almost always results in chronic active gastritis, many infected patients do not develop any complication, even those not showing clinical symptoms of infection [65]. This leads to the conclusion that some strains are more virulent than others [1], expressing, in different ways, specific bacterial products.

Other question that remains unclear, and that can be associated with these bacterium virulence factors, is why some tumors remain in the early stage and others are in advanced stage almost always in a short period of time? Are the different strains of *H. pylori* important to these changes? And, if the bacterium is eradicated, when this eradication is important? Is there a point of the development of the cancer when the eradication is not more important or when the bacterium presence does not make a difference?

In the present study we tried to understand some of these questions considering only one aspect of the development of the cancer, which were *H. pylori* strains presented in Brazilian patients with early and advanced distal type intestinal gastric adenocarcinoma. Considering the mentioned issues and a large number of studies that demonstrate that the cagPAI as one of the most important virulence factors of *H. pylori*, associated with higher grades of mucosa inflammation, we studied two genes that is in the cagPAI, the cagA and the cagT genes.

As regards to cagA gene, in an isolated analysis, our results were similar to those of in which strains cagA positive were related to the development of gastric cancer. cagA positive strains tend to be more virulent and induce higher levels of expression of cytokines such as interleukin 1b and 8 [66]. Some studies have shown that patients with strains that express CagA are three times more likely to develop gastric cancer (52,57,67] than those infected with cagA negative strains [56,68]. Besides, other study demonstrated that strains that express CagA are three times more likely to develop advanced gastric cancer than the early stage [54]. In the present study the same characteristics were observed and patients infected with cagA positive strains demonstrated a high risk of advanced gastric cancer development ($p=0.025$; $OR=3.023$, 95%CI). Besides, studies conducted in Western countries [69,70] and in Asian countries [71] reported that the most patients with gastric cancer are infected with *H. pylori* cagA positive strains.

One limitation for the comparisons of our results with others were that our study classified the two stages of the gastric cancer, the early and the advanced ones, and the most part of the studies consider only the gastric cancer disease, without classifying it in early or advanced stages. Besides, it was not our aim the study of the polymorphism of this gene, which are related to the EPIYA motifs, which can be important if we considerer the cagA gene in an isolated analysis, even though there has been limited information concerning clinical relevance of genetic variants outside the EPIYAs.

With our results, we can conclude that cagA gene is important for the development both of early and advanced gastric cancer, because it was presented in the most part of the strains in the two stages of the disease. Nevertheless, we can not conclude if it is important for the change of one stage in other (early in advanced stage) and we have also to consider that we do not really know if the bacterium presence is important or crucial after the beginning of the development of the disease. Some studies have demonstrated that the eradication of *H. pylori* when the precancerous lesions are present can be very important to prevent the cancer development, but, after this development beginning, we do not know if the regression of the early gastric cancer lesions can occur with the bacterium eradication.

Like the cagA gene, the cagT also belongs to the cagPAI and it is assumed that is related to the type IV secretion system, responsible for binding to cell receptors and inducing the release of interleukin-8 and also by ejecting the CagA protein [37]. The cagT gene has been linked to the development of peptic ulcer, and strains with the absence of this gene were generally related to chronic gastritis [63]. In this study, values were not found to be statistically significant between the two studied groups (p=0.323). However, the cagT gene was found, in the group as a whole, in 61.8% of the samples, which reflects an important result, showing that this gene, like cagA, or acting together with cagA, may be related to the gastric cancer development.

As regards to the comparison of the genotype cagAcagT, we reported again as a limitation for our study the fact that there are no studies that consider the early and the advanced stages of gastric cancer separately, so there were no relevant studies with which to compare the results from different stages of the same disease, gastric cancer. Further, we considered it unnecessary to make a comparison between these results and possible results from healthy individuals, because our aim was exactly to compare the strains presented in two stages of the same disease and not between the strains in the disease and in healthy volunteers.

For both groups, advanced and early, the most frequent genotype was cagA+cagT+ (62.07% and 35.48%, respectively). However, when comparison between the two groups was made, we found a statistically significance concerning the cagA+cagT+ and cagA-cagT+ strains (p=0.027). It can be considered very important because even though the genes cagA+ and cagT+ status were more frequent in both groups, the genotype cagA-cagT+ occurred with a higher frequency in the early gastric cancer group (advanced = 3.45%; early = 19.35%). Moreover, the genotype cagA+cagT+ occurred with a higher frequency in the advanced cancer group, a result that can be considered important too (advanced = 62.07%; early = 35.48%). We can suggest, with these results, that cagA gene positivity, independently of its polymorphisms, can be considered an essential virulence factor for the development of most severe gastric diseases, as gastric cancer.

Finally, as told before, the understanding of gastric carcinogenesis has advanced considerably over the past decades, especially with regards to insights into the role of *H. pylori* infection and the progression of chronic gastritis from premalignant stages to gastric cancer. Thereby, with the results obtained in the present study, cagA and cagT genes can be considered important *H. pylori* virulence factors implicated on the gastric cancer development.

Obviously, more studies are necessary to elucidate the *H. pylori* mechanisms of gastric tissue injury and we can also suggest that the identification of strains positive for cagA and cagT genes, besides others that are just considered virulence factors, can become very important and an useful tool to identify subjects most at risk for cancer, especially in places when this disease presents a higher incidence.

Author details

Bruna Maria Roesler* and José Murilo Robilotta Zeitune

*Address all correspondence to: brunaroesler@yahoo.com.br

Department of Internal Medicine, Center of Diagnosis of Digestive Diseases, Faculty of Medical Sciences, State University of Campinas, Campinas, Brazil

References

[1] Kusters, J. G., van Vliet, A. H. M., & Kuipers, E. J. (2006). Pathogenesis of *Helicobacter pylori* infection. *Clinical Microbiology Reviews*, 19(3), 449-490.

[2] Warren, J. R., & Marshall, B. J. (1984). Unidentified curved bacilli in the stomach of patients with gastritis and peptic ulceration. *Lancet*, 1(8390), 1311-1315.

[3] Goodwin, C. S., Armstrong, J. A., Chilvers, T., Peters, M., Collins, MD, Sly, L., Mc Connell, W., & Harper, W. E. S. (1989). Transfer of Campylobacter pylori and Campylobacter mustelae to Helicobacter gen. nov. as *Helicobacter pylori* comb. nov. and Helicobacter mustelae comb. nov., respectively. *International Journal of Systematic Bacteriology*, 39, 397-405.

[4] Dev, A. T., & Lambert, J. R. (1998). Diseases associated with *Helicobacter pylori*. *MJA*, 169(4), 220-225.

[5] Peek, R. M. Jr, & Blaser, M. J. (2002). *Helicobacter pylori* and gastrointestinal tract adenocarcinomas. Nature Reviews. *Cancer*, 2(1), 28-37.

[6] Ahmed, N., & Sechi, L. A. (2005). *Helicobacter pylori* and gastroduodenal pathology: new threats of the old friend. *Annals of Clinical Microbiology and Antimicrobials*, 4, 1-10.

[7] Gasbarrini, A., Franceschi, F., Armuzzi, A., Ojetti, V., Candelli, M., Sanz, Torre. E. S., De Lorenzo, A., Anti, M., Pretolani, S., & Gasbarrini, G. (1999). Extradigestive manifestations of *Helicobacter pylori* gastric infection. *Gut*, 45(1), 9-12.

[8] Figura, N., Franceschi, F., Santucci, A., Bernardini, G., Gasbarrini, G., & Gasbarrini, A. (2010). Extragastric manifestations of *Helicobacter pylori* infection. *Helicobacter*, 15(1), 60-68.

[9] Arnold, D. M., Bernotas, A., Nazi, I., Stasi, R., Kuwana, M., Liu, Y., Kelton, J. G., & Crowther, M. A. (2009). Platelet count response to H. pylori treatment in patients with immune thrombocytopenic purpura with and without H. pylori infection: a systematic review. *Haematologica*, 94(6), 850-856.

[10] Capurso, G., Lahner, E., Marcheggiano, A., Caruana, P., Carnuccio, A., Bordi, C., Delle, Fave. G., & Annibale, B. (2011). Involvement of the corporal mucosa and related changes in gastric acid secretion characterize patients with iron deficiency anemy associated with *Helicobacter pylori* infection. *Alimentary Pharmacology & Therapeutics*, 15(11), 1753-1761.

[11] Isaeva, G., S.h, Abuzarova. E. R., Valeeva, I.u. V., Pozdeev, O. K., & Murav'eva, E. V. (2009). *Helicobacter pylori* in patients with disorders of hepatobiliary system. *Zhurnal Mikrobiologii Epidemiologii I Immunobioogiil*, 2, 96-101.

[12] Pirouz, T., Zounubi, L., Keivani, H., Rakhshani, N., & Hormazdi, M. (2009). Detection of *Helicobacter pylori* in paraffin-embedded specimens from patients with chronic liver diseases, using the amplification method. *Digestive Diseases and Sciences*, 54(7), 1456-1459.

[13] Brown, L. M. (2000). *Helicobacter pylori*: Epidemiology and Routes of Transmission. *Epidemiologic Reviews*, 22(2), 283-297.

[14] Parsonnet, J. (1995). The incidence of *Helicobacter pylori* infection. *Alimentary Pharmacology & Therapeutics*, (2), 45 -51 .

[15] Moayyed, P., Axon, A. T., Feltbower, R., Duffett, S., Crocombe, W., Braunholtz, D., Richards, I. D., Dowell, A. C., Forman, D., & Leeds HELP Study Group. (2002). Relation of adult lifestyle and socioeconomic factors to the prevalence of *Helicobacter pylori* infection. *International Journal of Epidemiology*, 31(3), 624-631.

[16] Suerbaum, S., & Michetti, P. (2002). *Helicobacter pylori* infection. *The New England Journal of Medicine*, 347(15), 1175-1186.

[17] Parente, J. M. L., Silva, B. B., Palha-Dias, M. P. S., Zaterka, S., Nishimura, N. F., & Zeitune, J. M. R. (2006). *Helicobacter pylori* infection in children of low and high socioeconomic status in Northeastern Brazil. *American Journal of Tropical Medicine and Hygiene*, 75(3), 509-512.

[18] Rothenbacher, D., Bode, G., Berg, G., Gommel, R., Gonser, T., Adler, G., & Brenner, H. (1998). Prevalence and determinants of *Helicobacter pylori* infection in preschool children: a population-based study from Germany. *International Journal of Epidemiology*, 27(1), 135-141.

[19] Kodaira, M. S., Escobar, A. M. U., & Grisi, S. (2002). Aspectos epidemiológicos do *Helicobacter pylori* na infância e na adolescência. *Revista de Saúde Pública*, 36, 356-369.

[20] Drumm, B., Perez-Perez, G. I., Blaser, MJ, & Sherman, P. M. (1990). Intrafamilial clustering of *Helicobacter pylori* infection. *The New England Journal of Medicine*, 322(6), 359-363.

[21] Czinn, S. J. (2005). *Helicobacter pylori* infection: detection, investigation and management. The Journal of Pediatrics 3 S26., 146, S21.

[22] Sugiyama, T., & Asaka, M. (2004). *Helicobacter pylori* infection and gastric cancer. *Medical Eletron Microscopy*, 37(3), 149-157.

[23] Bornschein, J., & Malfertheiner, P. (2011). Gastric carcinogenesis. *Langenbecks Archives of Surgery*, 396(6), 729-742.

[24] Kabir, S. (2009). Effect of *Helicobacter pylori* eradication on incidence of gastric cancer in human and animal models: underlying biochemical and molecular events. *Helicobacter*, 14(3), 159-171.

[25] International Agency for Research on Cancer. (1994). Schistosomes, liver flukes and *Helicobacter pylori*.IARC Working Group on the Evaluation of Carcinogenic Risks to Humans. IARC monographs on the evaluation of carcinogenic risks to humans. *World Health Organization, International Agency for Research on Cancer*, 61, 1-241.

[26] Lauren, P. (1975). The two histological main types of gastric carcinoma: Diffuse and so-called intestinal type carcinoma. *Acta Pathologica et Microbiologica Scandinavica*, 64, 31-49.

[27] Nardone, G., Rocco, A., & Malfertheiner, P. (2004). Review article: *Helicobacter pylori* and molecular events in precancerous gastric lesions. *Alimentary Pharmacology & Therapeutics*, 20(3), 261-270.

[28] Correa, P., Haenszel, W., Cuello, C., Tannenbaum, S., & Archer, M. (1975). A model for gastric cancer epidemiology. *Lancet*, 2(7924), 58-60.

[29] Correa, P., & Houghton, J. (2007). Carcinogenesis of *Helicobacter pylori*. *Gastroenterology*, 133(2), 659-672.

[30] de Vries, A. C., Haringsma, J., & Kuipers, E. J. (2007). The detection, surveillance and treatment of premalignant gastric lesions related to *Helicobacter pylori* infection. *Helicobacter*, 12(1), 1-15.

[31] Bowles, M. J., & Benjamin, I. C. (2001). ABC of the upper gastrointestinal tract. Cancer of the stomach and pancreas. *BMJ*, 323(7326), 1413-1416.

[32] Han, F. C., Ng, H. C., & Ho, B. (2009). Stability of randomly amplified polymorphic DNA fingerprinting in genotyping clinical isolates of *Helicobacter pylori*. World Journal of Gastroenterology ' , 9(9), 2021-2024.

[33] Roesler, B. M., Oliveira, T. B., Bonon, S. H. A., Monici, L. T., Zeitune, J. M. R., & Costa, S. C. B. (2009). Restriction fragment length polymorphism of urease C and urease B genes of *Helicobacter pylori* strains isolated from Brazilian patients with peptic ulcer and chronic gastritis. *Digestive Diseases and Sciences*, 54(7), 1487-1493.

[34] Yamaoka, Y. (2008). Roles of the plasticity regions of *Helicobacter pylori* in gastroduodenal pathogenesis. *Journal of Medical Microbiology*, 57(5), 545-553.

[35] Censini, S., Lange, C., Xiang, Z., Crabtree, J. E., Ghiara, P., Borodovsky, M., Rappuoli, R., & Covacci, A. (1996). cag, a pathogenicity island of *Helicobacter pylori*, encodes type-I specific and disease-associated virulence factors. *Proceedings of the National Academy of Sciences of the United States of America*, 93(25), 14648-14653.

[36] Covacci, A., & Rappuoli, R. (2000). Tyrosine-phosphorylated bacterial proteins: Trojan horses for the host cell. *The Journal of Experimental Medicine*, 191(4), 587-592.

[37] Rohde, M., Puls, J., Buhrdorf, R., Fischer, W., & Haas, R. (2003). A novel sheated surface organelle of the *Helicobacter pylori* cag type IV secretion system. *Molecular Microbiology*, 49(1), 219-234.

[38] Backert, S., & Selbach, M. (2008). Role of type IV secretion in *Helicobacter pylori* pathogenesis. *Cellular Microbiology*, 10(8), 1573-1581.

[39] Odenbreit, S., Puls, J., Sedlmaier, B., Gerland, E., Fisher, W., & Haas, R. (2000). Translocation of *Helicobacter pylori* CagA into gastric epithelial cells by type IV secretion. *Science*, 287(5457), 1497-1500.

[40] Higashi, H., Tsutsumi, R., Muto, S., Sugiyama, T., Azuma, T., Asaka, M., & Hatakeyama, M. (2002). SHP-2 tyrosine phosphatase as na intracellular target of *Helicobacter pylori* CagA protein. *Science*, 295, 683-686.

[41] Franco, A. T., Israel, D. A., Washington, M. K., Krishna, U., Fox, J. G., Rogers, A. B., Neish-Hyams, Collier., Perez-Perez, L., Hatakeyama, G. I., Whitehead, M., Gaus, R., O'Brien, K., Romero-Gallo, D. P., Peek, J., & Jr , R. M. (2005). Activation of beta-catenin by carcinogenic *Helicobacter pylori*. *Proceedings of the National Academy of Sciences of the United States of America*, 102(30), 106464-10651.

[42] Murata-Kamiya, N., Kurashima, Y., Teishikata, Y., Yamahashi, Y., Saito, Y., Higashi, H., Aburatani, H., Akiyama, T., Peek, R. M., Jr Azuma, T., & Hatakeyama, M. (2007). *Helicobacter pylori* CagA interacts with E-cadherin and deregulates the β-catenin signal that promotes intestinal transdifferentiation in gastric epithelial cells. *Oncogene*, 26(32), 4617-4626.

[43] Amieva, M. R., Vogelmann, R., Covacci, A., Tompkins, L. S., Nelson, W. J., & Falkow, S. (2003). Disruption of the epithelial apical-junctional complex by *Helicobacter pylori* CagA. *Science*, 300(5624), 1430-1434.

[44] Suzuki, M., Mimuro, H., Suzuki, T., Park, M., Yamamoto, T., & Sasakawa, C. (2005). Interaction of CagA with Crk plays an important role in *Helicobacter pylori*-induced loss of gastric epithelial cell adhesion. *Journal of Experimental Medicine*, 202(9), 1235-1247.

[45] Franco, A. T., Johnston, E., Krishna, U., Yamaoka, Y., Israel, D. A., Nagy, T. A., Wroblewski, L. E., Piazuelo, M. B., Correa, P., & Peek, R. M. Jr. (2008). Regulation of gastric carcinogenesis by *Helicobacter pylori* virulence factors. *Cancer Research*, 68(2), 379-387.

[46] Brandt, S., Kwok, T., Hartig, R., Konig, W., & Backert, S. (2005). NF-kappaB activation and potentiation of proinflammatory responses by the *Helicobacter pylori* CagA protein. *Proceedings of the National Academy of Sciences of USA*, 102(26), 9300-9305.

[47] Figueiredo, C., van Doorn, L. J., Nogueira, C., Soares, J. M., Pinho, C., Figueira, P., Quint, W. G., & Carneiro, F. (2001). *Helicobacter pylori* genotypes are associated with clinical outcome in Portuguese patients and show a high prevalence of infections with multiple strains. *Scandinavian Journal of Gastroenterology*, 36(2), 128-135.

[48] Rota-Lima Pereira, CA, Blaya, J. C., & Nardi, C. N. B. (2001). Consensus and variable region PCR analysis of *Helicobacter pylori* 3' region of cagA gene in isolates from individuals with or without peptic ulcer. *Journal of Clinical Microbiology*, 39(2), 606-612.

[49] Nomura, A. M., Perez-Perez, G. I., Lee, J., Stemmermann, G., & Blaser, M. J. (2002). Relation between *Helicobacter pylori* cagA status and risk of peptic ulcer disease. *American Journal of Epidemiology*, 155(11), 1054-1059.

[50] Blaser, M. J., Perez-Perez, G. I., Kleanthous, H., Cover, T. L., Peek, R. M., Chyou, P. H., Stemmermann, G. N., & Nomura, A. (1995). Infection with *Helicobacter pylori* strains possessing cagA is associated with an increased risk of developing adenocarcinoma of the stomach. *Cancer Research*, 55(10), 2111-2115.

[51] Kuipers, E. J., Perez-Perez, G. I., Meuwissen, S. G., & Blaser, M. J. (1995). *Helicobacter pylori* and atrophic gastritis. Importance of the cagA status. Journal of the National Cancer Institute ' , 87(23), 1777-1780.

[52] Parsonnet, J., Friedman, G. D., Orentreich, N., & Vogelman, H. (1997). Risk for gastric cancer in people with CagA positive or CagA negative *Helicobacter pylori* infection. *Gut*, 40(3), 297-301.

[53] Wang, S. H., Zhu, H. F., He, BS, Zhang, Z. Y., Chen, Z. T., Wang, Z. Z., Wu, G. L., & cag, A. . H. (2007). pylori infection is associated with polarization of T helper cell immune responses in gastric carcinogenesis. *World Journal of Gastroenterology*, 13(21), 2923-2931.

[54] Roesler, B. M., Costa, S. C. B., & Zeitune, J. M. R. (2011). Virulence factors of *Helicobacter pylori* and their relationship with the development of early and advanced distal intestinal type gastric adenocarcinoma. *In: Paola Tonino (ed.). Gastritis and gastric cancer. New insights in gastroprotection, diagnosis and treatments. Rijeka, Croatia: InTech Publishers.*

[55] van Doorn, L. J., Figueiredo, C., Sanna, R., Plaisier, A., Schneeberger, P., de Boer, W., & Quint, W. (1998). Clinical relevance of the cagA, vacA, and iceA status of *Helicobacter pylori*. *Gastroenterology*, 115(1), 58-66.

[56] Yamaoka, Y., Kodama, T., Gutierrez, O., Kim, J. G., Kashima, K., & Graham, D. (1999). Relationship between *Helicobacter pylori* iceA, cagA and vacA status and clinical outcome: studies in four different countries. Journal of Clinical Microbiology ' , 37(7), 2274-2279.

[57] Hatakeyama, M. (2004). Oncogenic mechanisms of the *Helicobacter pylori* CagA protein. *Nature reviews Cancer*, 4(9), 688-694.

[58] Rizzato, C., Torres, J., Plummer, M., Munôz, N., Franceschi, S., Camorlinga-Ponce, M., Fuentes-Paraná, E. M., Canzian, F., & Kato, I. (2012). Variations in *Helicobacter pylori* cytotoxin-associated genes and their influence in progression to gastric cancer: implications for prevention. *PLoS ONE*, 7(1), 01-09.

[59] Goelz, S. E., Hamilton, S. R., & Vogelstein, B. (1985). Purification of DNA from formaldehyde fixed and paraffin embedded human tissue. *Biochemical and Biophysical Research Communications*, 130(1), 118-126.

[60] Saiki, R. K., Gelfand, S., Stoffel, S., Scharf, S. J., Higuchi, R., Horn, G. T., Mullis, K. B., & Erlich, H. A. (1988). Primer-directed enzymatic amplification of DNA with a termostable DNA polymerase. *Science*, 239, 487-491.

[61] Lage, A. P., Godfroid, E., Fauconnier, A., Burette, A., Butzler, J. P., Bollen, A., & Glupczynski, Y. (1995). Diagnosis of *Helicobacter pylori* infection by PCR: comparison with other invasive techniques and detection of cagA gene in gastric biopsy specimens. *Journal of Clinical Microbiology*, 33(10), 2752-2756.

[62] Faundez, G., Troncoso, M., & Figueroa, G. (2002). cagA and vacA strains of *Helicobacter pylori* from ulcer and non-ulcerative dyspepsia patients. *BMC Gastroenterology*, 2, 20-24.

[63] Mattar, R., Marques, S. B., Monteiro, MS, Santos, A. F., Iriya, K., & Carrilho, F. J. (2007). *Helicobacter pylori* cag pathogenicity island genes: clinical relevance for peptic ulcer disease development in Brazil. *Journal of Medical Microbiology* [Pt 1], 9 -14 .

[64] Peek, R. M., Blaser, MJ, Mays, D. J., Forsyth, M. H., Cover, T. L., Song, S. Y., Krishna, U., & Pietenpol, J. A. (1999). *Helicobacter pylori* strain-specific genotypes and modulation of the gastric epithelial cell cycle. *Cancer Research*, 59(24), 6124-6131.

[65] Blaser, M. J., & Atherton, J. C. (2004). *Helicobacter pylori* persistence: biology and disease. *The Journal of Clinical Investigation*, 113(3), 321-333.

[66] El -Omar, E. M., Carrington, M., Chow, W. H., Mc Coll, K. E., Bream, J. H., Young, H. A., Herrera, J., Lissowska, J., Yuan, C. C., Rothman, N., Lanyon, G., Martin, M., Fraumeni, J. F., & Jr Rabkin, C. S. (2000). Interleukin-1 polymorphism associated with increased risk of gastric cancer. *Nature*, 404(6776), 398-402.

[67] Huang, J. Q., Zheng, G. F., Sumanac, K., Irvine, E. J., & Hunt, R. H. (2003). Meta-analysis of the relationship between cagA seropositivity and gastric cancer. *Gastroenterology*, 125(6), 1636-1644.

[68] Husson, M. O., Gottrand, F., Vachee, A., Dhaenens, L., de la Salle, E. M., Turck, D., Houcke, M., & Leclerc, H. (1995). Importance in diagnosis of gastritis of detection by PCR of the cagA gene in *Helicobacter pylori* strains isolated from children. *Journal of Clinical Microbiology*, 33(12), 3300-3303.

[69] Crabtree, J. E., Farmery, S. M., Lindley, I. J., Figura, N., Peichl, P., & Tompkins, D. S. (1994). CagA/cytotoxic strains of *Helicobacter pylori* and interleukin-8 in gastric epithelial cell lines. *Journal of Clinical Pathology*, 47(10), 945-950.

[70] Blaser, M. J., Perez-Perez, G. I., Kleanthous, H., Cover, T. L., Peek, R. M., Chyou, P. H., Stemmermann, G. N., & Nomura, A. (1995). Infection with *Helicobacter pylori* strains possessing cagA is associated with an increased risk of developing adenocarcinoma of the stomach. *Cancer Research*, 55(10), 2111-2115.

[71] Mizushima, T., Sugiyama, T., Komatsu, Y., Ishituza, J., Kato, M., & Asaka, M. (2001). Clinical relevance of the babA2 genotype of *Helicobacter pylori* in Japanese clinical isolates. *Journal of Clinical Microbiology*, 39(7), 463-465.

Chapter 13

Gastric Cancer: Molecular Pathology State

Filomena Altieri, Paolo Arcari and Emilia Rippa

Additional information is available at the end of the chapter

http://dx.doi.org/10.5772/53757

1. Introduction

Despite the progressive decrease observed in the past fifty years, gastric cancer (GC) is the fourth of the world rankings incidence of various types of cancer and is the second as a cause of cancer-related death. There is distinct geographical variation in gastric cancer incidence with the highest rates reported from Japan, Korea and Eastern Asia. Other high incidence areas are Eastern Europe and parts of Latin America, while Western Europe, Africa, Australia and the US generally have low incidence rates. In the last decade there has been a downward trend in the incidence and mortality from this cancer. The reasons are to be found in the improvement of food both as regards its preservation procedures and the variability in the diet and for the decrease of infection by Helicobacter *pylori* (H. *pylori*). H. *pylori* infection is strongly associated with risk for stomach cancer. Likely, this association is supported by the strong link between this bacterium infections and precancerous lesions, including chronic atrophic gastritis and dysplasia. The development of gastric cancer is characterized by multistage process in which several alterations of genetic and epigenetic nature accumulate. These alterations are mainly related to abnormalities of growth factors and receptors, DNA mismatch repair genes, angiogenic factors, transcription factors, adaptor proteins, cell cycle regulators, and many other macromolecular cell components. All these abnormalities identify from one side the molecular and biological aspect of gastric cancer cells and from the other might suggest possible strategies for therapeutic intervention.

The most important epigenetic alterations are confined within the chromatin structure like chromatin remodeling, DNA methylation and histone modification. These molecular alterations are generally common in gastric cancer, independently from its classification (gastric or intestinal). Also genetic polymorphism represents a possible endogenous cause of cancer risk. However, it must be considered that genetic polymorphisms might influence the efficacy of gastric cancer therapy and the toxicity of anticancer drugs. Although the worldwide decline in incidence and recent diagnostic and therapeutic advances provided excellent survival for patients with early gastric cancer, the prognosis of patients with advances cancer is still poor. Over the past 15 years, integrated research, including genetic polymorphism and global analysis of gene expression has clarified detailed molecular mechanisms and the role of genetic and epigenetic abnormalities of cancer-related genes in the course of development and progression of gastric cancer. This review describes an outline of the molecular pathway of stomach carcinogenesis, as signaling pathways, H. *pylori*, epigenetic and oncogenic background of gastric cancer, and recent treatment modalities.

2. Risk factors and classification

The general decrease of gastric cancer frequency in developed countries is attributed to the changes in dietary habits and food preservation methods [1]. Chronic inflammation with gastric atrophy was shown to be the most important pathological entity with hypochlorhydria being the most important physiological abnormality. Alcohol and smoking are also thought to contribute to the etiology. Achlorhydria, pernicious anaemia and blood group A are also associated with a higher risk of gastric malignancy. However, following the discovery of H. *pylori* it is known that more than 80% of gastric cancer cases can be attributed to deregulation of signaling pathways caused by H. *pylori* infection [2]. Genetic syndromes are rare and families clustering of gastric cancer are usually attributed to common H. *pylori* infection. A family syndrome of gastric cancer due to germ-line mutation in E-cadherin has been described, and gastric cancer may be part of Lynch syndrome (HNPCC). Mutations and polymorphism of interleukin 1β (IL-1β) and Tumor Necrosis Factor α (TNFα) have been described in closer relatives of patients affected by gastric cancer, and considered predictive factors for cancer. Genetic polymorphism is an important endogenous cause and modulator of risk for developing gastric cancer. They include: 1) inflammatory responses to H. *pylori* infection such as variants of IL-1β and IL-1 receptor antagonist (IL-RA); 2) intrinsic variability of DNA repair processes; 3) function of carcinogen detoxification and antioxidant protection; 4) cell proliferation activity [3].

GC is characterized by two distinct histological type of adenocarcinoma (intestinal type and a diffuse type) each having different epidemiological and pathophysiological features [4]. The intestinal-type generally evolves through a relatively well-defined multistep process that starts from chronic gastritis and progresses to chronic atrophy, intestinal metaplasia and dysplasia [5, 6]. It is associated with H. *pylori* infections and certain dietary factors, such as high intake of salt, smoked meats and food preserved with nitrites or nitrates [7, 8]. Intestinal tumors consist of malignant cells that resemble functional glands of the gastrointestinal tract. They are well differentiated and occur more commonly in older patients, males and blacks. The diffuse-type has instead a poorer prognosis and develops from normal gastric epithelium through unknown genetic and morphological events. It comprises cells that lack cohesion and are no longer capable of gastric function and it is more frequent in younger patients [9]. Several common events are shared between the two histological GC subtypes whereas distinct differences also highlight the intriguing divergence in histogenesis. The etiology of these differences remains to be elucidated [10, 11].

3. H. *pylori* infection

The pathogenesis of gastric cancer remains poorly understood although it is evident that several environmental factors, such as H. *pylori* infection can be the cause leading to this disease.

H. *pylori* infection is associated with risk for both the intestinal and diffuse varieties of gastric cancer. In fact, the risk to develop gastric cancer is increased in patients with H. *pylori* infections probably as the result of a combination of genetic and environmental factors in which the infection by H. *pylori* is of particular relevance, especially when the inflammation involves the gastric body region with respect to the antrum [6, 12, 13]. Generally, this condition is associated to different degrees of atrophy and alterations of the secretory function that, in the long term, became associated to gastric carcinoma [14-16]. The positive correlation between H. *pylori* infection and development of gastric cancer is well established and proven in prospective controlled studies [17, 18], whereas in absence of infection, development of gastric carcinoma constitutes a rare event. Furthermore eradication of H. *pylori* leads to a substantial reduction the risk of gastric cancer. From a pathogenetic point of view, it is believed that H. *pylori* infection determines the release of free radicals, resulting in mitogen stimulation and the inflammatory response of the stomach epithelium. The pathogenesis is associated with two bacterial genes known as CagA (Cytotoxic Associated Gene-A) and VacA (Vacuolating cytotoxin gene-A). The CagA gene is a marker for about twenty genes capable of increase the turnover of gastric epithelium through the CagA protein release. As a result, the association with an increased risk of developing non-cardia gastric cancer seems to be associated to H. *pylori* strain CagA [19]. A key role seems to have the so-called nuclear factor kB (NF-kB) [20]. NF-kB activation is in fact not only limited to patients with H. *pylori* active infection,but its nuclear and cytoplasmic expression appears to be up-regulate in gastric adenocarcinoma compared to adjacent normal tissue. The key role that this protein plays is also confirmed by the correlation between its expression and tumor conditions: biological and clinical aggressiveness, lymphatic invasion, tumor size and metastasis [21].

Among the targets of CagA strain there is also RUNX3, a tumor suppressor in many tissues and frequently inactivated in gastric cancer. Recently, it has been shown that H. *pylori* infection inactivates RUNX3 in CagA-dependent manner: CagA directly associates with RUNX3 through the specific recognition between the PY motif of RUNX3 and the WW domain of CagA [22].

4. Molecular pathology

The bacterial, environmental and host genetic factors discussed above influence the development of gastric carcinoma. Genomic, proteomic and biotechnology could allow the identification of novel genes and molecules specifically up-regulated or down-regulated in gastric cancer. Advances in our understanding of the genetic and molecular bases of gastric cancer lead to improved diagnosis, personalized medicine and prevention of gastric cancer.

In the following section, we discuss some of the molecular mechanisms underlying the molecular pathway of stomach carcinogenesis and of the biological and clinical roles of recently identified genes involved in gastric cancer.

4.1 GKN1

Recently, a novel tissue-specific protein, gastrokine1 (GKN1), has been isolated from gastric mucosa cells of several mammalian species, including mouse [23]. The human GKN1 gene has been localized in a 6 kb region of the chromosome 2p13 and contains 6 exons [24]. GKN1 is found within the granules just under the apical plasma membrane, suggesting that it is a secreted rather than a membrane protein. GKN1 has been hypothesized to play an important role in maintaining the integrity of the gastric mucosa and mediating repair after injury. Oien et al. [25] demonstrated, by Northern blotting, that GKN1 mRNA was abundant only in normal human stomach, in all areas (cardia, body and antrum), but absent in gastric adenocarcinomas; gastro-oesophageal adenocarcinoma cell line and other normal and tumor gastro-intestinal tissues. Therefore, there is a transcriptional silencing of GKN1 gene in gastric cancer. Rippa et al. [26] recently demonstrated, by means of proteomic technology, that GKN1 protein is reduced in patients with *H. pylori*-positive chronic gastritis. In addition, from the analysis of 28 patients with gastric cancer, Nardone et al. [27, 28], showed the downregulation or the complete absence of the protein. Similarly, Shiozaki et al. [29] showed that transfection with GKN1 reduced colony formation in MKN-28 gastric carcinoma cells. These data suggest that GKN1 participates in the host response to *H. pylori* and may also function as gastric tumor-suppressor gene [30]. More recently, new interesting data about GKN1 are emerging. Jung Hwan Yoon et al. [31] observed in GKN1-transfected AGS cells the inhibition of the epithelial–mesenchymal transition (EMT), a biological process that allows a polarized epithelial cell to undergo multiple biochemical changes that enable it to assume a mesenchymal cell phenotype, including enhanced migratory capacity, invasiveness, and elevated resistance to apoptosis. Also, GKN1-transfected and recombinant GKN1-treated AGS cells showed decreased levels of reactive oxygen species (ROS) and of phosphatidylinositol 3-kinase (PI3K)/Akt pathway proteins, which are a major cascade mediating tumor metastasis, accompained by re-expression of E-cadherin (a cell adhesion molecule which prevents EMT) and decreased expression of cytoplasmic and nuclear b-catenin, slug, snail, fibronectin, and vimentin (EMT-related proteins). These data suggest that the GKN1 gene may play an important role in the progression of sporadic gastric cancers via inhibition of EMT and cancer cell migration. Xing et al. [32] showed instead that GKN1 is an autocrine/paracrine protein that inhibits cell growth due to senescence resulting from activation of p16/Rb and p21waf pathways. Furthermore, sustained activation of Ras/Raf/MEK/ERK signalling was characterised in gastric cancer cells and xenograft nude mouse model following GKN1 treatment. Therefore, this study provides molecular evidence that GKN1 induces also senescence of gastric cancer cells.

Our group has been studying the effect of GKN1 on gastric cancer cell lines (AGS and MKN28). We found by cytofluorimetry, Western blot and RT-PCR that overexpression of GKN1 in these cell lines stimulated the expression of Fas receptor. Moreover, compared to control cells, a significant increase of apoptosis, evaluated by TUNEL, was observed when GKN1 transfected cells were treated with a monoclonal antibody (IgM) anti-Fas. The activation of Fas expression was also observed by the overexpression of GKN1 in other cancer cell lines. GKN1-overexpressing gastric cancer cells exposed to FasL induced the activation of caspase-3 was as evaluated by Western blot and fluorescence assays [33]. In addition, MTT assay showed that recombinant GKN1 reduced cell proliferation of gastric cancer cells (AGS) compared to human embryonic kidney cell line (HEK 293) and non-gastric cancer cells, human lung epidermoid carcinoma cell line (H1355). Our data represent the first report for GKN1 as modulator of apoptotic signals and suggest that GKN1 might play an important role for tissue repair during the early stages of neoplastic transformation. In fact, it was seen that individuals with a lower expression of the protein have an increased risk to develop gastric diseases [34].

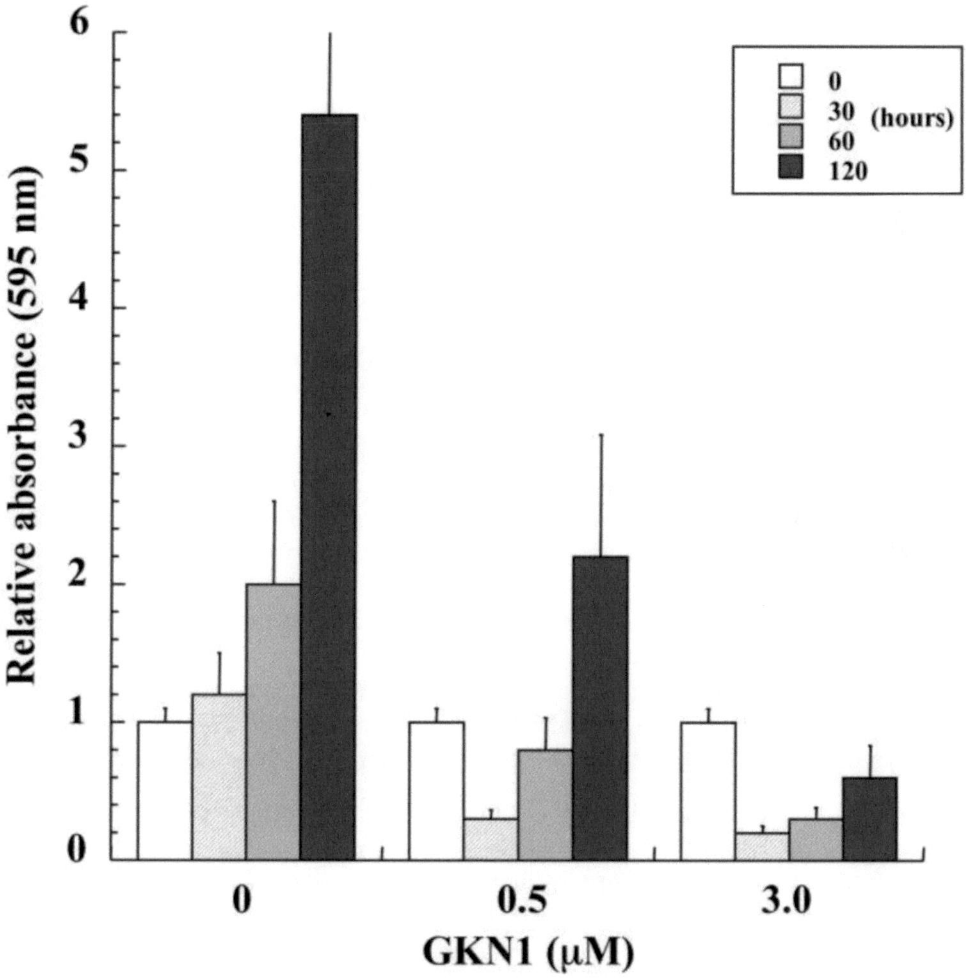

Figure 1. Effects of GKN1 on cell growth. AGS cell growth was evaluated using the MTT procedure after incubation of the cells with recombinant GKN1 at different times and concentrations. The data reported represent the average of three independent experiments.

Finally, regarding the mechanism by which *GKN1* gene is silenced in gastric cancer, this remains still unknown however, Hwan Yoon et al. [35] investigated this aspect in a sample group of 81 gastric carcinomas and 40 gastric adenomas: no mutation was detected in gastric tumours, hyper-methylation of *GKN1* gene promoter was found only in two tumours and DNA copy number of *GKN1* was significantly decreased in gastric cancer. However, epigenetic mechanisms could also contribute to silencing *GKN1* gene. Under this aspect, it would be important to clarify the causes of *GKN1* gene silencing and to determine whether this event might be involved in the development and progression of gastric cancer. Additional functional and translational studies of GKN1 will broaden our understanding of the pathogenesis of gastric cancer, and provide us with novel diagnostic and therapeutic modalities in gastric cancer.

4.2 E–cadherin and the Wnt system

The signal transduction pathway called Wnt is a central mechanism for regulating gene expression and is highly conserved in vertebrates and invertebrates. It includes a large family of ligands and plays a key role in many cellular processes, which ranging from regulation of embryogenesis control processes the proliferation of mature cells. In particular, it seems crucially involved in the processes of differentiation and proliferation of stem cell elements [36]. Central to these mechanisms is the process of regulation of expression of the β-catenin, an intracellular protein able to communicate on the surface of the cell with the system of cadherine, but also to act as nuclear transcription factor, including the Wnt/Wingless, epidermal growth factor (EGF), hepatocyte growth factor (HGF), and insulin-like growth factor (IGF) signaling pathways [37-40].

The Wnt signalling pathway can be activated trough the binding of Wnt ligands to their receptors Frizzled (Fz) and low-density lipoprotein receptor-related protein LRP5 and LRP6 (Figure 2). The binding induces an activation signal direct protein Dishevelled (DSH) and axin, that once activated, inhibit GSK3 kinase. Normally GSK3 phosphorylates β-catenin as part of a multiprotein complex that includes GSK3, APC and axin. The phosphorylation triggers the degradation of β-catenin through the process of ubiquitination (Figure 2, left panel). It follows that the inhibition Wnt-induced GSK3 interferes with the process of degradation of β-catenin and causes its cytoplasmic accumulation in a non-complexed form [41]. As consequence, β-catenin goes into the nucleus and regulates target gene transcription through association with the transcription factor TCF/ LEF (lymphoid enhancer binding factor) (Figure 2, right panel).

The translocation into the nucleus of β-catenin eventually leads to transcription of several genes including protagonists of carcinogenesis known protooncogenes such as c-myc and cyclin D1. In this regard, it is interesting that GSK3 can be inhibited through the PI3K/AKT pathway after toxin VacA stimulation [42]. This is a further element to support the correlation between infection by H. *pylori* and gastric carcinogenesis. Cell adhesion molecules may act as tumour suppressors such as E-cadherin whose gene is mutated in about 50% of diffuse type gastric carcinoma [43]. This homophilic cell adhesion molecule belongs to a family of cell-cell adhesion molecules with an important role in intercellular adhesion by establishing cell polarity, maintaining tissue morphology and cellular differentiation in normal cells [44, 45].

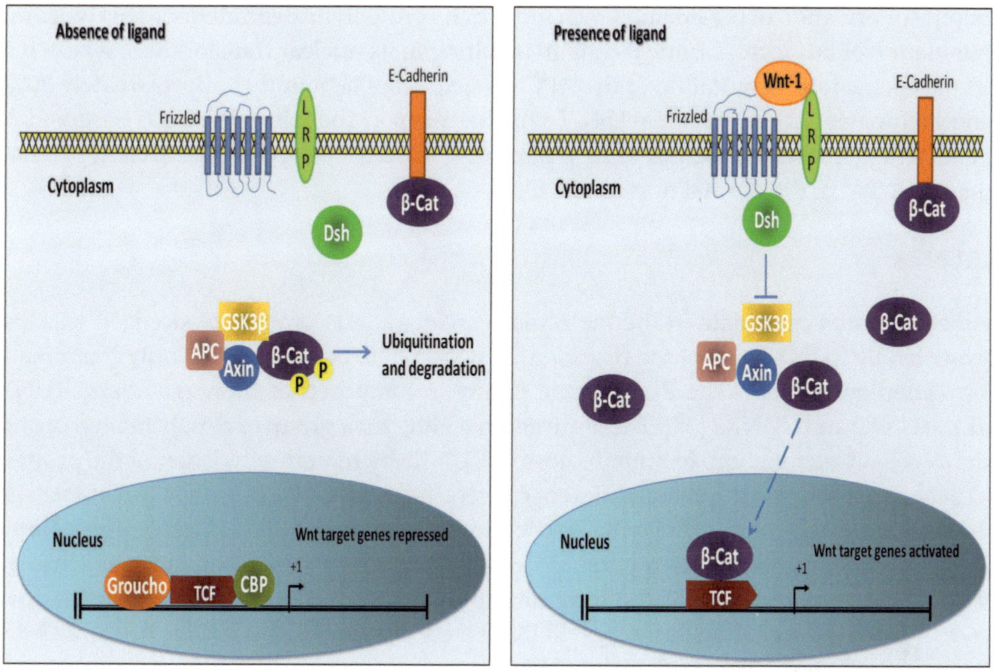

Figure 2. The Wnt signaling pathway. In the absence of Wnt ligand (left panel), the destruction complex (GSK3β, APC, Axin) creates a hyperphosphorylated β-catenin, which is a target for ubiqitination and degradation by the proteosome. Binding of Wnt ligand to a Frizzled/LRP-5/6 receptor complex (right panel) leads to stabilization of hypophosphorylated β-catenin, which interacts with TCF/LEF proteins in the nucleus to activate transcription. β-catenin normally binds to the intracellular domain of E-cadherin but the whole Wnt pathway is independent of E-cadherin expression.

E-cadherin binds to the actin cytoskeleton via a series of catenin proteins [46]. Therefore changes in E-cadherin expression have a direct effect on cell adhesion and therefore plays an important step in cancer development. Mutations in β-catenin and γ-catenin have also been observed in gastric cancer cell lines, and together with E-cadherin mutations appear to be involved in the development and progression of diffuse and schirrhous type cancers [47-49]. As the E-cadherin is responsible for the seizure of a major fraction of β-catenin in the compartment intracellular membrane, a loss of E-cadherin complexed to the cell membrane is associated with an increase in the share intracytoplasmic and nuclear of β-catenin [50]. In fact, this possibility is confirmed by immunophenotypic analysis of tumor diffuse gastric, where it often shows the increasing of nuclear β-catenin expression is associated with reduced of immunolocalization of membrane of the E-cadherin [51]. Recent data indicate that the simple down-regulation of E-cadherin, also obtained through epigenetic mechanism, alone would be sufficient to trigger the molecular carcinogenesis diffuse type of gastric cancer [52]. Despite the alterations of the E-cadherin seem limited to diffuse forms, also in carcinoma of intestinal type are observed alterations of the Wnt pathway that leads to an increase of cytosolic and nuclear β-catenin [53]. This accumulation of β-catenin can be explained by mutations in APC gene (Adenomatous Polyposis Coli) or in β-catenin gene itself. Both the situations lead to a hypophosphorylation of β-catenin, which reduces its proteolytic degradation. This is again an accumulation of intracytoplasmic β-catenin resulting in its nuclear translocation, where it can exert oncogenic role. A mutation of the APC gene appears be found in approximately 30% of adenocarcinomas of type intestinal [54]. To further support the role of Wnt, has observed that patients with germline mutations of APC present a risk of developing gastric cancer 10 times higher than that of the normal population [55].

4.3 RUNX3

Another potential candidate in the molecular carcinogenesis process of stomach cancers is represented by RUNX3, one of the first identified members of the RUNX family (mammalian Runt related genes) [56]. The RUNX gene family is composed of three members, RUNX1/ AML1, RUNX2 and RUNX3 [57]. These are genes coding for a group of closely related proteins with DNA binding function. In humans, loss of RUNX3 by hypermethylation of the promoter CpG islands is observed in several different cancers, including 64% of gastric carcinomas [58]. This loss reaches 90% in patients with gastric cancer in advanced stage. Gastric epithelium of RUNX3 knockout mice exhibits hyperplasia, reduced rate of apoptosis and reduced sensitivity to TGFβ1, thus suggesting that the tumour suppressor activity of RUNX3 operates downstream of the TGFβ signaling pathways. RUNX3 methylation is also a feature of 8% of chronic gastritis, 28% of intestinal metaplasia and 27% of gastric adenomas. These observations suggest RUNX3 is a target for epigenetic gene silencing in gastric carcinogenesis [59, 60]. Another element of great interest that correlates RUNX3 to H. *pylori* infection is represented by the fact that the H. *pylori* infection may down-regulate RUNX3 with an epigenetic mechanism [61]. In fact, it has been observed that during H. *pylori* infection there is the induction of nitric oxide production by macrophages resulting in methylation of the RUNX3 promoter. Recent results also show how the loss of expression of RUNX3 correlatessignificantly with the metastatic spread of cancer by adversely affecting the prognosis [62].

4.4 Genomic instability

In gastric cancer the loss of genomic stability represents a key molecular step that occurs early in the carcinogenesis process and creates a permissive environment for the accumulation of genetic and epigenetic alterations in tumor suppressor genes and oncogenes. It iswidely accepted that gastric cancer can follow at least two major genomic instability pathways, chromosome instability (CIN) and microsatellite instability (MSI). CIN is defined as the loss of chromosomal material during dysfunctional chromosome replication, repair or segregation [63]. MSI, which results from an erroneous DNA mismatch repair system, has been well known to be involved in the carcinogenesis of hereditary nonpolyposis colon cancers and some of sporadic colorectal cancers [64, 65]. A variable fraction from 15% to 50% of sporadic gastric cancer ischaracterized by MSI as a result of genetic inactivation or mainly Mismatch Repair (MMR) genes epigenetics, including hMLH1 and hMSH2. The inactivation of MMR genes is not itself a transforming event and additional genetic changes are required for progression to malignancy. In particular, in gastric cancer MSI is observed with the presence of mutations in repetitive sequences of genes involved in the regulation of cell growth (TGF-βRII, IGF-IIR), in apoptosis (BAX) and DNA repair (hMSH6, hMSH3). These mutations can alter the gene expression and give an advantage in cell growth and in clonal expansion. GC with MSI represents a tumor subset with clinico-pathological specific features. In particular, MSI GC is an intestinal gastric cancer, with antral location, low prevalence of vascular invasion or lymph node infiltration and better prognosis.

5. The molecular aspect of gastric cancer as rational for new therapeutic targeted strategies

In recent years it has strengthened the tendency to identify therapeutic strategies different from classical chemotherapeutic approach. The reviewed signaling pathways are relevant contributors for gastric carcinogenesis and encompass a multitude of potential therapeutic targets. In particular, there are growing efforts designed to identify the molecular mechanisms whose inhibition can significantly reduce the clinical aggressiveness of tumor malignacy. This innovative approach has achieved major successes in rare neoplastic diseases such as chronic myeloid leukemia and gastrointestinal stromal tumors (GIST) where it was possible to effectively inhibit constitutionally activated receptor tyrosine kinase such as the KIT gene [66, 67]. Except for the inhibition of HER2 in breast carcinoma, the same success has not yet been achieved in other tumors hence the need to further investigate on the existence of new potential molecular targets. Under this aspect, GC is not an exception indeed it represents a disease for the possible application of targeted therapies.

5.1 HER 2

HER2 (Human Epidermal Growth Factor Receptor 2) also known as Neu, ErbB-2, CD340 (cluster of differentiation 340) or p185 is part of a large family of receptors of tyrosine kinase activities. Along with HER1, also known as EGFR, up-regulation of HER2 is an important event in molecular carcinogenesis of many cancers. Ligand binding to EGFR extracellular domain leads to its activation, with subsequent homodimerization leading to the phosphorylation of its intracellular tyrosine kinase domain. This will initiate a series of intracellular signals, including activation of the central Ras/Raf/mitogen activated protein kinases (MAPK) signaling pathway (Figure 3). Up to now, the best model known is constituted by breast carcinoma in which HER2 is amplified in about 20% of cases [68]. This amplification is correlated to an increase of the expression of the protein and thus in growth advantage [69]. The prognostic negative role played by the amplification of HER2 in breast cancer is balanced by the possibility to interfere with that oncogenetic mechanism through the use of molecular therapies targeted with humanized monoclonal antibodies (i.e. Trastuzumab) [70]. On the basis of the results obtained in the treatment of breast cancer and counting on the fact that gastric carcinomas show amplification of HER2 in approximately 20% of cases, clinical trials have been designed that demonstrated significant improvement in progression-free survival disease for patients with HER2 overexpression, treated with trastuzumab, particularly when associated to conventional chemotherapy [71-73]. It is interesting to note how the aberrations of HER2 are practically exclusive of gastric (and cardial) adenocarcinomas of intestinal type, while they are decidedly not represented in the forms of the diffuse type. As in the case of E-cadherin alterations, there is a correlation between morphological and molecular mechanism in the diffuse forms. The EGFR/MAPK pathway has also shown to be activated in gastric carcinomas with microsatellite instability [74].

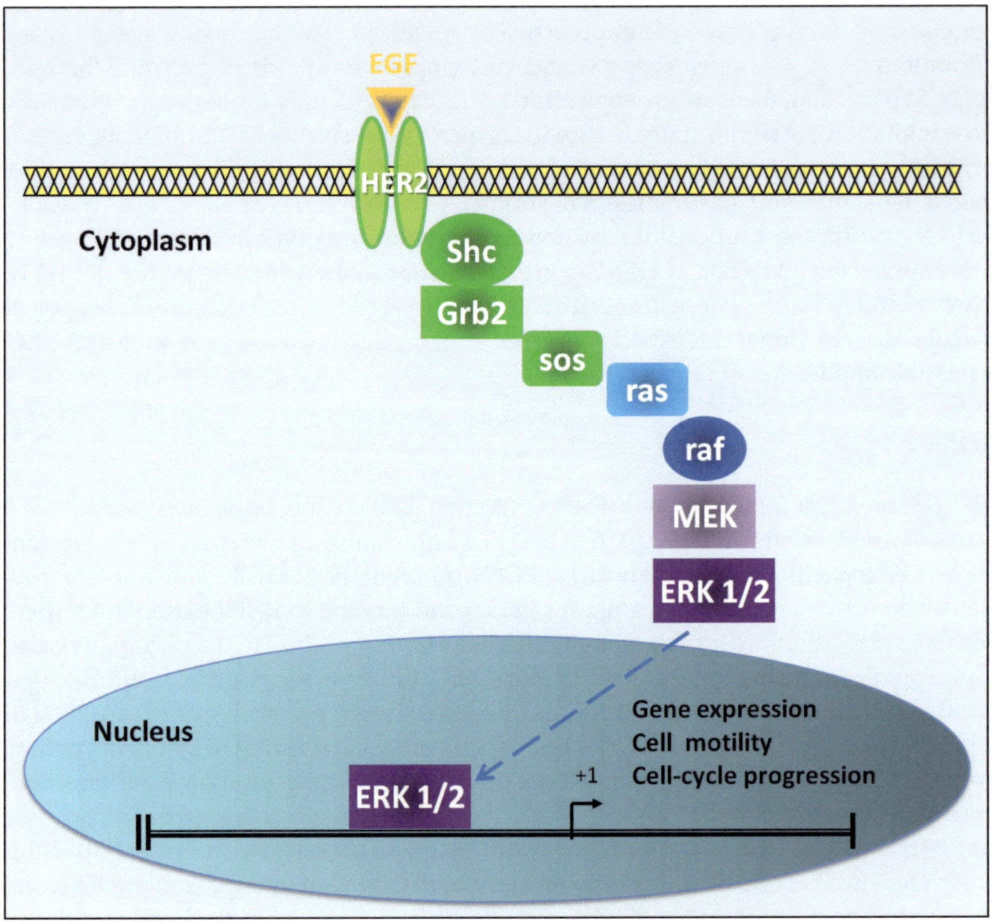

Figure 3. HER2 signaling pathway. Binding of EGF to HER2 initiate a series of intracellular signals, including activation of the central Ras/Raf/mitogen activated protein kinase (MAPK) signaling pathway.

5.2 VEGF

The mechanisms of angiogenesis have recently received a lot of interest in oncology and the inhibition of tumor angiogenesis has become a therapeutic option even feasible in gastric cancer [75]. The vascular endothelial growth factor (VEGF) is a dimeric heparin-binding glycoprotein and it is characterized by the ability to exert a powerful mitogenic action on endothelial cells, promoting their growth both in the primary tumor and in metastases, in the latter case after having stimulated the migration from home neoplastic primitive and secondary levels. A very recent study has shown a direct relationship between VEGF concentrations and new blood vessel development; gastric mucosal neovascularization was also reported to be significantly higher in the antrum of patients with H. *pylori*-positive gastritis versus non-infected individuals [76]. Experimental studies using different approaches clearly demonstrate that VEGF promotes tumor growth, angiogenesis, and metastasis formation [77, 78]. Overexpression of VEGF levels has been actually observed in the serum of gastric cancer patients compared with normal control and the increase of the expression seems to be correlated with the tumor stage and mass and is a negative prognostic factor [79]. However, there are limited data regarding the clinical and prognostic significance of serum VEGF (sVEGF) levels in gastric cancer patients. The fact that for some years it was possible to interfere with the neoangiogenesis using a recombinant humanized antibody directed against VEGF (bevacizumab) constitutes an element of great clinical interest. Recent is a publication of data from the first Phase II study conducted on patients with advanced or metastatic gastric cancer treated with a combination of bevacizumab, docetaxel and oxaliplatin. Using primary endpoint of progression-free survival, complete responses were observed in 5%, partial response in 37% and stabilization of disease in another 37% of cases. These data certainly encourage randomized trials to definitively clarify whether the inhibition of angiogenesis can be a very effective way in the treatment of gastric cancer.

5.3 mTOR

The mammalian target of rapamycin (mTOR) pathway has become a major focus of preclinical and clinical cancer research [80]. mTOR is a central regulatory kinase that increases the production of proteins involved in key cellular processes such as cell growth and proliferation, cell metabolism, and angiogenesis [81-83]. mTOR increases translation of proteins that drive cell growth and cell division, such as cyclin D1, and decreases translation of negative regulators of cell cycle progression [84]. It plays a role in cellular metabolism too by stimulating the surface expression of nutrient transporters [85]. mTOR consists in a double molecular complex (mTORC1 and mTORC2). mTORC1 is regulated by two components of the complex tuberous sclerosis (TSC1 and TSC2), which are controlled by the PI3K/AKT. mTORC2 instead regulates AKT cascade. Recently, because of their function in cell proliferation, these molecular complexes were considered ideal target for the design of drugs in oncology [86].

The efficiency of this approach has obtained a first success in a group of rare tumors known as PEComi [87]. However, significant results seem to be possible in the context of solid tumors. In fact, recent data show that the activation of mTOR in gastric cancer represents a key event observed in approximately 50% of cases [88]. Hence, the first attempts to use mTOR inhibitors to improve the efficiency of systemic therapies [89, 90].

6. Conclusions

In this review, we have summarized reports on genes, proteins and factors involved in gastric carcinogenesis based on currently available literature. Gastric carcinoma results from a complex interaction between bacterial, environmental, host-genetic and molecular mechanisms. It is evident that gastric cancer is the consequence of a multistep process involving different genetic and epigenetic changes in numerous genes. Host genetic background and environmental factors also play an important role in the pathogenesis of the disease. The majority of genetic alterations contributing to the malignant transformation were observed in growth regulatory genes, and in genes involved in cell cycle progression and arrest. In recent years, the analysis of molecular carcinogenesis gastric epithelial neoplasm has certainly provided information of great importance. It is understood that the molecular mechanisms involved in carcinogenesis of intestinal type are different from those prevailing in the development of diffuse one. The element of greater importance from a clinical point lies in the fact that the elucidation of these mechanisms is the prerequisite for exploring innovative therapeutic approaches. While the conventional forms of treatment seem to have reached the limit of effectiveness, it is possible that use of targeted therapies based on solid preclinical rational can translate into tangible clinical benefit. The reviewed signaling pathways are relevant contributors for gastric carcinogenesis and encompass a multitude of potential therapeutic targets. In addition to these signaling-related targets we included new data on

GKN1 as being involved in gastric cancer susceptibility phenotype.

Acknowledgements

This work was supported by funds from PON Ricerca e Competitivita` 2007–2013 (PON01_02782).

Author details

Filomena Altieri[1], Paolo Arcari[1,2] and Emilia Rippa[1]

1 Department of Biochemistry and Medical Biotechnologies, University of Naples Federico II, Naples, Italy

2 CEINGE, Advanced Biotechnologies Scarl, Naples, Italy

References

[1] Crew, K. D, & Neugut, A. I. Epidemiology of gastric cancer. World J Gastroenterol (2006)., 12(3), 354-362.

[2] Houghton, J, & Wang, T. C. Helicobacter *pylori* and gastric cancer: a new paradigm fo inflammation-associated epithelial cancers. Gastroenterology. (2005). , 128(6), 1567-1578.

[3] Yasui, W, Oue, N, Kitadai, Y, & Nakayama, H. Recent advances in molecular pathobiology of gastric carcinoma. In: The diversity of gastric carcinoma. Springer-Verlag (2005)., 2005, 51-71.

[4] Lauren, P. The Two Histological Main Types of Gastric Carcinoma: Diffuse and So-Called Intestinal-Type Carcinoma. An Attempt at a Histo-Clinical Classification. Acta Pathologica et Microbiologica Scandinavica (1965)., 64, 31-49.

[5] Correa, P. Helicobacter *pylori* and gastric carcinogenesis. Am J Surg Pathol (1995). SS43., 37.

[6] Correa, P. Human gastric carcinogenesis: a multistep and multifactorial process-First American Cancer Society Award Lecture on Cancer Epidemiology and Prevention. Cancer Research (1992)., 52, 6735-6740.

[7] Hamilton, J. P, & Meltzer, S. J. A review of the genomics of gastric cancer. Clin Gastroenterol Hepatol (2006)., 4(4), 416-425.

[8] Yamashita, K, Sakuramoto, S, & Watanabe, M. Genomic and epigenetic profiles of gastric cancer: potential diagnostic and therapeutic applications. Surg Today (2011)., 41(1), 24-38.

[9] Panani, A. D. Cytogenetic and molecular aspects of gastric cancer: clinical implications. Cancer Lett, (2008)., 266(2), 99-115.

[10] Costa, N. R, Sousa, A, Teixeira, C, Castro, J, Guimaraes, N, & Santos-silva, F. Oncogenic Signaling in Gastric Cancer. Rijeka: In Tech; (2011).

[11] Hudler, P, Vogelsang, M, & Komel, R. Genetic Instability in Gastric Cancer. Rijeka: In Tech; (2011).

[12] Goldstone, A. R, Quirke, P, & Dixon, M. F. Helicobacter *pylori* infection and gastric cancer.Journal of Pathology(1996)., 179, 129-137.

[13] Nabewera, H. M, & Logan, R. P. Epidemiology of Helicobacter *pylori* infection: transmission, translocation and extragastric reservoirs. J Physiol Pharmacol (1999). , 50, 711-722.

[14] Forman, D, Newell, D. G, & Fullerton, F. Association between infection with Helicobacter *pylori* and risk of gastric cancer: evidence from prospective investigation. BMJ (1991). , 302, 1302-1305.

[15] Parsonnet, J, Friedman, G. D, Oremtreich, N, & Vogelman, H. Risk for gastric cancer in people with CagA positive or CagA negative Helicobacter *pylori* infection. Gut (1997). , 40, 297-301.

[16] Watanabe, T, Tada, M, & Nagai, H. Helicobacter *pylori* infection induces gastric cancer in Mongolian gerbils. Gastroenterology (1998). , 115, 642-648.

[17] Uemura, N, Okamoto, S, Yamamoto, S, Matsumura, N, Yamaguchi, S, Yamakido, M, Taniyama, K, Sasaki, N, & Schlemper, R. J. Helicobacter *pylori* infection and the development of gastric cancer. New England Journal of Medicine (2001). , 345, 784-789.

[18] Fukase, K, Kato, M, Kikuchi, S, Inoue, K, Uemura, N, Okamoto, S, Terao, S, Amagai, K, Hayashi, S, & Asaka, M. Effect of eradication of Helicobacter *pylori* on incidence of metachronous gastric carcinoma after endoscopic resection of early gastric cancer: an open-label, randomised controlled trial. Lancet (2008). , 372(9636), 392-397.

[19] Blaser, M. J, & Berg, D. E. Helicobacter *pylori* genetic diversity and risk of human disease. Journal of Clinical Investigation (2001). , 107, 767-773.

[20] Isomoto, H, Mizuta, Y, Miyazaki, M, Takeshima, F, Omagari, K, Murase, K, Nishiyama, T, Inoue, K, Murata, I, & Kohno, S. Implication of NF-kappaB in Helicobacter *pylori*-associated gastritis. American Journal of Gastroenterology (2000). , 95, 2768-2776.

[21] Sasaki, N, Morisaki, T, Hashizume, K, Yao, T, Tsuneyoshi, M, Noshiro, H, Nakamura, K, Yamanaka, T, Uchiyama, A, Tanaka, M, & Katano, M. Nuclear factor-kappaB p65 (RelA) transcription factor is constitutively activated in human gastric carcinoma tissue. Clinical Cancer Research (2001).

[22] Tsang, Y. H, Lamb, A, Romero-gallo, J, Huang, B, & Ito, K. Peek jr RM, Ito Y and Che LF. Helicobacter *pylori* CagA targets gastric tumor suppressor RUNX3 for proteasomemediated degradation. Oncogene (2010). , 29(41), 5643-5650.

[23] Martin, T. E, Powell, C. T, Wang, Z, Bhattacharyya, S, Walsh-reitz, M. M, Agarwal, K, & Toback, F. G. A novel mitogenic protein that is highly expressed in cells of the gastric antrum mucosa. AJP Gastrointesinal and Liver Physiology (2003). GG343., 332.

[24] Yoshikawa, Y, Mukai, H, Hino, F, Asada, K, & Kato, I. Isolation of two novel genes, downregulated in gastric cancer. Japanese Journal of Cancer Research (2000). , 91, 459-463.

[25] Oien, K. A, Mcgregor, F, Butler, S, Ferrier, R. K, Downie, I, Bryce, S, Burns, S, & Keith, W. N. Gastrokine 1 is abundantly and specifically expressed in superficial gastric epithelium, down-regulated in gastric carcinoma, and shows high evolutionary conservation. Journal of Pathology (2004). , 203, 789-797.

[26] Rippa, E, Martin, G, & Rocco, A. La Monica G, Fiengo A, Siciliano RA, Cacace G, Malori A, Nardone G, Arcari P. Changes of protein expression in Helicobacter *pylori*-infected human gastric mucosa. Current Topics in Peptide & Protein Research (2007). , 8, 35-43.

[27] Nardone, G, Rippa, E, Martin, G, Rocco, A, Siciliano, R. A, Fiengo, A, Cacace, G, Malorni, A, Budillon, G, & Arcari, P. Gastrokine 1 expression in patients with and without Helicobacter *pylori* infection. Digestive and Liver Disease (2007). , 39, 122-129.

[28] Nardone, G, Martin, G, Rocco, A, & Rippa, E. La Monica G, Caruso F, Arcari P. Molecular expression of gastrokine 1 in normal mucosa and in Helicobacter *pylori* related preneoplastic and neoplastic gastric lesions. Cancer Biology and Therapy (2008). , 7, 1890-1895.

[29] Shiozaki, K, Nakamori, S, Tsujie, M, Okami, J, Yamamoto, H, Nagano, H, Dono, K, Umeshita, K, Sakon, M, Furukawa, H, Hiratsuka, M, Kasugai, T, Ishiguro, S, & Monden, M. Human stomachspecific gene, CA11, is down-regulated in gastric cancer. Internal Journal of Oncology (2001). , 19, 701-707.

[30] Du, J. J, Dou, K. F, Peng, S. Y, Wang, W. Z, Wang, Z. H, Xiao, H. S, Guan, W. X, Liu, Y. B, & Gao, Z. Q. Down-regulated full-length novel gene GDDR and its effect on gastric cancer. Zhonghua Yi Xue Za Zhi (2003). , 10, 1166-1168.

[31] Yoon, J. H, Kang, Y. H, Choi, Y. J, Park, I. S, Nam, S. W, Lee, J. Y, Lee, Y. S, & Park, W. S. Gastrokine 1 functions as a tumor suppressor by inhibition of epithelial-mesenchymal transition in gastric cancers. Journal of Cancer Research and Clinical Oncology (2011). , 137, 1697-1704.

[32] Xing, R, Li, W, Cui, J, Zhang, J, Kang, B, Wang, Y, Wang, Z, Liu, S, & Lu, Y. Gastrokine 1 induces senescence through Rb pathway activation in gastric cancer cells. Gut (2011). , 16.

[33] Rippa, E. La Monica G, Allocca R, Romano MF, De Palma M, Arcari P. Overexpression of gastrokine 1 in gastric cancer cells induces fas-mediated apoptosis. Journal of Cellular Physiology (2011). , 226, 2571-2578.

[34] Moss, S. F, Lee, J. W, Sabo, E, Rubin, A. K, Rommel, J, Westley, B. R, May, F. E, Gao, J, Meitner, P. A, Tavares, R, & Resnick, M. B. Decreased expression of gastrokine 1 and the trefoil factor interacting protein TFIZ1/GKN2 in gastric cancer: influence of tumor histology and relationship to prognosis. Clinical Cancer Research (2008). , 14(13), 4161-4167.

[35] Yoon, J. H, Song, J. H, Zhang, C, Jin, M, Kang, Y. H, Nam, S. W, Lee, J. Y, & Park, W. S. Inactivation of the Gastrokine 1 gene in gastric adenomas and carcinomas. Journal of Pathology (2011). , 223, 618-625.

[36] Katoh, M, & Katoh, M. WNT signaling pathway and stem cell signaling network. Clinical Cancer Researh (2007). , 13, 4042-4045.

[37] Kemler, R. From cadherins to catenins: cytoplasmic protein interactions and regulation of cell adhesion. Trends in Genetics (1993). , 9, 317-321.

[38] Desbois-mouthon, C, & Cadoret, A. Blivet-Van Eggelpoel MJ, et al. Insulin and IGF-1 stimulate the beta-catenin pathway through two signalling cascades involving GSK-3beta inhibition and Ras activation. Oncogene (2001). , 20(2), 252-259.

[39] Moon, R. T, Bowerman, B, Boutros, M, & Perrimon, N. The promise and perils of Wnt signaling through beta-catenin. Science (2002). , 296(5573), 1644-1646.

[40] Lu, Z, Ghosh, S, Wang, Z, & Hunter, T. Downregulation of caveolin-1 function by EGF leads to the loss of E-cadherin, increased transcriptional activity of beta-catenin, and enhanced tumor cell invasion. Cancer Cell. (2003). , 4(6), 499-515.

[41] Huang, H. He X.Wnt/beta-catenin signaling: new (and old) players and new insights. Current Opinion in Cell Biology (2008). , 20, 119-125.

[42] Nakayama, M, Hisatsune, J, Yamasaki, E, Isomoto, H, & Kurazono, H. Hatakeyama Azuma T, Yamaoka Y, Yahiro K, Moss J, Hirayama T. Helicobacter *pylori* VacA-induced inhibition of GSK3 through the PI3K/Akt signaling pathway. Journal of Biological Chemistry (2009). , 284, 1612-1619.

[43] Becker, K. F, Atkinson, M. J, Reich, U, Becker, I, Nekarda, H, & Siewert, J. R. Hofle r H. E-cadherin gene mutations provide clues to diffuse type gastric carcinomas. Cancer Research (1994). , 54, 3845-3852.

[44] Wijnhoven, B. P, & Dinjens, W. N. Pignatelli M. E-cadherin-catenin cell-cell adhesion complex and human cancer. British Journal of Surgery (2000). , 87, 992-1005.

[45] Smith, M. E, & Pignatelli, M. The molecular histology of neoplasia: the role of the cadherin/catenin complex. Histopathology (1997). , 31, 107-111.

[46] Tucker, E. L, & Pignatelli, M. Catenins and their associated proteins in colorectal cancer. Histology and Histopathology (2000). , 15, 251-260.

[47] Kawanishi, J, Kato, J, Sasaki, K, Fujii, S, Watanabe, N, & Niitsu, Y. Dysfunction of E-cadherin due to mutation of beta-catenin in a scirrhous gastric cancer cell line. Nihon Rinsho. (1995). , 53(7), 1590-1594.

[48] Shibata, T, Ochiai, A, Kanai, Y, Akimoto, S, Gotoh, M, Yasui, N, Machinami, R, & Hirohashi, S. Dominant negative inhibition of the association between beta-catenin and c-erbB-2 by N-terminally deleted beta-catenin suppresses the invasion and metastasis of cancer cells. Oncogene (1996). , 13(5), 883-889.

[49] Caca, K, Kolligs, F. T, Ji, X, Hayes, M, Qian, J, Yahanda, A, Rimm, D. L, Costa, J, & Fearon, E. R. Beta- and gamma-catenin mutations, but not E-cadherin inactivation, underlie T-cell factor/lymphoid enhancer factor transcriptional deregulation in gastric and pancreatic cancer. Cell Growth Differentation Journal (1999). , 10(6), 369-376.

[50] Oliveira, C, Senz, J, Kaurah, P, Pinheiro, H, Sanges, R, Haegert, A, Corso, G, Schouten, J, Fitzgerald, R, Vogelsang, H, Keller, G, Dwerryhouse, S, Grimmer, D, Chin, S. F,

Yang, H. K, Jackson, C. E, Seruca, R, Roviello, F, Stupka, E, Caldas, C, & Huntsman, D. Germline CDH1 deletions in hereditary diffuse gastric cancer families. Human Molecular Genetics (2009). , 18, 1545-1555.

[51] Cheng, X. X, Wang, Z. C, Chen, X. Y, Sun, Y, Kong, Q. Y, Liu, J, Gao, X, Guan, H. W, & Li, H. Frequent loss of membranous E-cadherin in gastric cancers: A cross-talk with Wnt in determining the fate of beta-catenin. Clinical and Experimental Metastasis (2005). , 22, 85-93.

[52] Humar, B, Blair, V, Charlton, A, More, H, & Martin, I. Guilford P. E-cadherin deficiency initiates gastric signet-ring cell carcinoma in mice and man. Cancer Research (2009). , 69, 2050-2056.

[53] Ebert, M. P, Fei, G, Kahmann, S, Müller, O, Yu, J, Sung, J. J, & Malfertheiner, P. Increased beta-catenin mRNA levels and mutational alterations of the APC and beta-catenin gene are present in intestinal-type gastric cancer. Carcinogenesis (2002). , 23, 87-91.

[54] Fang, D. C, Luo, Y. H, Yang, S. M, Li, X. A, Ling, X. L, & Fang, L. Mutation analysis of APC gene in gastric cancer with microsatellite instability. World Journal of Gastroenterolology (2002). , 8, 787-791.

[55] Offerhaus, G. J, Giardiello, F. M, Krush, A. J, Booker, S. V, Tersmette, A. C, Kelley, N. C, & Hamilton, S. R. The risk of upper gastrointestinal cancer in familial adenomatous polyposis. Gastroenterology (1992). , 102, 1980-1982.

[56] Otto, F, Lübbert, M, & Stock, M. Upstream and downstream targets of RUNX proteins. Journal of Cellular Biochemistry (2003). , 89, 9-18.

[57] Ito, Y. Oncogenic potential of the RUNX gene family: 'overview'. Oncogene (2004). , 23, 4198-4208.

[58] Li, Q. L, Ito, K, Sakakura, C, Fukamachi, H, Inoue, K, Chi, X. Z, Lee, K. Y, Nomura, S, Lee, C. W, Han, S. B, Kim, H. M, Kim, W. J, Yamamoto, H, Yamashita, N, Yano, T, Ikeda, T, Itohara, S, Inazawa, J, Abe, T, Hagiwara, A, Yamagishi, H, Ooe, A, Kaneda, A, Sugimura, T, Ushijima, T, Bae, S. C, & Ito, Y. Causal relationship between the loss of RUNX3 expression and gastric cancer. Cell (2002). , 109, 113-124.

[59] Kim, T. Y, Lee, H. J, Hwang, K. S, Lee, M, Kim, J. W, Bang, Y. J, & Kang, G. H. Methylation of RUNX3 in various types of human cancers and premalignant stages of gastric carcinoma. Laboratory Investigation (2004). , 84, 479-484.

[60] Sakakura, C, Hasegawa, K, Miyagawa, K, Nakashima, S, Yoshikawa, T, Kin, S, Nakase, Y, Yazumi, S, Yamagishi, H, Okanoue, T, Chiba, T, & Hagiwara, A. Possible involvement of RUNX3 silencing in the peritoneal metastases of gastric cancers. Clinical Cancer Research. (2005). , 11(18), 6479-6488.

[61] Katayama, Y, Takahashi, M, & Kuwayama, H. Helicobacter *pylori* causes runx3 gene methylation and loss of expression in gastric epithelial cells, which is mediated by ni-

tric oxide produced by macrophages. Biochemical and Biophysical Research Communications (2009). , 388, 496-500.

[62] Hsu, P. I, Hsieh, H. L, Lee, J, Lin, L. F, Chen, H. C, Lu, P. J, & Hsiao, M. Loss of RUNX3 expression correlates with differentiation, nodal metastasis, and poor prognosis in gastric cancer. Annals of Surgical Oncology (2009). , 16, 1686-1694.

[63] Lengauer, C, Kinzler, K. W, & Vogelstein, B. Genetic instability in colorectal cancers. Nature (1997). , 386, 623-627.

[64] Thibodeau, S. N, Bren, G, & Schaid, D. Microsatellite instability in cancer of the proximal colon. Science (1993). , 260, 816-819.

[65] Ionov, Y, Peinado, M. A, Malkhosyan, S, Shibata, D, & Perucho, M. Ubiquitous somatic mutations in simple repeated sequences reveal a new mechanism for colonic carcinogenesis. Nature (1993). , 363, 558-561.

[66] Casali, P. G, Jost, L, Reichardt, P, Schlemmer, M, & Blay, J. Y. ESMO Guidelines Working Group. Gastrointestinal stromal tumours: ESMO clinical recommendations for diagnosis, treatment and follow-up. Annals of Oncology (2009). suppl 4): 64-67.

[67] Warren, R. S, Yuan, H, Matli, M. R, Gillett, N. A, & Ferrara, N. Regulation by vascular endothelial growth factor of human colon cancer tumorigenesis in a mouse model of experimental liver metastasis. Journal of Clinical Investigation (1995). , 95, 1789-1797.

[68] Slamon, D. J, Clark, G. M, Wong, S. G, Levin, W. J, Ullrich, A, & Mcguire, W. L. Human breast cancer: correlation of relapse and survival with amplification of the HER-2/neu oncogene. Science (1987). , 235, 177-182.

[69] Nicholson, R. I, Gee, J. M, & Harper, M. E. EGFR and cancer prognosis. European Journal of Cancer (2001). S, 9-15.

[70] Slamon, D. J, Leyland-jones, B, Shak, S, Fuchs, H, Paton, V, Bajamonde, A, Fleming, T, Eiermann, W, Wolter, J, Pegram, M, Baselga, J, & Norton, L. Use of chemotherapy plus a monoclonal antibody against HER2 for metastatic breast cancer that overexpresses HER2. New England Journal of Medicine (2001). , 344, 783-792.

[71] Jørgensen, J. T. Targeted HER2 treatment in advanced gastric cancer. Oncology (2010). , 78, 26-33.

[72] Pinto, C. Di Fabio F, Siena S, Cascinu S, Rojas Llimpe FL, Ceccarelli C, Mutri V, Giannetta L, Giaquinta S, Funaioli C, Berardi R, Longobardi C, Piana E, Martoni AA. Phase II study of cetuximab in combination with FOLFIRI in patients with untreated advanced gastric or gastroesophageal junction adenocarcinoma (FOLCETUX study). Annals of Oncology (2007). , 18, 510-517.

[73] Liu, X, Guo, W. J, Zhang, X. W, Cai, X, Tian, S, & Li, J. Cetuximab enhances the activities of irinotecan on gastric cancer cell lines through downregulating the EGFR path-

way upregulated by irinotecan. Cancer Chemotherapy and Pharmacology (2011). , 68(4), 871-878.

[74] Corso, G, Velho, S, Paredes, J, Pedrazzani, C, Martins, D, Milanezi, F, Pascale, V, Vindigni, C, Pinheiro, H, Leite, M, Marrelli, D, Sousa, S, Carneiro, F, Oliveira, C, Roviello, F, & Seruca, R. Oncogenic mutations in gastric cancer with microsatellite instability. European Journal of Cancer (2011). , 47(3), 443-451.

[75] El-Rayes, B. F, Patel, B, Zalupski, M, Hammad, N, Shields, A, Heilbrun, L, Venkatramanamoorthy, R, & Philip, P. A phase II study of bevacizumab, oxaliplatin, and docetaxel in locally advanced and metastatic gastric and gastroesophageal junction cancers. Annals of Oncology (2010). , 21(10), 1999-2004.

[76] Tuccillo, C, Cuomo, A, Rocco, A, Martinelli, E, Staibano, S, Mascolo, M, Gravina, A. G, Nardone, G, Ricci, V, & Ciardiello, F. Del Vecchio Blanco C, Romano M. Vascular endothelial growth factor and neo-angiogenesis in H. *pylori* gastritis in humans. Journal of Pathology (2005). , 207(3), 277-284.

[77] Stegmeier, F, Warmuth, M, Sellers, W. R, & Dorsch, M. Targeted cancertherapies in the twenty-first century: lessons from imatinib. Clinical Pharmacology & Therapeutics (2010). , 87, 543-552.

[78] Claffey, K. P, & Brown, L. F. del Aguila LF, Tognazzi K, Yeo KT, Manseau EJ, Dvorak HF. Expression of vascular permeability factor/vascular endothelial growth factor by melanoma cells increases tumor growth, angiogenesis, and experimental metastasis. Cancer Research (1996). , 56, 172-181.

[79] Karayiannakis, A. J, Syrigos, K. N, Polychronidis, A, Zbar, A, Kouraklis, G, Simopoulos, C, & Karatzas, G. Circulating VEGF levels in the serum of gastric cancer patients: correlation with pathological variables, patient survival, and tumor surgery. Annals of Surgery (2002). , 236, 37-42.

[80] Bjornsti, M. A, & Houghton, P. J. The TOR pathway: a target for cancer therapy. Nat Rev Cancer (2004). , 4(5), 335-348.

[81] Edinger, A. L, & Thompson, C. B. Akt maintains cell size and survival by increasing mTORdependent nutrient uptake. Molecular Biology of the Cell (2002). , 13, 2276-2288.

[82] Fingar, D. C, Richardson, C. J, Tee, A. R, Cheatham, L, Tsou, C, & Blenis, J. mTOR controls cell cycle progression through its cell growth effectors S6K1 and 4E-BP1/ eukaryotic translation initiation factor 4E. Molecular and Cellular Biology (2004). , 24, 200-216.

[83] Patel, P. H, Chadalavada, R. S, Chaganti, R. S, & Motzer, R. J. Targeting von Hippel-Lindau pathway in renal cell carcinoma. Clinical Cancer Research (2006). , 12, 7215-7220.

[84] Hay, N, & Sonenberg, N. Upstream and downstream of mTOR. Genes Development. (2004)., 18, 1926-1945.

[85] Wullschleger, S, Loewith, R, & Hall, M. N. TOR signaling in growth and metabolism. Cell (2006)., 124, 471-484.

[86] Faivre, S, Kroemer, G, & Raymando, E. Current development of mTOR inhibitors as anticancer agents. Nature Reviews Drug Discovery (2006)., 5, 671-688.

[87] Wagner, A. J, Malinowska-kolodziej, I, Morgan, J. A, Qin, W, Fletcher, C. D, Vena, N, Ligon, A. H, Antonescu, C. R, Ramaiya, N. H, Demetri, G. D, Kwiatkowski, D. J, & Maki, R. G. Clinical activity of mTOR inhibition with sirolimus in malignant perivascular epithelioid cell tumors: targeting the pathogenic activation of mTORC1 in tumors. Journal of Clinical Oncology (2010)., 28, 835-840.

[88] Yu, G, Wang, J, Chen, Y, Wang, X, Pan, J, Li, G, Jia, Z, Li, Q, Yao, J. C, & Xie, K. Overexpression of phosphorylated mammalian target of rapamycin predicts lymph node metastasis and prognosis of chinese patients with gastric cancer. Clinical Cancer Research (2009)., 15, 1821-1829.

[89] Donnell, O, Faivre, A, Burris, S, Rd, H. A, Rea, D, Papadimitrakopoulou, V, Shand, N, Lane, H. A, Hazell, K, Zoellner, U, Kovarik, J. M, Brock, C, Jones, S, Raymond, E, & Judson, I. Phase I pharmacokinetic and pharmacodynamic study of the oral mammalian target of rapamycin inhibitor everolimus in patients with advanced solid tumors. Journal of Clinical Oncology (2008)., 26, 1588-1595.

[90] Matsuzaki, T, Yashiro, M, Kaizaki, R, Yasuda, K, Doi, Y, Sawada, T, Ohira, M, & Hirakawa, K. Synergistic antiproliferative effect of mTOR inhibitors in combination with 5-fluorouracil in scirrhous gastric cancer. Cancer Sci (2009)., 100, 2402-2410.